DATE DUE

DEMCO 38-296

Sick, Not Dead

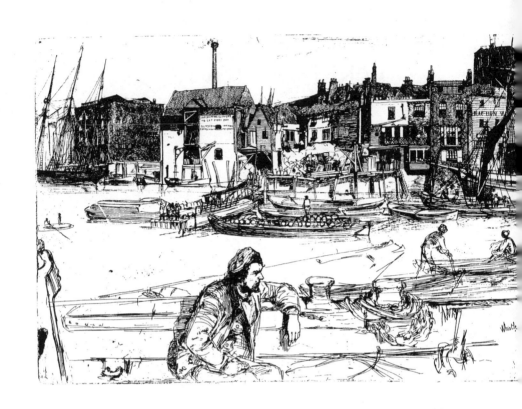

The Health of

British Workingmen

Sick, Not Dead

during the

Mortality Decline

James C. Riley

THE JOHNS HOPKINS UNIVERSITY PRESS

Baltimore and London

© 1997 THE JOHNS HOPKINS UNIVERSITY PRESS
All rights reserved. Published 1997
Printed in the United States of America on acid-free paper
06 05 04 03 02 01 00 99 98 97   5 4 3 2 1

THE JOHNS HOPKINS UNIVERSITY PRESS
2715 North Charles Street
Baltimore, Maryland 21218-4319
The Johns Hopkins Press Ltd., London

Library of Congress Cataloging-in-Publication Data will be found at the end
of this book.
A catalog record for this book is available from the British Library.

Frontispiece: "Black Lion Wharf," etching, 1859,
by James McNeill Whistler

ISBN 0-8018-5411-3

To the memory of
Walter Cooper and
to Dorothy Cooper

'Tis a good thing to belong to a good Club, and 'tis our duty to make provision for sickness, when in health, if possible.

WILLIAM HART, "Autobiography"

Contents

Illustrations

Tables

Preface and Acknowledgments

THIS BOOK BEGAN in a snit. I was waiting at the Southampton offices of the Ancient Order of Foresters Friendly Society—the AOF—for a chance to ask the order's historian a few questions, and I was growing impatient. The secretary in whose office I was waiting may have noticed that my patience was wearing thin. She suggested looking at the order's directories on the bookshelves behind me. I had seen directories before and believed them all to contain lists of the names and officers of local units of the friendly society, so I turned to these thinking I already knew their contents. The first few in the series confirmed my expectations. But the AOF historian continued to be occupied by other things, so I looked further.

Beginning in 1872, the AOF volumes became thicker. They included not merely a list of local units, called *courts,* but also data about sickness in each court. The additional data appeared each year thereafter through 1922. It was immediately evident that these directories would reveal two things that could not otherwise be learned about the health experience of friendly society members. They would provide a year-to-year portrayal of sickness and death, whereas all other sources provide such data only for the occasional periods for which statisticians and actuaries tabulated sickness. And the AOF directories would show whether and to what degree patterns of health varied across Britain.

From that snit emerged an application to the National Endowment for the Humanities for money to support the research I wanted to do, specifically to microfilm the AOF directories and to code what they had to say about sickness. From that grant—NEH RH-20934-90-Riley—came this book. Dan Jones, program officer in the Division of Research Programs, helped me plan and revise an application.

Many other people, too, contributed to this book. The first group of them I do not know and never met. They are the people who organized local archives in Britain and elected to include among the materials they collected the records of friendly societies. Without their willingness to save those records, I would have been unable to track experience to the local courts and their members. At the initial stage of the funded part of this project, the part for which I had a specific design, and assisted by the guide to British archives compiled by Janet Foster and Julia Sheppard,[1] I wrote to all the local archives in Britain asking for help in finding sources. The archivists responded generously. Hundreds wrote back to describe their holdings, sometimes at length. On the basis of those descriptions I planned research itineraries that added much to what I had found earlier in a more haphazard scheme of visiting local archives and record offices. Moreover, the archivists were unfailingly helpful in person. Even though they were always enormously busy, they found time to think more about the kinds of materials I needed and to make further suggestions about manuscripts to consult. The local archives of Britain and the archivists are a national treasure.

Other people helped me by advising how to carry out the work I wanted to do and by reading passages, chapters, or the whole text of earlier drafts, calling errors to my attention and suggesting ideas I had not had myself. For this kind of help I want to thank my colleagues at Indiana University, especially George Alter, Ann Carmichael, and Jeanne Peterson. Roger Schofield advised me about literacy and the census. Naomi Williams explained how to conceptualize the geographical analysis I wanted to make, helped with drawing maps, and offered suggestions about an earlier draft. For the advice they gave me about earlier drafts and how best to approach the problems this research presented, I want to thank Tim Cuff, Stan Engerman, Eilidh Garrett, Anne Hardy, David James, Bill Becker, John Lyons, Alice Reed, Elyce Rotella, Barry Smith, and Humphrey Southall. Michelle Facos helped me search for a cover illustration.

I want to thank Jacqueline Wehmueller, my editor at Johns Hopkins, for her enthusiasm for this project, and Katherine Kimball for such expert copyediting. I hope that the manuscript's referees will read the book and understand how much I appreciate their learned and skillful advice.

Walter Cooper, the AOF historian I waited to see in Southampton, let me examine the Foresters records he had collected and used his microfilming equipment to photograph relevant parts of the directories. When I visited him in Woodbridge I found only one hotel, which I could not afford. Dorothy Cooper insisted I stay in their home so I could study the material

1. Foster and Sheppard, *British Archives*.

her husband had collected. Walter died before I finished this book, which is dedicated to his memory and to Dorothy.

In Bloomington, Indiana University's Population Institute for Research and Training provided office space and equipment for turning plans into reality. Martha Zuppann took charge of hiring and supervising the workers who coded and proofread data and devised a training program to teach student-workers how to enter information. Randy Johnson worked out problems with data entry and visited some collections to collect material. Many students worked at entering and proofreading data; their labor was essential to this project. Michelle Buttacavoli, Angela Dortch, Greg Farrar, Seneka Johnson, Chris Knowlton, Jeff Leising, Kent Lemley, Jennifer Mandel, Rafael Marin, Barb Richard, Rachael Ritzmann, Celeste Schaefer, Dayatra Smith, and Laura Waldron coded data from the directories. Rich Brandi, Michael Caldwell, Jennifer Chisholm, Helen Choi, Fred Cummins, Kevin Hughes, Scott Locke, Cynouai Matthias, Doug Miller, and David Mutchnik worked on other parts of the project. I am deeply grateful for their interest in this work.

Introduction

LIFE IS MAPPED by special events, among them birth, baptism, entry into adulthood, marriage, old age, and death. These ceremonies and passages mark noteworthy personal experiences, some of them happy. Another type of experience stands in a parallel territory. It consists of a series of passages across the threshold from wellness into sickness, and from there to either recovery or death. If the entries into sickness are unhappy events, the reemergences into wellness, which in any life are exactly as numerous as the passages into sickness, minus one, are pleasing. They allow a resumption of activities, and they allow personal growth to resume. Sickness focuses the sufferer's attention on discomfort, but wellness lets a person concentrate on other things. Sicknesses are significant events and significant parts of experience. But they do not as readily create a record of themselves as do the other significant events that map our lives, which are often celebrated and recorded. As time passes the memory of each sickness fades. Before long, people recall only some of their sicknesses, and those often as specific diseases or injuries rather than as events. Oddly, it is especially the recoveries that first pass from our recollection. Thus, we do not ordinarily create a record of our sicknesses or our wellnesses; even in the short run, we often remember them inaccurately.[1]

Still, people try to preserve certain insights about sickness: what made us sick, and what made us well? What is the individual meaning of each sickness, and what is the meaning of the cumulative record of our sicknesses? Memories of these sicknesses are not the same as records, and they do not give sicknesses the status of historical events, which baptisms, marriages, deaths, and other of life's special events possess. Hence, these memories are not adequate to allow historians to explore the territory

1. In the ongoing health surveys now conducted in Britain and the United States, respondents are asked to recall sickness episodes during only the preceding fourteen days. For any longer period, it is feared, memories will be inaccurate.

of sickness and thereby to satisfy our curiosity about other people's sicknesses.

Whereas death is dramatic, sickness is too often tiresome. It is, of all conversational topics, perhaps the one from which people flee most eagerly. Doctors and nurses earn our respect not only because they keep irregular hours and study so hard to learn what they need to know but also because they voluntarily listen to people complain about their health. Sickness is a territory of diminished moral status. Wellness is not merely the absence of sickness but also the absence of the moral stigma sometimes associated with sickness.[2] People often want to deny that they are sick and thereby deny that they suffer the spiritual malaise associated with sickness. The sick—even people with incapacitating long-term disabilities—often claim to be in good health.[3]

As a topic, sickness is too important to allow us to shy away from it in our interpretations of past experience. Moreover, its importance has grown. Premature death constituted the singular health problem of the nineteenth century, when death rates were high. In the second half of the twentieth century, sickness has become an issue of equivalent concern. Health care is, in developed countries, the largest industry and the biggest single item in national accounts. In the United States the health sector is more than twice as large as its nearest rival, and growing. Yet its importance is not just a question of cost. Ill health, construed as either the events of disease and injury or the time of sickness, has continued to bulk large in human experience, even while death has been pushed chiefly into the territory of old age. Some moral philosophers and historians have responded to the continuing importance of ill health by studying specific diseases. In 1979, on the eve of the AIDS epidemic, Susan Sontag examined the ways in which cancer has replaced tuberculosis as the disease people most fear and the one which carries the most profound stigmas.[4] Among the most powerful historical investigations with this orientation is Anne Hardy's study of the rise of preventive medicine in Britain in the second half of the nineteenth century.[5] Like those studies, this book directs attention away from death and toward health. But here the focal point is not so much disease as the patterns of sickness.

Two of the most engagingly informative books in the recent medical

2. Twaddle, *Sickness Behavior and the Sick Role*, 1.
3. Calnan, *Health and Illness*, 28, 139.
4. Sontag, *Illness as Metaphor.*
5. Hardy, *Epidemic Streets.*

history of Britain, written by Irving Loudon and Ann Digby, draw attention to the social history of nineteenth-century doctors and of medical care.[6] This book seeks to complement those studies by addressing the social history of workingmen, as patients and prospective patients. What did these men want from their doctors?

In this parallel territory, ill-health time accumulates. For people who live into old age, it ultimately accounts for months and years of life as well as for a certain number of passages. In the most abrupt summation of life, what is prized is not the number of years that have been lived but the number of years lived in wellness—not life expectancy but health expectancy. The preeminent reason for exploring patterns of sickness is to see that sickness time is, like the age at death, open to manipulation. Over time, populations have accumulated varying amounts of sickness time. No particular sum of it is assigned to us.

This book addresses sickness and wellness among ordinary working people living in Britain in the nineteenth and the early twentieth centuries. Like every other history, this one has more than one meaning. Its direct subject is the study of certain features of health patterns among the central ranks of the working population in that place and time. Its indirect subject is the experience of sickness in any place and time and, more especially, the issue of discovering more about how to promote circumstances in which people are sick less often and for a shorter time. The risk of sickness, of long sickness as well as short, is as open to human control as the risk of death. Thus, it is feasible to plan and promote for the future a great morbidity decline, analogous to the great decline of mortality that has been under way since the late eighteenth century. Imagine a future in which the expected life span continues to increase and wellness time increases faster than sickness time.

SOURCES

Three types of records have proved especially useful for investigating patterns of sickness. Some people kept a running account of their lives, often including their sicknesses. They explored what made them sick and what made them well; they recounted what they did to take care of themselves while sick and to make themselves well. The nineteenth century was a great age of curiosity about self, which received expression in autobiogra-

---

6. Loudon, *Medical Care and the General Practitioner*; Digby, *Making a Medical Market*.

phies, some written by workingmen. Accounts of this sort will be useful here, but they are not numerous enough to stand as a principal source.

At a certain point in sickness, governed by motives and stimuli that are poorly understood, people decide to supplement the comfort they derive from discussing a sickness with relatives and friends, and from medicating themselves, with the advice and care of a medical practitioner. Thus, the ledgers and the more personal records that nineteenth-century doctors and pharmacists accumulated about the people who consulted them constitute another source about the history of people's sicknesses. But these, too, are not the principal sources.

The principal sources consist instead of records that working people created without an intention specifically of marking their sicknesses. In nineteenth- and early-twentieth-century Britain, many men and women joined friendly societies, cooperative associations that provided their members with compensation for part of the wages they lost during bouts of sickness and paid their heirs the cost of a respectable burial. Often, the friendly societies also hired a doctor to treat the members, and sometimes their spouses and children. Before 1911, when national insurance was introduced, people made these provisions for themselves, bearing directly the costs of sickness insurance. Their insurance cooperatives had counterparts on the European continent, usually called mutual associations or simply sick clubs. Wherever such societies existed, they held business meetings and recorded minutes, kept ledgers, drafted rules, and in other ways created a paper trail. In the process, they fashioned an orderly record of the decisions they made about policy and the payments they made and received. These records allow us to recapture some of the features of sickness patterns and of the provisions working people made to avoid sickness and to assist their recovery when sick.

For Britain, these records, preserved chiefly in county and municipal archives, constitute one of the most abundant sources about working-class activities that was generated by working people themselves. For each local sick club they present an account of sicknesses and wellnesses, of discussions and debates about the rules of sickness and their interpretation, of decisions made about engaging doctors and appraising their services.

Workingmen are the principal topic of this study, chiefly because the national friendly societies, such as the Foresters, did not admit women until the 1890s. But enough of the evidence explored here speaks to the experience of women to make worthwhile the attempt, throughout this book, to distinguish things that can be said about men alone from those things that can be said about men and women or about women alone.

In our personal histories, sicknesses mark themselves for several reasons. They bring periods of discomfort, perhaps even serious physical or emotional distress, accompanied by signs and symptoms worth remarking and remembering. They interrupt ordinary activities: work, recreation, social and sexual intercourse, eating, sometimes even sleeping. They give people something to talk about. The sick complain to family members and friends about the way they feel. They ask for advice about how to make themselves feel better or to get well. They sometimes seek professional advice, paying for medical attendance and even entering a hospital. Sickness puts people in touch with the unfamiliar, with doctors who know more than their friends and relatives about how to recognize and differentiate sickness, perhaps even how to relieve it. And, of course, for the doctoring we have to pay, which is a thing made more difficult by the degree to which being sick in the first place has robbed us of the chance to work and earn income. These are all issues worthy of attention that do not ordinarily give rise to records. Friendly society materials shed light on such events.

Sickness has many implications. It is not merely a time when people feel far enough below par that they suspend many of their ordinary activities. During sickness the sick and the people around them also suspend the usual rules of conduct and behavior. The sick are not merely allowed to complain about the way they feel, they are encouraged to do so. That is their first line of reaction to sickness. Their testimony may provide evidence about how to deal with the sickness, especially how to medicate it. For society, the sum of the sick—the proportion of people who at any given time are sick—is not merely a gauge of distress and the suspension of ordinary activities. It is also a measure of income not won and of expenditures that must in consequence be forgone. What is more, sickness has long been acknowledged as the kind of experience that warrants extra expenditures. It is a justification for buying medications, which in the nineteenth century, and still at the end of the twentieth century, is the second line of reaction to sickness. Over-the-counter medicaments existed and still exist in abundance precisely because people so often try to medicate themselves into recovery. When self-medication does not suffice, or perhaps as a coincidental bid for wellness, the sick may call on medical experts and expert caregivers. Indeed, an entire industry emerged around this demand for medical services and care. Each year in nineteenth-century Britain thousands of people worked to train themselves to provide medical care, and tens of thousands of men and women earned their livelihoods by giving such care. The medical infrastructure also required hospitals, infirmaries, dispensaries, and the household space in which the sick convalesced, although rarely as yet for working people a separate sickroom. It was not nearly as big a business then as it has become, in terms of the proportion of all spending allocated to health. But it was already an important subsector of economic activity.

The relationship between the sick person and the caregiver requires oversight and regulation, a code of etiquette. How shall the sick and their doctors behave toward one another? How often shall they meet together to explore the sickness? How much pay has the caregiver earned? What, to a working man who is sick, is it worth to consult a doctor? What amount of compensation from a working man, woman, or child suffices to draw a doctor out for a house call, perhaps at night in bad weather? Friendly society records also address these questions, sometimes directly and sometimes indirectly.

Mutual association records exist for many places and periods. Such associations formed a part of medieval confraternities. Guilds created sick funds, initially taking up a collection for the colleague who had fallen sick or for the heirs of the colleague who had died. Over time, that business became formal: premiums were levied in anticipation of future sicknesses and deaths. The guilds and the journeyman's associations that accompanied them saved or invested their income in order to meet future demands. In the process, they acquired from experience a knowledge of which ratios between premiums and benefits worked out best. They also learned something about the relationships between age, on one hand, and sickness and death risks, on the other. They learned, for example, and in quantitative rather than qualitative terms, how much likelier people are to die in old age than in mature adulthood. They learned also that the average length of sickness episodes increases with age. They learned, sometimes painfully, that it was not enough to balance revenues with expenditures each year when the members were young adults. Instead, the society had to accumulate reserves, which would cover the higher costs of sickness and death for older members.

Mutual associations unattached to guilds became commonplace among independent working people in the eighteenth century in Britain and western Europe. They thrived until, in the twentieth century, governments assumed the financial responsibilities that these societies had met and levied taxes in place of the societies' premiums. In the interim, and for

somewhat longer in places where the mutual association movement remained strong despite government involvement, such as Cuba and Australia, self-help provided the principal means by which ordinary working
people anticipated the financial costs of sickness and death. Self-help existed so that working people could share among themselves the costs of
medical care, of the wages lost during bouts of sickness, and of burial.
These were nonprofit organizations whose goal was to accumulate reserves large enough to meet future costs the size of which could not be
anticipated precisely but which could be forecast by looking at past experience. Britain, therefore, is not the only land for which a history of sickness
can be recaptured from the records of sick clubs.

WHAT DO THE SOURCES REPORT?

Sickness becomes a historical event only when the sufferer records it or
calls someone else's attention to it. Many of the actions people take to call
attention to their sicknesses are informal, in the sense both that they follow
implicit rules and standards of behavior and that there is no particular
likelihood that the action will be recorded. In nineteenth-century records,
loved ones rarely remarked the sicknesses of their intimates. In their autobiographies, working people and members of the elite alike paid closer
attention to their own sicknesses than they did to the sicknesses of their
spouses or children, much less other people.

The rules and standards that people follow in deciding whether to consult a medical practitioner are largely informal, when they are not part of
an insurance system. But the consultation itself is a formal thing, in that the
doctor usually creates a record of it following a certain form. A consultation with a doctor is usually taken to certify sickness, but it is not sickness
itself. That is, the consultation is a signal of sickness; the episode began
before the doctor was consulted, and, especially when the patient lacks
insurance, it is very likely to continue after the last consultation. Moreover,
many people forgo consulting a doctor when they are sick.

The sicknesses of friendly society members come to our attention because the men who suffered them entered a claim, the payment of which
marks the initiation and conclusion of the episode. These episodes might
be called either claims or sicknesses, but it is preferable to call them sicknesses when the issues focus on health rather than on insurance practice.

In their sickness ledgers, friendly societies recorded the date of initiation and conclusion of the claims they paid. To the national organization of the Ancient Order of Foresters (AOF), however, they reported the aggregate number of days of sickness experienced by members of the local unit during a calendar year, without reporting the number of sickness episodes. Information about the incidence of sickness and the duration of specific episodes can be recovered only from the ledgers of local courts. What can be recovered from AOF directories is the prevalence of sickness each year. Modern health surveys measure prevalence by asking respondents about sickness in the previous few days, as few as three days in Japan's survey or as many as fourteen in the British and U.S. health surveys. Such short periods of observation mean that many of the episodes of sickness surveyed began before the survey period and continued after the survey ended. Hence information will be truncated. In the AOF directories, however, coverage is continuous from 1872 until 1922. Since this analysis stops in 1910, the only truncation within this record occurs at 1872, in the loss of information about sicknesses under way in 1871 that continued into 1872, and at 1910, in the loss of information about episodes that continued into 1911. What is measured, therefore, is the period prevalence of sickness, with a period of unusually generous length. Whereas the period of British and U.S. health surveys is fourteen days, the period here consists of thirty-nine years. Thus, what is under observation here could be called the period prevalence of sickness claims. I shorten that to "sickness time."

THE CONSTRUCTION OF SICKNESS

Sickness is at once a physiological, an emotional, and a cultural construct. Forces outside of ourselves, an array of disease and injury hazards, and forces within ourselves, albeit only partially under our explicit control, help us decide when we have passed the threshold from wellness into sickness. At the initiation of sickness, the balance of these forces favors disease and injury hazards, which alert us to the passage into sickness by the physical and mental changes they induce. But at the conclusion of a sickness episode, the balance among these forces may be more evenly distributed. Often the symptoms of disease and injury fade gradually rather than abruptly, so that it is more difficult to decide when a sickness has ended than when one has begun. Similarly, cultural forces, which consist of the promptings and rules we learn about what to count as sickness and wellness and also about how to express ourselves as being sick, have greater definition at the initiation of an episode than at its conclusion. The rules about when sickness begins are more specific than the rules about when sickness ends, the more so when money is involved. For emotional maladies, especially those unaccompanied by blatant physiological signs or symptoms, the conclusion of sickness is still more uncertain than its initiation.

The way we think about sickness urges us to focus on its initiation and on the hazards associated with its initiation, such as exposure to someone with a communicable disease, risk-laden behavior at work or play, or environmental hazards. Here, falling sick is still an important issue; but the conclusion of sickness assumes more importance than is usually granted it, because so many of the questions that can be pursued deal with how long sicknesses last and because, as sickness durations rise, the length of episodes assumes greater importance as an economic as well as a cultural force. More time in sickness means, of course, less time spent at the ordinary activities of life. More time in sickness also means a greater demand for health services and health facilities.

If sickness is at once a physiological, emotional, and cultural construct, if its initiation is not entirely lacking in problematic qualities and its conclusion is often rife with them, then it follows that a specific definition of *sickness* must be difficult to provide. That, indeed, is one reason historians have paid so much more attention to mortality than to morbidity. Compared with life, death is a clear-cut state, which cannot be said of sickness compared with health. Aside from some uncertainty about how to recognize the moment of death, death poses no temporal problems, whereas for sickness it is necessary not merely to distinguish it from wellness but also to be cognizant of its duration. The problem of arriving at an all-encompassing definition of sickness that is anything more than vague is probably intractable. Fortunately, such a definition is not required in order to proceed with this investigation. What is needed is a description and explanation of the definition used by friendly societies in nineteenth- and early-twentieth-century Britain, a definition that focused on the most ordinary activity of adults: work. Friendly societies paid benefits to men and women who were too sick to work. That need introduces the problem of definition in a certain form, and it also introduces the need to reconstruct features of friendly society practice, especially the practice of the Ancient Order of Foresters, that impinge on the matter of defining sickness.

The threshold at which the Foresters deemed themselves sick must have varied from one person to another, as the threshold seems to vary today. It must also have varied in an orderly manner, as it does today; although some people applied strong or weak criteria and stood at either end of the spectrum, most applied criteria in the middle of the spectrum. The threshold may also have differed from what it is today. Many commentators believe that, in the past, people took sickness more seriously and applied stronger criteria than we do today; they tolerated more discomfort and pain before considering themselves sick. That opinion is, by its very nature, difficult to confirm or overturn, although the evidence assembled here calls it into question and tends to undermine its more extreme versions. In the nineteenth century, as today, people took time off from work for ailments ranging from minor colds to life-threatening ailments. Moreover, the annual record of sickness in the AOF makes it possible to explore many factors that might be suspected of influencing people's judgments about their health. Were changes in sickness rates, as reported in the AOF directories, influenced by factors other than health?

In the AOF operating definition, sickness began when members found they could not work and ended when they recovered the ability to work. Both threshold crossings, at entry into and exit from sickness, required the confirmation of a fellow member and, with increasing frequency from the 1840s, also the corroborating opinion of a doctor. This differentiation between wellness and sickness on the basis of the ability to work is a threshold of wide and long-standing use,[7] but it is only one definition of sickness. We might draw different conclusions if we knew how often and how long friendly society members complained about bad health or how often and how long they were hospitalized. What matters is the consistency of the threshold relating health to the ability to work, as well as the safeguards that friendly societies adopted to protect themselves from abuse of the benefits they paid. Hence, it is important not to compare on the same terms sickness rates derived from the application of different thresholds.

TRENDS IN SICKNESS AND MORTALITY

Friendly society coverage of the risks of both death and sickness posed a contradiction. On the side of death and burial insurance, the longer a person lived the later was it necessary to pay burial costs and the longer the time during which more money could be earned from premiums and in-

7. Waitzkin, "Critical Theory of Medical Discourse," 222.

vestments. A declining trend of mortality favored high earnings and, because the friendly societies were nonprofit organizations, higher earnings favored lower premiums. But the longer people lived the greater the likelihood that they would fall sick or spend more time in sickness. Old age meant at once a more compressed demand for burial benefits and higher outlays for sickness. Members living longer lives meant that the sick club needed to possess reserves adequate to pay these eventual costs. The imprecisely known scale of such future payments favored higher premiums and great caution in spending money.

This was the dilemma the friendly societies faced at the end of the nineteenth century. As friendly society officials saw it, this was above all a dilemma about premiums. Forecasts based on past experience were turning out more favorably for burial costs but less favorably for sickness costs, and each had its effect on the premiums members would have to pay. For the larger British society, including friendly society members, however, this dilemma posed a choice in health policy between programs and actions calculated to reduce mortality and those calculated to reduce sickness time.

During the last three decades of the nineteenth century and into the twentieth century, the average sickness episode became more prolonged, holding everything else constant.[8] Friendly societies members increasingly remained sick, where previously they had recovered or succumbed to their diseases and injuries. For adults, the great mortality decline under way in the nineteenth century was preeminently a deferral of the moment of resolution of sickness, in either recovery or death. For adults, the central fact of the mortality decline was not that, overall, people died in smaller proportions but that they more often survived the specific diseases and injuries that afflicted them. The mortality decline might have occurred because proportionally fewer people fell sick in the first place. This book shows that the incidence of sickness declined, but less sharply than the incidence of mortality, while the average duration of sickness episodes and aggregate sickness time increased. That people were sick more rather than less of the time—that they were sick rather than dead—means that their health was improving; the unambiguous sign of that lies in the decline of the lethality of specific diseases. In Britain's health transition, life spans first became longer and more occupied with sickness, marked by somewhat fewer episodes that lasted much longer.

At that moment important parts of potential survival time remained to

8. Thus the extensive new data examined and analyzed for this book confirm findings reported earlier from actuarial studies. See Riley, *Sickness, Recovery, and Death.*

be conquered. Hence, it still made sense at the end of the nineteenth century to focus the attention of changes in public policy and personal behavior toward reducing the death rate still further. That effort would succeed. Life expectancy for a male aged twenty rose from 39.5 years at the mid-nineteenth century to 44.2 years in 1910–12; between 1910–12 and 1989–91, it increased further to 54.3 years.[9] But the main problem of public and individual health policy a century later, at the end of the twentieth century, could already be discerned: how can sickness time, especially the sickness time associated with old age, be reduced? How can longer lives of wellness be promoted? If it has been possible to subdue so much of the risk of death before old age as has been done in the last two hundred years, is it not also possible to subdue the risk of nonlethal diseases and injuries? This study seeks to address these questions by formulating them as they confronted people in Britain at the end of the nineteenth century rather than by examining their present-day manifestation, an ongoing rise in disability.[10]

If death rates were declining but sickness time rising, how did the two trends interact? How did the forces and policies that can be linked to one trend play out in the development of the other? That is the final question raised in this book. The answer draws on a combination of evidence from the 1891 census of England and Wales and the experience of friendly society members in the years around 1891. The aim of this book is not merely to discover some things not yet known about the forces operating in these parallel but contradictory worlds of mortality and morbidity at that time and in that place. It is also to work out how to pose this issue of sickness versus death in clear terms that lend themselves to analysis in the present and to the redirection of public policy and personal behavior in ways that will promote for the twenty-first century longer lives with less sickness time.

SICKNESS THEORY

Some of the issues treated in this book have theoretical properties or implications. First, death rates show a strong association with age. So also

9. Farr, *English Life Table,* cli, dealing with 1838–54; Great Britain, Office of Population Censuses and Surveys, *English Life Tables No. 14,* 6, for the period 1910–12; Great Britain, *Annual Abstract of Statistics 1994,* 41, for the period 1989–91.
10. Bebbington, "Expectation of Life without Disability"; Riley, "Morbidity Trends in Four Countries," esp. 414.

do both the incidence of sickness episodes and the amount of time spent in sickness. Nineteenth-century statisticians and actuaries searched for laws of mortality and morbidity. Their work laid the foundation for understanding the regularities in experience in these two areas across time and among communities. This book seeks to carry that discussion forward by examining the relation between age and sickness time in more detail, by focusing attention on the accumulation of sickness time over the life course, and by looking at the relation between mortality and morbidity. Sickness time increased during the period under close scrutiny, 1872–1910, while wellness time also increased. Since the average age of the population rose and sickness rates are higher at higher ages, the population's sickness expectation increased more rapidly still. In 1910, Britain's population experienced far more sickness time than it had in 1870. In one sense it was a frailer population than it had been, succumbing to more sickness time. In another sense it was a hardier population, surviving longer.

Second, the friendly society definition of sickness as the incapacity to work raises a number of questions about the basis on which people assume a sick role. People who believe that they have fallen sick may complain to their friends, medicate themselves, or consult a doctor. They may also suspend their ordinary activities, which for adults center on work. Anthropologists and sociologists have done much to explore how people identify sickness stimuli and respond to them; historians need to attend to these issues, too, because strong assumptions about the past guide the way they are discussed. Some commentators assume, without offering evidence, that the stimuli needed to persuade people that they may be sick have weakened over time. That is, they assume that people have become more prone to regard deviations from the way they ordinarily feel as sickness and to behave as though they are sick. Unsupported assumptions about the past constitute a challenge to historians. Can we really imagine the past? Does it resemble the way we imagine it?

Third, when is a sickness legitimate? If it is true that people have become more likely to deem deviations from well-being to be sickness, does this mean that we have altered the threshold between wellness and sickness in a way that qualifies many of our present sicknesses as trivial or false? Is the commonplace nature of sickness in the modern world to some degree merely an affectation? Difficult as it is to collect objective data about this, many aspects of the experience of friendly society members speak to the matter of legitimacy. Those working people were the models many commentators have in mind when they puzzle over shifting thresholds. Each of us, reading about the sicknesses those people experienced, can form an opinion about the comparative legitimacy of their sicknesses and our own.

Fourth, for individuals and for populations, patterns of health early in life influence later health. For men working in specific occupations and for working people in general, the quantity of sickness experienced earlier, the relative survival of members of their cohort, and the characteristics of the communities in which they lived all mattered not just for the moment but also for the future.

WHOSE HEALTH CAN BE SCRUTINIZED?

Historians have often interpreted legislative reports about the friendly societies, official statistics, and some friendly society documents, chiefly rules.[11] The sources used most here are, instead, the minutes of friendly society meetings, the financial and membership records kept by individual clubs, the magazines published by the societies, and the annual directories put out by the national friendly societies, especially the Ancient Order of Foresters. As a group, friendly societies appealed to workingmen in Britain. The AOF stood in the middle of the hierarchy of friendly societies, drawing as members men from across the ranks of working people. Its members practiced a wide range of trades. Few of the Foresters were foresters. At various times in the period 1872–1910, the AOF was the largest or the second-largest friendly society. Its operations were centered in Britain, but local units could be found throughout the world where British people had settled, and a few had been formed elsewhere. Together with the Oddfellows, who resembled the Foresters, the AOF occupied a prominent place in national life, representing the friendly society view of working people's interests, providing social insurance, and forming a community of working people.

The most sharply drawn interpretation of working-class health now

11. Gosden, *Self-Help,* and *Friendly Societies in England,* provide the best institutional history, though only up to 1875. Crossick, *Artisan Elite,* 174–98, gives a social history of the friendly society movement in an important community. No general European history of this working-class movement has been written, but there is a growing body of scholarly work on mutual associations in individual countries. For example, see Mitchell, "Function and Malfunction of Mutual Aid Societies."

Finlayson, *Citizen, State, and Social Welfare in Britain,* discusses the friendly societies within the context of voluntarism in general in nineteenth-century British life.

available, F. B. Smith's *The People's Health, 1830–1910*, describes the poor and the working poor of Britain as people frustrated by ill health and under the heels of institutions, elites, and forces outside their power.[12] Smith's portrayal of the people's health and status is sharply at odds with the picture I draw here, in which working people are seen as well more often than sick and as men and women in control of their lives.

The chief reason for the contrast, I think, is that Smith's principal sources, medical journals and official accounts, report about the poor from the perspective of elite observers, who could hardly fail to be appalled by what they saw. My principal sources, in contrast, were generated by working people who did not have in mind a point of contrast and who, whatever they may have felt in the depths of their hearts, did not craft a record of misery. They were not much impressed by how far the circumstances of their lives contrasted with those of the elite. A second reason Smith's description differs so sharply from my own must be that he focuses on people in desperate circumstances, whereas my sources relate the experiences of people at work or, at worst, out of work because of sickness and in receipt of friendly society benefits. Smith looks at the health of the poor, old and young; I have looked at the health of the central ranks of working people, all adults. A third reason for the contrast lies in our respective forms of naiveté. Smith searched out striking stories that relate poor health, inadequate medical attendance, adulterated food, failures of sanitary reform, and the like. For my part, I became seduced by the narratives of the friendly society sources, which are narratives of men and women who optimistically claim their own influence and importance.

Manual workers and their families accounted for three-quarters or somewhat more of the population of Britain in the late nineteenth and early twentieth centuries.[13] They stood between the poor, some of whom would have engaged in manual labor had they held jobs, and the elite, itself a diverse group extending from merchants and members of the professions to large-scale landowners and peers of the realm. Although they occupied its central ranks, working people were not representative of the whole population. They were distinctive, in the view they held of themselves and in the view that others, above and below, held of them. Their health experience was also distinctive, insofar at least as that can be determined from such indexes as death rates, which show that a mortality hierarchy

12. Smith, *The People's Health*, 170–77, 321, passim.
13. See, e.g., McKibbin, *Ideologies of Class*, vii; and Benson, *Working Class in Britain*, 3.

was already in place in the nineteenth century, from expressed attitudes about health, or from body measurements.[14] Members of the elite faced lower mortality risks than working people, skilled workers lower risks than unskilled workers, and working people lower risks than the non-working poor.

Given these differences in mortality, there is no reason to think that the rate of sickness among working people should capture the rate among either the poor or the rich. Nevertheless, it is probably true that the trends of sickness discerned among working people in the long run reflect trends under way in other social groups. In that limited sense, the health of working people can speak for the health of the population at large, just as the mortality trend of working people closely approximates the mortality trends of lower and higher social groups.

Working people cultivated ties outside the family and the household through several modes of association. At work, they were part of one cultural and friendship group. They belonged to another in their neighborhood and perhaps also to a third among friends and relatives who neither worked with them nor lived nearby. Among their organizations, two were most commonplace: the church and the friendly society.[15] In 1898, 4.2 million people, mostly workingmen, belonged to registered friendly societies in the United Kingdom, compared with the no more than 1.6 million who belonged to labor unions.[16] If the number who belonged to unregistered societies was known, the disparity would be greater still. Even in the years after 1910, when labor unions were thriving and friendly societies were fading, working people belonged to friendly societies in larger numbers than to any other secular organization. Unlike most churches, friendly societies were usually under the control of working people.

The German observer J. M. Baernreither remarked in 1889 that English workingmen thought their unions more important than their friendly soci-

---

14. For an introduction to the literature on and the problem of socioeconomic inequalities in health, see Blaxter, "Fifty Years On—Inequalities in Health." Oddy, "Health of the People," surveys the nutritional status of working people, especially working-class children, showing deficits in height. Regarding attitudes, contrast Bruce Haley's description of the health concerns of the middle class and the elite, especially the cultural elite, in *Healthy Body and Victorian Culture*, 11–13, passim, with the pragmatic working-class attitudes revealed below. Reinhard Spree explores socioeconomic differences in health in Germany in much the same period covered by this book. See his *Health and Social Class in Imperial Germany.*
15. On the part of friendly societies within voluntary societies in general, see Morris, "Voluntary Societies and British Urban Elites."
16. Gilbert, *Evolution of National Insurance*, 162 n. 5.

eties because the unions helped them obtain higher wages.[17] Nevertheless, many more of them belonged to friendly societies, which offered fellowship and collective financial security. In Wales more men and women belonged to registered friendly societies in 1876 than attended church and chapel.[18] If the workingman's first resort in times of hardship was his family,[19] the next most important source of assistance was the friendly society. Although only part of the working class belonged to friendly societies, the societies provided benefits each year to far larger numbers of men than did poor law authorities or any other source outside the family.

Those benefits took two forms. First, members who missed work because they were sick earned compensation for part of the wages they lost. Second, at the death of a member survivors received a lump sum intended to pay for burial costs. Sick pay mattered most to the individual's or the family's economic well-being; without it even a short sickness might have brought destitution. But sick pay was never as much as wages, and thus it provided only partial aid. For working-class men and women and their families, for whom the central fact of life was too often a low and unpredictable income, self-help alleviated the threat of financial crisis but did not resolve it.[20] The most oft-remarked attraction of friendly societies to working people lay in the security that sickness benefits provided against reliance on workhouse and parish relief, toward which many working people felt strong aversion.[21] Burial pay mattered, too, for it ensured another form of respectability: friendly society members and their wives would be interred properly—an important consideration in a society where people counted dignified burial as a weighty matter.[22]

Self-help constituted a line of defense in a nation that acknowledged only a small fiscal interest in the health and well-being of its inhabitants, working people or not, and against employers who often took a detached

17. Baernreither, *English Associations of Working Men,* 155–56. The first edition appeared in 1889.

18. Jones, "Women and Computers," 2.

19. Anderson, *Family Structure in Nineteenth-Century Lancashire,* 136–61, esp. 147–48, offers one view; Dupree, *Family Structure in the Staffordshire Potteries,* 271–345, gives another.

20. Johnson, *Saving and Spending,* 232. For a detailed treatment of how common low wages were in British cities, see Treble, *Urban Poverty in Britain,* esp. 13–90.

21. E.g., Snell, *Men, Movements, and Myself,* 6–7; Grey, *Cottage Life in a Hertfordshire Village,* 67–68; and Cox, *Among the Doctors,* 12, recalling his working-class childhood. See also Kiesling, "Duration of Downturns and Self-Insurance."

22. Richardson, *Death, Dissection, and the Destitute,* 275–78.

or, worse, an antagonistic attitude toward ill or injured employees. Friendly societies protected working people from dependence on such employers.

In recent years some historical observers, disenchanted with British social democracy, have taken a fresh look at the friendly societies. For David Green and Keith Joseph, who have written in the most vigorous terms on this matter, Victorian self-help in the friendly society format seems preferable to today's social welfare.[23] It is true that when friendly societies were strong the men and women who belonged saved in advance in order to help themselves when they were sick, and that is an admirable thing. Anyone who wants to recall the friendly societies to their former glory must, however, resolve three large problems, to which neither Green nor Joseph has attended.

First, many men and women, among them those most in need of aid, did not belong to friendly societies. How should these people be included?

Second, people require help for many reasons other than sickness, but the friendly societies found it difficult to draw people into more comprehensive insurance plans. That is, the friendly socieites constituted a voluntary community, which some chose not to join, and those who joined wished to pay as little as they could for a narrow range of essential services rather than to pay more for a broader range of desirable services. Who will fund the necessary services that people elect not to pay for themselves?

Third, these societies depended for their spirit and their integrity on the type of community and the popular attitudes that existed in those times. Rebuilding self-help is not just a matter of reviving the friendly societies, which still exist and seem to be eager to have more members. For modern culture, perhaps the most alarming feature of the friendly societies is the degree to which they depended on the willingness of friends and acquaintances to hold one another under surveillance and, correspondingly, the willingness of friends and acquaintances to be held under surveillance. The sick had to be watched to see that they were indeed sick and to see that they did not resume the activities of wellness before they went "off the funds" (i.e., stopped making claims for benefits). Whatever rights of privacy Victorians thought they possessed, privacy had to be surrendered to belong to a friendly society. Would people surrender their privacy today; would they be willing either to watch or to be watched?

23. Green, *Working-Class Patients;* Joseph, "Friendly Societies That Smile on Self-Help," 16.

The friendly societies as they were constituted in nineteenth-century Britain also offer some noteworthy advantages. They held down the costs of medical care by bargaining with doctors and by forming their own clinics. Because so many of them were small and local, they were personal rather than impersonal organizations. They thrived because their members volunteered so much time to serve the purposes of the club and because others served for meager pay. In that way the members acquired a stake in their community, forming bonds of friendship based not on mutual support for a sports team or a shared preference for the same tavern but instead on the visible contributions they made to assist the community. And, unlike some modern insurers and health maintenance organizations, the friendly societies did not try to expel their sickest members.

I am skeptical about both the possibility and the desirability of reviving the friendly societies. I admire working people in nineteenth-century Britain for all that they did for themselves. But I do not think that their version of self-help can serve as a historical model for the present. It worked better than no help at all. But too many of the circumstances of nineteenth-century working life were still deplorable, despite the friendly societies, and deploring them is one way that we can discuss the present. In Britain in those times, too much was left to private interests, and too little was done to safeguard and assist the weak.

HOW THIS INVESTIGATION IS ORGANIZED

Sickness remains one of the least carefully scrutinized aspects of the past. Much more is known about medical theory, in the past and the present, than about the experience of sickness. The private records of the friendly societies make it possible to peer behind the curtain at sickness and to turn the shameless historian's gaze in two directions. First, we can investigate the medical, political, and moral terms of sickness as those things preoccupied working people in Britain in the nineteenth and early twentieth centuries. Second, we can explore certain quantitative dimensions of sickness, especially its trends and regional differences in its scale.

These two issues make up, respectively, the central topics of the two parts of this book. Part 1 is introduced by a description of the friendly societies and the Ancient Order of Foresters, their appeal and their ethos, in chapter 1. Chapters 2–4 take up the medical, political, and moral repercussions of sickness. More especially, they address how workingmen dealt with their doctors. The minutes of friendly society meetings and the rules that governed these societies show how the terms of this new relationship were worked out. They reveal the character of the relationship, and they deal in detail with the matter of cost. The sick clubs were training grounds where men and women learned what doctors expected of them. Because of the sick clubs, millions of men and women joined the ranks of people who regularly called a doctor when they were sick.

The clubs were also training grounds for doctors, who learned something about humility. Workingmen manipulated the economic relationship to their own advantage, teaching their doctors what it meant to submit to the forces of the market. In the privacy of their club rooms, the men sometimes aired their worries and grievances about health and about their doctors. If they could not confidently confront their doctors in public or in the midst of a medical consultation, they could still speak their minds at the club. In the collective force of the club room, and ultimately in the collective force of the friendly society movement, they could devise and execute strategies for manipulating not just the fees that they paid their doctors but also the attention that doctors gave working-class patients. They could demand and obtain consultations that took place mostly in their own homes, and they could expect their doctors to provide the medicaments they wanted. When first formulated, the terms of treatment and of trade between working people and their doctors favored working people. In previous studies, much useful attention has been focused on the supply of doctors. Here, attention falls more on the supply of paying patients and the terms of the agreements struck between doctors and these largely new patients from the working class.

A pattern of laments about doctors and doctoring drew my attention to a central change in the confidence with which working people dealt with their social superiors. Abruptly in the 1890s, friendly society members across Britain lost their nerve. No longer were they willing to defy the people who advised them about health, finances, and rules. Formerly, they had challenged doctors to deliver medical care on terms set by working people, judged independently and sometimes rejected the advice of actuaries about how to govern their clubs, and in other ways stood up to the people who wanted to advise and direct them. But that independent spirit collapsed in the 1890s.

Part 2 investigates the dimensions of sickness in Britain, its trends and regional differences, and searches for explanations of regional patterns. It is introduced in chapter 5 by an investigation of how the friendly society

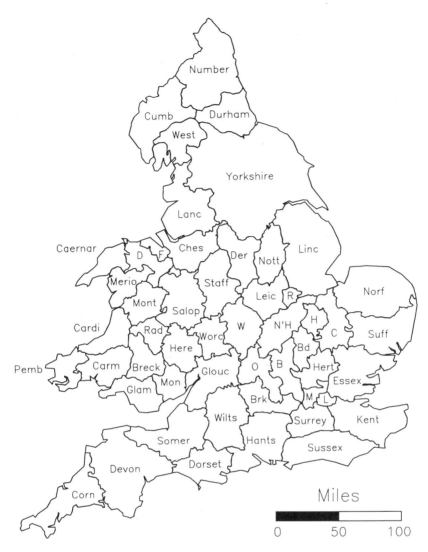

Map 1.1. England and Wales
Source: Data from Bickmore and Shaw, *The Atlas of Britain and Northern Ireland,* 188–99; *The Ordnance Survey Gazetteer of Great Britain.*

B	Buckinghamshire	Glam	Glamorgan	Norf	Norfolk
Bd	Bedfordshire	Glouc	Gloucestershire	Nott	Nottinghamshire
Breck	Brecknock	Hants	Hampshire	Number	Northumberland
Brk	Berkshire	Here	Herefordshire	O	Oxfordshire
C	Cambridgeshire	Hert	Hertfordshire	Pemb	Pembroke
Caernar	Caernarvon	H	Huntingdonshire	R	Rutland
Cardi	Cardigan	L	London	Rad	Radnor
Carm	Carmarthen	Lanc	Lancashire	Salop	Shropshire
Ches	Cheshire	Leic	Leicestershire	Somer	Somerset
Corn	Cornwall	Linc	Lincolnshire	Staff	Staffordshire
Cumb	Cumberland	M	Middlesex	Suff	Suffolk
D	Denbigh	Merio	Merioneth	W	Warwickshire
Der	Derbyshire	Mon	Monmouthshire	West	Westmorland
Devon	Devonshire	Mont	Montgomery	Wilts	Wiltshire
Dorset	Dorsetshire	N'H	Northhamptonshire	Worc	Worcestershire
F	Flint				

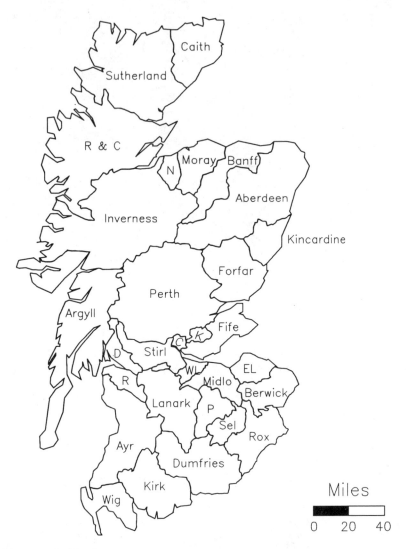

Map 1.2. Scotland
Source: Data from Bickmore and Shaw, *The Atlas of Britain and Northern Ireland,* 188–99; *The Ordnance Survey Gazetteer of Great Britain.*

Caith	Caithness	Midlo	Midlothian	Rox	Roxburgh
C	Clackmannan	N	Nairn	Sel	Selkirk
D	Dumbarton	P	Peebles	Stirl	Stirling
EL	East Lothian	R&C	Ross and Cromarty	WL	West Lothian
K	Kinross	R	Renfrew	Wig	Wigtown
Kirk	Kirkcudbright				

definition of sickness worked in practice, how a claim captures sickness, and the implications insurance coverage had for sickness behavior. Chapters 6–9 deal with issues that can be quantified. Actuarial studies of friendly society sickness in specific periods, especially 1866–70, 1871–75 and 1893–97, show that aggregate sickness time increased, holding age constant. Statistics from the AOF directories confirm that impression and reveal how the sickness trend changed from year to year and from place to place. The records of a single AOF court, located in Abthorpe, a Northamptonshire village, add some important information about the incidence of sickness. Because the secretaries who compiled records sometimes reported causes of sickness in the early twentieth century, some steps can be taken toward creating a picture of the sickness profile for adult males. Chapter 7 searches out differences between that profile and the profile of causes of death in England and Wales.

Thousands of local units made up the AOF, and the directories report the sickness time accumulated in each court in each year. Those assessments comprise the data needed to study regional differences in health experience, in chapter 8. Some parts of Britain were favored in morbidity, and some were unfavored. Over time most counties retained the relative position they held in the 1870s, but a few gained or lost standing. In contrast, Scotland and Wales lost position, compared to England. Differences in the patterns of health in individual courts in the nine years centered on 1891, a census year, provide an opportunity to search for characteristics in the locale that can be associated statistically with morbidity and mortality. By showing that mortality and sickness time moved in opposing directions across the period 1872–1910, chapter 6 suggests that different forces should be expected to have promoted each trend. That expectation is confirmed in chapter 9, where many of the characteristics of communities are shown to have been associated with sickness time and mortality in conflicting ways. Less sickness time, like lower mortality, was a desirable goal. Chapter 9 suggests, however, that the two goals were in large measure inconsistent with one another. The community characteristics associated with lower mortality rates were rarely associated also with less sickness time. From 1870 to 1910 and beyond, Britain followed a path toward diminishing mortality. But it also followed a path toward increasing sickness time.

PART ONE

The Medical, Political, and Moral Economies of Friendly Society Members

CHAPTER I

The Friendly Societies: What They Were, What They Did

IN THE EARLY MODERN era, working people began to institutionalize the traditional but informal arrangements by which they often assisted each other at the death or during the sickness of a family breadwinner. Whereas formerly they had passed the hat to help a friend, in the institutional form they regularly paid in small sums to build up a sick fund. The new arrangements required a selection of officers to administer the fund, a strongbox with a lock, and a place to keep the strongbox. In time it seemed desirable also to keep a ledger of contributions to the fund and benefits paid from it, to draft rules establishing conditions of membership and assistance, and to replace rule-of-thumb estimates of how much would have to be collected in order to pay promised benefits with sound calculations, based on experience. Keeping accurate records became all the more important. In Britain sick funds came to be called friendly societies, signifying their role in providing assistance outside the family but within a community. When a member fell sick, the friendly societies paid out benefits each week through the steward, an officer who visited the sick. Although the societies had other appealing features, the principal reason people joined was to obtain benefits for the wages they no longer earned while sick.

From the late seventeenth century—but with special fervor in the last decades of the eighteenth century—well-meaning members of the elite began to call for the formation of organizations of this type. Daniel Defoe liked the mutual compact organized among sailors at Chatham to promote the idea of saving when healthy in anticipation of the financial hazards of sickness and old age, and he urged it as a model. Between 1752 and 1797

other observers of British working people picked up Defoe's idea, trans-
forming it into advice about what working people should do for themselves.[1] For some, the point was to urge, or require, working people to
become provident in order to relieve wealthier people from having to pay
the taxes necessary to assist the improvident. For others, the point was less
to safeguard the rich from paying taxes than to cultivate among working
people desirable attitudes and practices. But focusing on the literature of
advice misses the point. Those who promoted the formation of friendly
societies took their lead from working people, who were already doing
what the out-of-touch elite wished them to do. This idea traveled up rather
than down the social ladder.

In 1797, by Frederick Eden's estimate, there were 7,200 societies with
648,000 members, a figure that relies on the multiplier of 90 (648,000 /
7,200 = 90).[2] Five years later reports from overseers of the poor suggested
9,672 societies with 704,350 members, a figure that indicates slightly
fewer than 73 members in each.[3] In 1801, Britain's population counted
some 2.3 million males aged twenty or more; these estimates suggest that
friendly societies already enrolled about 30 percent of the eligible population, although only part of that proportion belonged to clubs providing
sickness as well as burial benefits.[4]

The question of scale is difficult to address with precision from the
outset, and that remains true into the twentieth century. Some friendly
societies registered with the Registrar General of Friendly Societies, making themselves eligible for tax benefits but submitting to the regulations of
the registrar, while other societies did not.[5] Some counts were made of the
membership of registered societies, but none was made of unregistered
societies (even though some observers, like Frederick Eden, meant to include them). Several authorities, most recently Paul Johnson, have tried to
reconstruct membership and to estimate the number of members eligible
for sickness as well as burial benefits as distinct from the number who
belonged to societies supplying only burial benefits. All these efforts, ranging from C. G. Hanson's generous to Johnson's restrictive figures, deal

---

1. Gosden, Self-Help, 4–12, reviews this advice.
2. Eden, Observations on Friendly Societies, 8; Rule, Experience of Labor in Eighteenth-
Century Industry.
3. Gosden, Self-Help, 12.
4. See Mitchell, British Historical Statistics, 11, for the figure of 4.4 million males. The
calculation of males twenty years and older uses the proportion in 1841, the first census year
in which ages were given.
5. On the regulation of friendly societies, see Gosden, Friendly Societies in England, 173–
97; and Supple, "Legislation and Virtue."

with large uncertainties. Johnson reports that, in 1901, 5.47 million adult males belonged to two classes of registered societies, affiliated and ordinary.[6] That proportion made up 54.5 percent of the adult male population of England and Wales. Of those, he believes that 4.14 million, or 41.2 percent of adult males, insured for sickness as well as burial, which he takes to show a smaller gain over earlier membership proportions than previous scholars had suggested.

Recent research has confirmed the view that substantial numbers of people belonged to friendly societies already at the beginning of the nineteenth century and that the significant development during the nineteenth century was not the growth of membership per se but rather a shift of membership from independent to affiliated societies.[7] Affiliated societies united local units under a regional or national umbrella. Johnson's interpretation is consistent with this view. But his numbers are suspect. Johnson excludes from consideration the members of numerous unregistered societies, trade union societies, and other benefit groups that provided sickness coverage.[8] As a result, his estimate of 41.2 percent understates the proportion of men who enjoyed sickness and burial coverage at the end of the nineteenth century, although the size of the understatement is difficult to establish. Around 1900, near the peak of the self-help movement, probably half or more of adult males belonged to societies providing sickness and burial coverage.[9]

In fact, all these estimates understate the scale of the friendly societies, because they compare the membership of organizations serving the working class with the entire adult male population, whereas the appropriate comparison would be with the social and income groups among which membership was commonplace.[10] If working people made up three-quarters of the population, as many authorities suggest, and if at least half of adult males belonged to societies offering sickness benefits, then the proportion of workingmen who enjoyed sickness benefits came not to one-

6. Johnson, *Saving and Spending,* 49–57; Hanson, "Welfare before the Welfare State."
7. Jones, "Did Friendly Societies Matter?"
8. Hardy, "Friendly Societies," 255–60, lists the types of societies. Brown, *Meagre Harvest,* 42–74, passim, discusses the sickness benefit element of the National Agricultural Labourers' Union; Southall, "Neither State nor Market," discusses provision of sickness benefits by the union of steam-engine workers; and Boyer, "What Did Unions Do in Nineteenth-Century Britain?" discusses union sickness funds and reports (320) that 612 thousand union members were eligible for sickness benefits in 1893.
9. Digby and Bosanquet, "Doctors and Patients," 78, suggest this proportion for working people who had access to contract medical care, chiefly through friendly societies, in 1905.
10. This point is made by Thompson, *Rise of Respectable Society,* 201.

half but to two-thirds. Friendly society membership and access to its sickness and burial benefits was characteristic of men in the British working class in the second half of the nineteenth century.

Children were first recruited into sick clubs in large numbers in the 1820s and 1830s, when some Sunday schools organized sick funds for teachers and students.[11] By the 1870s, the Foresters and the Oddfellows enrolled children of eight or ten in juvenile clubs, which served as a source of assistance for working children who fell sick and as a recruitment device for the affiliated sick clubs. When they reached eighteen, the children, it was hoped, would join the adult club. Women working at home rarely joined societies, but women who joined while in the workforce did not always leave when they married or gave up their jobs. Even so, for women the friendly society movement remained limited chiefly to independent clubs until the 1890s, when the affiliated societies began to recruit women.[12] Thus although many children and women belonged, friendly societies served chiefly adult males.

As friendly society authorities eagerly pointed out, both members and those dependent on them were represented. Although information is unavailable about numbers of dependents, it is important to see the membership as reflecting not merely the insurance needs of working people but also those of their dependents. Sometimes, the dependents' wages could be insured or access to medical care gained through a society. But more often the benefits dependents received consisted only of what the societies did to maintain the household's income flow by paying benefits to its head.

Since many British working people did not belong to friendly societies, the question naturally arises as to whether the characteristics of members and nonmembers differed. Were they part of the divisions within the working class that so troubled Friedrich Engels? Johnson, like some earlier authorities, including John Frome Wilkinson, Eric Hobsbawm, Bentley Gilbert, and Geoffrey Crossick,[13] argues that members differed in an important way because friendly societies appealed especially to skilled workers,[14] people often characterized, because of their high wages or their

11. Laqueur, *Religion and Respectability*, 172–74.
12. *Foresters' Miscellany*, May 1889, 223, reports that more than 4.5 million unmarried women worked in Britain at that time.
13. Wilkinson, *Friendly Society Movement*, 183–201; Hobsbawm, *Workers: Worlds of Labor*, 227; Gilbert, *Evolution of National Insurance*, 166; Crossick, *Artisan Elite*, 175, 181, 186 (but see also 182–84 for reservations).
14. Johnson, *Saving and Spending*, 55, 60.

residence outside the crowded central city, as part of a labor aristocracy.[15] Some nineteenth-century observers made a similar argument on the basis of their belief that men earning less than some twenty shillings a week could not afford to pay friendly society premiums. That is certainly true of some individual friendly societies, and it is true also of most friendly societies in certain locales, such as Kentish London.[16] It appears also to have some value for characterizing the early years of the friendly society movement, up to the middle of the nineteenth century.

But for Britain as a whole and for the second half of the nineteenth century, this view is persuasively contradicted by what local historians have found from the rosters of individual clubs, which show the occupations of members. Dot Jones's research on the occupations of Welsh club members shows that laborers often belonged and were sometimes the single largest occupational group.[17] Hilary Marland, focusing on sick clubs in two West Riding towns, concluded that the societies represented a cross section of the working class, a position taken earlier by E. P. Thompson.[18] In Cambridge, too, Elizabeth Edwards found that friendly society membership was not a badge of skilled workers.[19] And in rural East Riding, according to David Neave, agricultural laborers and other workers usually (but inaccurately)[20] described as unskilled often belonged to friendly societies. Neave remarks further how different is the picture of friendly societies inferred from the records of local clubs, which emphasize how many men in poorly paid occupations belonged, from the conclusions

15. Hobsbawm, "Labour Aristocracy in Nineteenth-Century Britain." Gray, *Aristocracy of Labour in Nineteenth-Century Britain,* esp. 20–29, and *Labour Aristocracy in Victorian Edinburgh,* esp. 43–90, argues that the distinction is appropriate but also that it is a distinction not simply between skilled and unskilled workers but also of an elite within each trade. Drawing on the writings of Thomas Wright, Alastair Reid questions the value of this concept, pointing out the many ways in which skilled workers resembled laborers. Reid, "Intelligent Artisans and Aristocrats of Labour." Henry Pelling himself made the same point in "Concept of the Labour Aristocracy," 55.

16. Whether it applies to Essex farmworkers is unclear. Brown, *Meagre Harvest,* 36, 146, argues both that farmworkers did not join the Oddfellows because the premiums were too high and also that they did join, their entrance fees being paid by benefactors.

17. Jones, "Did Friendly Societies Matter?" 337–38, and "Self-Help in Nineteenth-Century Wales," 22.

18. Marland, *Medicine and Society in Wakefield and Huddersfield,* 177–83; Thompson, *Making of the English Working Class,* 419. Although he described friendly society members as chiefly the more prosperous of workers, E. J. Hobsbawm also used the statistics of the Oddfellows to describe the working class in general. Hobsbawm, *Labouring Men,* 71, 135.

19. Edwards, "Friendly Societies," 189–92.

20. See the point made by Snell, *Men, Movements, and Myself,* 8. An agricultural laborer himself in his youth, he regarded such workers as highly skilled.

based on official and printed sources.[21] Even Samuel Strudwick, the composite fictional character created to introduce British schoolchildren to the hard life of farm laborers in the Victorian era, belonged to a benefit club, although he earned only thirteen shillings a week.[22] A broad-based friendly society membership existed well before 1870, when the detailed analysis given here begins.

Studies by friendly society actuaries, who examined the mixture of members in hazardous and nonhazardous trades and, in the process, accumulated data about the numbers in individual occupations or groups, also show the broad reach of self-help across the working classes. For 1893–97, Alfred Watson calculated that people working in agriculture, chiefly farm laborers, made up 13.6 percent of the Oddfellows, a figure quite close to the 11.9 percent of males in England and Wales working in agriculture according to the 1891 census.[23]

The AOF never published tables showing the occupations of members. Their actuary, F. G. P. Neison Jr., wanted to add data on occupational risks to his 1882 report, but the AOF executive council, believing enough had already been spent on the project, refused to spend anything more. Hence, Watson's survey of the Oddfellows in 1893–97, which focuses on hazardous occupations, provides the most extensive data available for comparing the occupations of friendly society members to those of men in England and Wales in general. Table 1.1 shows the results of this comparison, reallocating the occupations of males aged ten and over as reported in the 1891 census to Watson's categories, which attempted to appraise health hazards and thus grouped most occupations in a nonhazardous category called "other."[24] In some hazardous occupations men joined the Oddfellows in slightly smaller or larger numbers than their proportion in the population at large. But the comparison is more remarkable for the congruence of proportions. Not only did the Oddfellows and other friendly societies enroll many men who had poorly paying jobs, but also the occupational mix among the Oddfellows who held jobs that friendly society records

21. Neave, *Mutual Aid in the Victorian Countryside*, 7, passim.
22. Huggett, *Day in the Life of a Victorian Farm Worker*, 49, 60.
23. Watson, *Sickness and Mortality Experience*, 30–33. The proportion is based on years of life at risk. For census results, see Mitchell, *British Historical Statistics*, 104. Male indoor domestics rarely joined friendly societies, but female servants often did. Regular members of the armed forces also did not ordinarily join.
24. Watson reports years of life exposed to risk rather than numbers of men, but the proportions are not affected by that approach. He also makes the comparison easier by listing specific trades included within each general category. But he does not report their proportions within the category.

Table 1.1
OCCUPATIONS OF ODDFELLOWS, 1893–1897, AND OF MALES (AGE 10+)
IN ENGLAND AND WALES, 1891

	Proportion in the IOOF (percent)	Proportion in England and Wales (percent)
Agriculture	13.6	11.9
Building	8.1	6.4
Railways	1.7	1.8
Seafaring and fishing	1.4	2.2
Quarrying	0.9	2.0
Iron and steel	3.6	5.3
Mining	5.9	6.0
Other	64.9	64.5

Source: Data from Watson, Sickness and Mortality Experience, 30–33; Great Britain, Parliamentary Papers, 1893–94, CVI, vii–ix.

showed to be hazardous resembled the mix in the overall male population.

Individual societies tended to occupy niches within the hierarchy of working-class life. The Oddfellows stood slightly higher in the wage hierarchy than did most other friendly societies,[25] just above the Foresters. Unregistered clubs often enrolled the worst-paid workers of village and town, while, at the other extreme, a few societies excluded lower-wage earners, those practicing hazardous trades, or people who acknowledged that they drank. The Royal Standard Benefit Society required a weekly wage of at least twenty-four shillings, the Hearts of Oak for a time excluded miners, and the Rechabites limited its membership to teetotalers.[26] The Foresters and the Oddfellows, the two societies whose records figure most prominently in this study, applied none of these exclusions, though local units may sometimes have done so. At the time, both societies were regarded as especially representative of the working classes, and the evidence reported here confirms that impression.[27]

Although friendly societies, taken as a whole, appealed to a cross section of the working-class population, their members were not necessarily char-

25. Wilkinson, Friendly Society Movement, 194; Gray, Labour Aristocracy in Victorian Edinburgh, 122–26.

26. Johnson, Saving and Spending, 61.

27. See Watson's remarks about the Oddfellows in Rusher, "Statistics of Industrial Morbidity," 78. The same broad mix of occupations appears among the sixty members of friendly societies whose height and weight were measured for John Beddoe in 1866 (John Beddoe Collection, DM2). Those sixty men were slightly shorter than average Englishmen of the same ages, but they weighed more and had a larger body mass index, 23.09, compared to the English average, 22.86. Riley, "Height, Nutrition, and Mortality Risk Reconsidered."

acteristic of working people. Society leaders, who described their colleagues in favorable terms, often spoke of members as a select class of men,
meaning not that they earned higher wages but that they were morally
superior. They were men characterized by "prudent foresight and eleva-
tion of mind."[28] Friendly society members anticipated financial risks and
prepared for them in advance. Whether a risk-averse attitude actually
distinguished members from nonmembers who otherwise resembled them
is also unlikely. Most men joined in their early twenties, a time in life when
risk calculations count less than peer acceptance. They were often recruited by friends and workmates, which suggests that attitudes toward
risk mattered less than friendship networks in determining who would join
a friendly society and who would not.[29]

Certainly, the societies' members differed from the general population.
People of higher-than-petit-bourgeois status were rarely inclined to join a
friendly society, although a few self-made men remained members after
they had risen above club peers. Friendly societies also did not intend to
appeal to the poor—those who could not afford to pay the contributions
necessary to secure friendly society benefits. By the late nineteenth century,
the societies charged weekly premiums of at least four to six pence for
basic sickness and burial benefits. These were amounts a workingman
with commonplace skills making sixteen to twenty shillings a week might
pay without great difficulty, for they amounted to between 1.7 and 3.1
percent of such wages.[30] But even these low premiums were often beyond
the reach of people without jobs or employed only sporadically. Many men
and women joined friendly societies only to leave them when they could no
longer pay premiums, a phenomenon the societies called secession. Typically, those members who left—seceded—did so within a few years of
joining, thus in their early or middle twenties, and because they could not
pay.[31] Irregular employment, a common enough problem, prevented some
working people from joining or maintaining their memberships. One leading cause of departure from a friendly society was, therefore, a transition
into poverty.

28. Committee of the Highland Society of Scotland, *Report*, 55–56. Also Neison, *Contributions to Vital Statistics*, v, xiii.

29. The issue of selection is discussed in chapter 5 and appendix 1.

30. Reeves, *Family Life on a Pound a Week*, mentions how often families with wage
incomes of eighteen to twenty shillings a week belonged to burial societies.

31. For an exception, see Marcroft, *Marcroft Family*, 62–63. Marcroft, who belonged,
apparently at different times, to the Oddfellows and the Rechabites, left because he did not
think the benefits were worth the expense and because he wanted to save on his own account.
He dropped out of his union at the same time.

Southwood Smith argued in 1830 that ill health caused poverty.[32] That trap was precisely what friendly society membership was meant to avoid by supplying benefits that would save the sick from poverty. Hence, friendly society members, those who fell sick before they exhausted their ability to pay premiums, were meant to escape the trap. But some men and women fell into poverty first, losing the wherewithal to pay friendly society premiums and thereby losing also that safeguard. For them, poverty might cause ill health; except in rare cases of charitable generosity there would be no relief offered from their old sick club.[33]

Late-nineteenth-century commentators sometimes divided the poor into two categories, primary and secondary. To the category of primary poverty were assigned people who could not afford the necessities of life; few such people belonged to friendly societies, except those who fell temporarily into such poverty but were assisted by their colleagues. To the category of secondary poverty were assigned people whose earnings were sufficient but whose expenses left them in danger of destitution.[34] Many friendly society members belonged to this category, even though the small sums they paid to sick clubs must sometimes have forced them to do without other things. Friendly societies appealed chiefly to people with jobs, including many whose circumstances made them seem poor to such observers as Charles Booth, Seebohm Rowntree, and Fred Scott.

Divisions within the working class complicate the matter of deciding to whom the friendly societies appealed.[35] In London, for example, Booth estimated the poor to account for 30.7 percent of the population, of whom most were poor either because they worked regularly but did not earn enough to escape Booth's threshold or because too often they lacked work.[36] Many of the poor, certainly, belonged to friendly societies: for example, members who were drawing long-term benefits for sickness because those benefits were paid at such a low level as to qualify these men as poor, by Booth's standard or Rowntree's. (The friendly societies usually paid full benefits for the first six months of a long episode, half benefits for the next six months, and quarter benefits thereafter.) Booth numbered between 23 and 45 percent of the poor as members of East London friendly

32. See Youngson, *Scientific Revolution in Victorian Medicine*, 22. For the context of Smith's remarks, see Flinn, "Introduction."
33. Burn, *Autobiography of a Beggar Boy*, 155, recalls an instance in which he was helped out by the Oddfellows even though his premiums were not paid up.
34. Treble, *Urban Poverty in Britain*, 11–12.
35. On such divisions, see Chinn, *They Worked All Their Lives*, 1–6.
36. Booth, *Life and Labour of the People in London*, 2:20–21.

societies, apparently not counting people in dividing societies, which appealed especially to those whose economic position was marginal.[37]

Setting the poverty level at, respectively, 18s. and 21s. 8d. a week, Booth and Rowntree automatically included full-pay beneficiaries of the Hearts of Oak, which paid a generous 18s. a week, and of the Foresters, which were paying 10 or 12s. at the end of the century, and of course all those friendly society members on benefits for lengthy periods and receiving only half or quarter pay.[38] Booth's group must also have included many men who had, at one time or another, belonged to a friendly society but, finding it difficult to keep up their contributions, had been expelled for nonpayment. Men in such circumstances could rejoin a society, as long as they were under the ceiling age, usually forty. But their poorly paid or irregular employment made it difficult to keep up membership. It was especially people in such circumstances who benefited from the introduction of national insurance in 1912 and its medical benefits in 1913. Thereafter, they received sickness benefits and medical care without having to save in advance, except indirectly, by paying contributions and taxes.

In fact, Booth's threshold for distinguishing the poor from working people does not coincide very closely with the threshold that distinguished people who could not afford to keep up friendly society membership from those who could. The group he designates as poor includes many more people than the proportion, then somewhat less than 3 percent, benefiting from poor relief, but it also includes many people belonging to and benefiting from provident organizations.

WHAT FRIENDLY SOCIETIES DID
FOR WORKING PEOPLE

A history of the friendly societies' asylum in Cambridge sums up the appeal of these organizations:

> if the poor man have no provision [against sickness], he and his family must soon feel the pressure of want: even if by rigid economy he may have been enabled to lay by a small sum, it must soon be exhausted: by degrees he is com-

---

37. Ibid., 1:106–10. In dividing societies, any balance accumulated each year was meted out in proportion to claims made during the year, and no assets were held for future liabilities. In contrast, most friendly societies accumulated assets against the expectation that claims would rise as members aged and that they would rise at a faster rate than members would be willing to augment their premiums.

38. Rowntree, *Poverty: A Study of Town Life*, 110; Booth, *Life and Labour of the People in London*, 1:33.

pelled to dispose of his little stock of furniture, on which all the comforts of his home depend; and if illness be prolonged, or frequent, he is ultimately driven to take refuge in the workhouse, by which event his wounded feelings inflict far more suffering than his personal privations.[39]

That was the view of social superiors, who spoke with confidence about the attitudes and feelings of working people.

Working people put the case differently. They certainly stressed the importance of financial security. But when they explained why friendly societies appealed to them, the men and women who belonged also emphasized fellowship. Friendly societies provided their members with a circle of friends who came to their aid in trying times and kept them from being forced to go on relief. Sickness was one of the most common hazards working people faced that forced them onto poor relief,[40] but most members who fell sick escaped that fate. Members could count on being visited when sick, on receiving benefits, and on other signs of fraternal affection. For example, they turned out for a brother's funeral to show the world how many friends he had had and to console his survivors. "There are few men who do not consider consolation as a necessary appendage to friendship," intoned the *Foresters' Miscellany* in 1871.[41] Both the sentiment and its ponderous phrasing are typical.

Membership also conveyed respectability, which Crossick labels "one of the most pervasive of mid-Victorian social concepts."[42] It conveyed respectability not on grounds of the individual's characteristics, which were often insufficient to persuade workers that they earned the respect of society, but on grounds of membership in a group which, collectively, earned that respect. Among themselves, in meetings and in the pages of their periodicals, friendly society members could talk about singular things: the antiquity of their clubs and the nobility of the members. Foresters sometimes called themselves a "noble army."[43] The friendly society provided a guarantee of independence, in the form of the financial security that allowed a man or a woman to have no fear of being forced onto relief.[44] It was at once insurance against both the poverty that sickness might bring and the prospect of relief under the New Poor Law.

Strictly speaking, that guarantee of independence was something of an

---

39. *Cambridge Victoria Friendly Societies' Asylum*, 5.
40. Treble, *Urban Poverty in Britain*, 94.
41. *Foresters' Miscellany*, Jan. 1871, 285.
42. Crossick, *Artisan Elite*, 135. See also Tholfsen, *Working-Class Radicalism*, 216–22.
43. E.g., *Foresters' Miscellany*, July 1869, 403.
44. Howkins, *Reshaping Rural England*, 63–64, quotes opinions of some working people on the workhouse.

exaggeration. Some friendly society members who suffered long illnesses were forced onto relief or into public or charitably funded institutions, while the society and poor law authorities argued over who was liable for providing support. But in the typical case friendly society membership did provide financial security in the form of cash payments too high to allow the recipient to qualify for poor relief, however one may judge their sufficiency for keeping a man and his family at an acceptable standard of living.[45] Alternately, when a fellow member suffered reverses that did not qualify him for benefits, members often helped out by making a special collection or drawing on the benevolent fund that most clubs accumulated. When Joseph Gutteridge's son died of smallpox at a time when the family lacked the resources to pay for his burial, the Oddfellows of his lodge took up a collection.[46]

Charles Marshall illustrated the keen appeal of financial security in a story he wrote for the *Foresters' Miscellany* in 1873.[47] As the story goes, a building laborer named Charles Williams one day asked his wife, Anne, whether the sovereign he had managed to set aside should be used to join the Foresters. His wife thought that a good idea but thought it better still to buy the children some new clothes. She was, in Marshall's imagination, a feckless woman for whom appearance counted more than security. Williams gave in to her whim in order to avoid her unpleasantness. Later Williams fell, suffering internal injuries. Anne called the doctor, only to learn that her husband would be laid up for a long time and might never recover. She feared being forced onto poor relief. But to her surprise some of her husband's fellow workers brought her twelve shillings and promised each week to do the same again. Without her knowledge her husband had joined the Foresters. She was overcome with relief. Having faced the prospect of asking for poor relief, she was so relieved that her husband had joined the AOF that she reformed herself. Friendly society recruiters told stories like this to explain why men should join.

How large the risk of financial dependence loomed for men who did not belong to friendly societies is now difficult to specify. It is possible to recount stories both of nonmembers who contracted a disease or were

45. For unmarried members, benefits accrued while the individual was on public assistance and were paid upon recovery, with or without liability by the individual to the public institutions that had provided relief. See, e.g., AOF, *Second Quarterly Report of the Forty-First Executive Council,* 39–40.
46. Chancellor, *Master and Artisan in Victorian England,* 132.
47. Marshall, "Charles Williams's Accident." To the same effect, Marshall, "Do You Belong to a Benefit Society?"

injured and were forsaken by their relatives, friends, and employers, and of men who received aid from those sources.

James Smith, a Dundee stonemason, lived in the era of the friendly societies but gives no indication in his memoirs of having joined one. Born in 1805, he married twice, had six children, earned as much as £87 4s. 11d. in a single year (1847), suffered a long disability, and wrote at length about his confidence in his God, the ailments he suffered, the sources of his income in hard years, and the memorable moments of his life. He includes a coy reference to being deceived by a widow who took him for a gentleman and pretended herself to be a lady, though neither was true, and the story of the joyous day of a family picnic, on which began a long bout of problems with his ankles that incapacitated him. His problem, diagnosed initially as rheumatism, prompted a long and varied course of treatment, including the amputation of a big toe. When he fell sick in 1849, Smith had been working one day a week for the Dundee Bank, carrying parcels to Edinburgh for a wage of 16s. a week. Though the bank obliged him to return to Dundee, cutting short a period of convalescence at his sister's home near Banff, it was also generous and patient in helping him out. From 1849 until April 1854, though he did no work for the bank, Smith received 8s. a week, which made up the bulk of the family earnings in those years.[48] After the bank stopped helping him, Smith was supported by his son John, who for a time shared his wages with his parents, by the earnings of his wife, who took jobs in domestic service, and by church charity. He never recovered enough to return to work but lived until at least 1869.

If Smith's part-time employer can only be called generous, his situation was atypical. Employees of the Great North of Scotland Railway appear often to have been discharged when they were ill or injured for lengthy periods, even though they were on leave without pay.[49] The treatment another man received from his employer moved Dr. John Johnston, a general practitioner in Bolton, to make an entry in his diary titled "How a master treats men crippled in his Employ":

Speaking to the manager of the mill in wh[ich] JR lost his left arm a few weeks ago I said "I suppose you will find him something to do in the mill." He said: "I dont know what he could do. He couldnt follow his own trade & *he would be no use to us*[.]" "Then," I said, "I suppose you will give him some compensation for the loss of his arm?" To this he replied: "I don't know

48. Memoirs of James Smith, 49–59.
49. Great North of Scotland Railway Passenger Department papers, register of staff off duty, vol. 2, 1902–13.

that we shall. We've paid him his wages up to now, and we didnt give any compensation to the two other men who lost their arms here—for this is the third case that has happened at our mill."[50]

Not everyone was as hardhearted as Johnston's unnamed mill operator. Some employers provided compensation either from their own resources or through works clubs they partially funded.[51]

At first glance, the growth of the friendly societies from the 1830s would seem to be an argument for the growing need for assurance against the risk of financial dependence. Perhaps this was an effect of a change in labor markets, in which men had fewer opportunities to find jobs that carried with them a network of supportive neighbors, friends, and employers. Perhaps it was an outgrowth of the greater average distance that separated people in an increasingly mobile society from the places where they had been born and from their parents and siblings. But it is at least as likely that the growth of friendly societies was driven by the increasing degree to which working people could afford to spend what the societies charged for wage insurance and medical services and, therefore, that the friendly societies were a product of rising discretionary resources rather than of a rising need for assurance against financial dependence.

THE FORESTERS' AND THE FRIENDLY SOCIETIES' ETHOS

"The Ancient Order of Foresters is eminently an outcome and a symbol of latter-day civilization."[52] So opens the history of the order written by T. Ballan Stead, former national head of the order and permanent secretary, and republished each year from 1886, with emendations, in the AOF directory. Elizabeth Edwards accuses the friendly societies of pretentiousness.[53] It is an accurate charge. Friendly society leaders blustered about the importance of their organizations not because, on the national scene, the friendly societies were dominant institutions but because the members and leaders of these organizations wished to be taken as more important than they were.

50. Johnston Papers, ZJO/3/4, 1894–95.
51. See, e.g., Great Northern Railway Locomotive Friendly Society papers, minutes, DS9/10/1.
52. AOF, Directory, 1903, viii.
53. Edwards, Friendly Societies, 2–3.

Thus, they bragged about the financial resources at their disposal. On a per capita basis the assets of the friendly societies were as modest as the wages of working people. Only in the aggregate were these assets as important as friendly society officials proclaimed. The thirty-three societies represented at the National Conference of Friendly Societies in 1899 claimed 3,481,672 members and assets of £23.7 million, or £6 16s. 2d. per capita.[54] Friendly society investments in the public debt, real estate, savings banks, and other directions did something to sustain the low interest rates that prevailed in late-nineteenth-century Britain, if not so much because of the scale of their assets as because the friendly societies were so often cautious in their investment choices and managed their portfolios in ways that did little to promote higher interest rates. Not until 1901 did the national organization encourage the formation of investment funds, which searched out secure but higher-yielding investments.

Friendly societies claimed national political influence. Political leaders took care to join, usually as honorary members, and willingly spoke at national meetings. How far their attentiveness to the societies translated into political power is another matter, one put to the test in debates over the views of friendly society leaders on the National Insurance Act of 1911. The societies found they had less power than they had thought, even that their organizations could be made objects of ridicule.[55]

For local friendly society members themselves, especially in villages and towns, the symbol of their importance was for some years the annual procession, in which officers and members marched, wearing their regalia. Like Stead's opening statement in the AOF history, the processions asserted that the friendly societies and workingmen, too, had a public ritual and thus could legitimately claim a position of importance in a society where such rituals seemed, to working-class outsiders at least, to constitute the outward manifestation of power and position. Quickly enough, however, participation in the processions declined. Perhaps public reaction to these processions, revealed by the often sneeringly patronizing tone of newspaper articles describing them, which Edwards quotes, taught club members that ritual was not enough. Perhaps members were dismayed at how much their club day threatened to become an occasion for listening to speeches about how working people should emulate the moral values of the middle and upper classes of Britain. Read about in the memoirs of

54. AOF, *Directory*, 1903, xlv.
55. Gilbert, *Evolution of National Insurance*, 377.

members of the elite, who gave speeches, or in newspaper accounts of the speeches, it seems plausible to argue that the moral values of the elite penetrated the working class through the friendly societies.[56] In friendly society minutes, however, club day activities have the appearance not of allowing working people to learn what the elite wanted of them but of letting the people who watched the procession learn about working people.

Stead, who worked for workingmen but also patronized them, thought that the function of the friendly societies was to "bind men together in bonds of keenest sympathy, and teach them how exquisite is the pleasure of 'relieving distress, aiding the weak, and comforting the mourner.'"[57] He did not understand that the friendly societies were an outgrowth of the needs and aspirations of workingmen or that leaders like himself were products of the friendly societies rather than their causes. Like so many people within the national leadership of the societies and among outside observers and critics, the point seemed to be to use the societies to teach workingmen something. Yet much of the history of the friendly societies, told from the perspective of their individual units, is a story of conflicts between would-be teachers and reluctant students. For a long time members spiritedly resisted the advice of their national officers, as they did also the advice of community leaders who thought they knew better than working people what was best for them.[58]

Because national leaders were so much apart from members, the history of the AOF that Stead wrote has remarkably little to do with what matters here. As a history it stresses names and dates, of course, and seeks to find a part for every region in Britain in the order's experience by organizing the narrative around national meetings, which were held each year in a different town. For ordinary members one of the most commonplace experiences of membership was the submission of a claim for sickness benefits and the receipt of benefits. Stead barely mentions this feature of AOF history.

Many friendly society leaders wished to believe that the origins of the societies they led were lost in the mists of time, made obscure by the old-regime government's opposition to organizations among working people. Stead admitted that the AOF could not trace its origins to Robin Hood, as

56. Howkins, "Taming of Whitsun."
57. AOF, *Directory*, 1903, viii.
58. On the ideology of friendly society members and their independent spirit, see Neave, *Mutual Aid in the Victorian Countryside*, 86–96; Kirk, *Growth of Working-Class Reformism*, 207–20; and Tholfsen, *Working-Class Radicalism*, esp. 11 and 288–305.

its symbols and ritual implied, but in the same thought claimed nearly as much antiquity. The origins of mutual aid are, indeed, lost in the mists of time, but the AOF and its fellow affiliated friendly societies were products of the nineteenth century. The AOF itself formed in 1834 among a splinter group of courts belonging to the Royal Order of Foresters, which had been formed some time earlier. The splinter group objected to the arbitrary and authoritarian manner of the governing leaders of the Royal Foresters. In sum, the AOF owed its formation to the willingness of workingmen to defy their leaders. For a long time defiance marked its meetings. In individual courts members rejected the advice from national officers and their social betters, preferring to make their own mistakes; and at national meetings delegates often resisted the recommendations of AOF officials, especially about financial issues.

The Royal Foresters regarded "life as a journey 'through the Forest of this world,' and so they called themselves Foresters."[59] The order's ritual and regalia pursued the theme of forestry, giving a distinctive character to the society. Like other friendly societies, the Foresters emphasized ritual, piety, and the reaffirmation of moral values in their inaugural documents. As time passed these features retreated, giving way to a stress on fellowship and on the community of working people assisting one another.

The AOF grew rapidly for a time after 1834. By 1871, 5,650 courts had been organized, of which 3,658 remained active, mostly in England and Wales but also a few in Ireland, more in British colonies, and elsewhere. During the 1870s the order expanded rapidly in Scotland. Of the 3,658 active courts, all but two reported to headquarters in time to be included in the 1872 directory.[60] Many courts had a brief history. The AOF was willing to constitute a court when as few as eight men joined, but not many courts with such small memberships survived. Other courts disappeared by amalgamating, some broke away from the AOF in disputes, and some failed financially.[61]

For many workingmen in the AOF, participation in the local, regional, and national organization was a matter of pride. Some courts and officers failed in their duties, but it is more remarkable that so many thousands of men took so much trouble to fulfill their tasks: keeping the extensive ledgers and minutes of each court, reporting each year to the national

59. Cooper, *Ancient Order of Foresters Friendly Society*, 2, quoting 1790 founding documents from the Royal Order of Foresters.

60. However, not all supplied information on all points. Those failing to supply data in given years have been excluded from analysis.

61. In 1863–74, an average of 14.9 courts were closed each year, and 15.8 were amalgamated with other courts. AOF, *Fourth Quarterly Report of the Forty-First Executive Council*, 82.

organization, visiting the sick, recruiting new members, and otherwise tending to business. Internal checks of the AOF directories and the records of individual courts show also that court officers took care to keep and report accurate records. As an innkeeper in Matlock mused one day in 1985, "Me old Dad spent a lot of time keeping the records of his court."

In the nineteenth century friends and relatives no longer sufficed as support in times of distress. To supplement the aid they gave, working people turned to organizations of their own, especially to friendly societies. These societies enrolled a large minority of workingmen at the beginning of the nineteenth century and up to two-thirds of them at the century's end. In the early 1800s most of their members belonged to local societies, which lost ground during the century to national friendly societies, with which local units affiliated. In the affiliated societies the men of a village or neighborhood retained control over the club, but they allied it with a national organization able to contribute sound actuarial advice, one that also allowed members to move about Britain without having to give up what they had invested in a friendly society. The researches of local historians show that by the 1870s membership of friendly societies comprised a cross section of Britons who worked with their hands, including many people whose employment was irregular.

In the way they described themselves, friendly society members seem likeliest to have differed from their peers not in the wages they earned, their attitudes toward risk, or their qualities of character and mind but in their desire for respectability. Men joined friendly societies at the beginning of their working lives, apparently because of the influence of friends and workmates rather than their own individual attitudes. Within the societies they cultivated a collective sense of self-worth and independence. In this respect they made themselves into a distinctive group. But in the more conventional terms of analysis, where jobs, level of income, and residence count, friendly society members stood within—indeed they made up—the central ranks of working people. In the middle of the hierarchy of friendly society pay and occupational status stood the Foresters. Arthur Munby, notorious for his close scrutiny of the working classes, especially muscular workingwomen, explained that visiting a Foresters' anniversary celebration in London "is of all the others the scene and the time to see the English working classes."[62]

62. Quoted by Hudson, *Munby, Man of Two Worlds*, 71.

CHAPTER 2

The Friendly Societies' Medical Economy

JAMES SMITH, a Dundee stonemason, turned forty in 1845. He suffered from gravel, which he had tried for a long time to treat himself. Smith wrote to his brother in northern Scotland, where there was a "clever" doctor who sent him a prescription. The Dundee druggist to whom he took the prescription told Smith that he had seen this medication tried repeatedly and without success. The druggist recommended instead that Smith try several beverages, including small beer, ale, porter, and buttermilk, to discover which made him pass the most urine and then drink as much of that beverage as he could. That might, the druggist claimed, lead him to pass the small grain or grains that had formed in his kidneys. "I then set to work you may suppose & found that Butter Milk was the most powerfulest on the Kidneys." Friends and children fetched buttermilk from the country every day. But this therapy, too, failed.

Smith's sickness reached a crisis one night, when he could not urinate because the pain was so severe. The next morning he made his weekly trip to Edinburgh, carrying parcels for the Dundee Bank. Passing a hotel on his way to the wharf, Smith decided to have a glass of gin. He then crossed the Firth of Tay and took a stage coach for Edinburgh, suffering terribly. Boarding a second ferry at Kirkcaldy to cross the Firth of Forth, however, he went to the water closet and passed urine. "Something had come away after I was on deck. I thought I should see, so I went down & found a stone." He suffered no more from gravel, though for years he suffered a pain in his left side.[1]

Smith does not say what he thought had cured him, but he seems to attribute his cure to the chance consumption of a glass of gin on the morning after his crisis. Perhaps he thought it was the combination of gin

1. Memoirs of James Smith, 45–46.

45

plus a rough stagecoach ride and then a stormy passage from Kirkcaldy. What is more pertinent about Smith's bout with gravel is how it typifies what medical treatment was for working people of his day.

In the eighteenth and early nineteenth centuries, manual laborers did not usually consult formally trained medical practitioners, either physicians or surgeons, unless they were destitute. The poor on parish relief received some attention from formal practitioners, given gratis or under contract to poor law authorities. Under the old poor law, people judged eligible for relief received financial help when they were sick, infirm, or old as well as when they were unemployed or earned too little, and if they needed a doctor, nurse, or midwife, parish authorities paid the bill. Under the 1834 law, the poor law union bore the same responsibility for providing medical attendance for the sick. A relieving officer decided on eligibility for assistance and sent all those needing attendance to the union's medical officer, who provided care and medicine in return for a fixed stipend or moved the sick poor into the union's workhouse, which increasingly acquired the character of a hospital. In the eyes of poor law authorities, paupers were not numerous. A substantial fraction of paupers qualified for medical relief, but paupers in all forms—the destitute and infirm elderly, lunatics, the blind, orphans, and others—never constituted more than a small fraction of the populace.[2] Formal medical practice focused on the middle and upper classes.

For the working class—skilled artisans, industrial workers, and unskilled laborers alike—contact with formal medicine occurred chiefly through chemists and apothecaries who dispensed medications, selling both the components of prescriptions they mixed and medicinal substances that working people wanted but could not grow or make for themselves. Working people bought drugs from apothecaries on their own advice or because the apothecary suggested a certain treatment. For other medical services working people relied on informal practitioners, who lacked training or were medical autodidacts, and on friends and family members. Members of the family nursed one another and often called on the family's store of folk wisdom to identify maladies and select medications for them.[3] James Smith consulted a doctor, but by mail rather than in

2. Hodgkinson, *Origins of the National Health Service*, 6–7, 465–66, passim; Lane, "Provincial Practitioner and His Services to the Poor"; Lane, "Eighteenth-Century Medical Practice"; Henriques, *Before the Welfare State*, 46, 62 n. 66.

3. Porter and Porter, *Patient's Progress*, 33–52, passim; Porter and Porter, *In Sickness and in Health*, esp. 258–72; Loudon, *Medical Care and the General Practitioner*, 13–18; Fissell,

person. He relied most heavily on a local druggist and ultimately seems to have been cured by chance rather than by a course of therapy.[4]

Eighteenth- and early-nineteenth-century men and women from all social classes believed that maladies could and should be medicated. There was also widespread acceptance of certain ideas about treatment. Treatments were expected to yield a noticeable humoral response: patients dosed themselves in order to void, vomit, or sweat, and they took the expected effect as a promising sign that recovery would follow.[5] Yet people did not ordinarily turn to physicians or surgeons to identify their ailments, select humoral remedies, or otherwise be treated.[6] Smith evidently preferred the druggist's remedy to that proposed by his medical correspondent—he does not say whether he actually had the prescription filled—but in any case he believed that medicine, rather than Nature, would effect a cure.[7] When a cure came, his implied explanation for it cites beliefs typical in humoral theory. Changes in the nonnaturals—in this instance a glass of gin and perhaps also a rough journey, something he drank and some physical activity—promoted a cure.

FRIENDLY SOCIETIES AND ACCESS
TO FORMAL PRACTITIONERS

In Britain workingmen began regularly to consult formal medical practitioners between the late eighteenth and the mid-nineteenth centuries. They preferred surgeons, who in the same period increasingly shifted their practice from the treatment of injuries and external lesions to general medicine.[8] This transition from consulting apothecaries to seeing surgeon-general practitioners is evident in some working-class autobiographies. To

---

Patients, Power, and the Poor, 16–73; Waddington, *Medical Profession,* 181–82; Horn, *Labouring Life in the Victorian Countryside,* 185–88; Schofield, *Medical Care of the Working Class;* Chamberlain, *Old Wives' Tales,* 70–71, 84–93. See also the sketch of working-class medicine given by Stead, "New Era in Medical Aid." [Brodie], *Autobiography,* 37–39, describes the practice of a London chemist around 1800.

4. Later in his life, when he was laid up for years at a time, Smith often consulted doctors.

5. See, e.g., the remedies offered by a London chemist, as identified by [Brodie], *Autobiography,* 39.

6. Loudon, *Medical Care and the General Practitioner,* 65.

7. Later, in 1853, Smith went to Edinburgh for treatment of a swollen and stiff ankle, which had incapacitated him since 1849. A doctor there told him no man could help him, only Nature. But when he returned to Dundee, Smith began an apparently self-prescribed course of treatment, drinking cod-liver oil. Memoirs of James Smith, 56.

8. On the blurred lines between practitioners, see Digby, *Making a Medical Market,* 28 ff., and on the transition to surgical general practice, 107–27.

David Binns, of Halifax, Yorkshire, and his circle of relatives and acquaintances, it was becoming customary by the middle of the nineteenth century to call a doctor when someone was sick.[9] This transition is apparent also in the city directories that listed tradesmen. In Bristol, for example, changes can be traced through the city directories published from 1791 onwards. There were at the time twenty-two surgeons and surgeon apothecaries, nine physicians, and thirty-four apothecaries, druggists, and chemists practicing in the city. Apothecaries were more numerous than surgeons and physicians taken together. But already by 1814 the structure of formal medicine had been transformed. That year's directory listed sixty-four surgeons, some mixing the practice of surgery with dispensing medicines, twenty-three physicians, and twenty-eight apothecaries.[10]

The numerical dominance of surgeon–general practitioners continued to grow into the nineteenth century, in substantial measure because surgeons successfully took over much of the trade in dispensing medicines but in part also because individuals who earlier had designated themselves apothecaries and dispensing chemists began to call themselves surgeons instead. In Leicester the apothecary John Moore was appointed in 1829 to attend members of the Bond Street Friendly Society. He remained in service until 1868, but by 1836 he was called "doctor," and later, "surgeon."[11] At the end of the nineteenth century apothecaries retained an important role in the medical world of working-class patients, who called on them to fill prescriptions and to obtain medications that patients selected for themselves and presumably to ask for advice about self-treatment.[12] But general practitioners took over a substantial portion of the service of identifying sicknesses and selecting therapies that had been performed by apothecaries or by patients and their friends.

Above all, the growing access of working people, especially working men, to formal practitioners is evident from friendly society records. Led-

9. Autobiography of David Binns, 1203/4. See also the frequent mention of contacts with doctors in [Mountjoy], *Life, Labours, and Deliverances of a Forest of Dean Collier*, 29.

10. Loudon, *Medical Care and the General Practitioner*, 134–36, distinguishes surgeons and apothecaries from chemists and druggists and notices a sharper rise in the proportion of the latter in Bristol and elsewhere. In any case, the point of a shift toward practitioners serving working people stands.

11. Leicester Bond Street Friendly Society papers, DE1884/1, minutes, Oct. 12, 1829, and May 23, 1836. Moore also served as Leicester medical officer of health in the 1850s.

12. See pharmacists' prescription books, D/DM/273/1–33, among which I examined books 12, 13, and 14; and Francis and Co. prescription books, DD/DM/196/1–38; the comments on popular remedies in Almond, "Sutton-in-the-Isle," essay 4, "Maladies and Remedies"; and the remarks of Roberts, whose family sold medications, in *Classic Slum*, 97–100.

gers frequently show payments to doctors for contract services. Minutes relate discussions about hiring or discharging a doctor. Rules relate the terms under which members could elect to pay extra for medical care and sometimes also address the responsibilities of the club doctor to the members.[13] With the provident dispensaries, where uninsured working people often found treatment and to which some sick clubs subscribed, the friendly societies made consulting a doctor a customary rather than an unusual thing for working people to do.[14]

Some scholars have stressed how growth in the size of the middle class provided the basis for growth in the number of general practitioners.[15] Evidence from friendly society records suggests that the number of general practitioners increased also because the working class more often demanded medical services from licensed practitioners. Friendly societies pioneered medical contacts based on contract services and group coverage. Charging small monthly or quarterly fees, which members paid when they were sick and well, the club accumulated enough money to hire a surgeon on retainer, paying usually for attendance and medicines.[16] Before the end of the nineteenth century most of the men in registered societies paid the one-half to one pence a week required for contract medical services. Even in the rural counties in the south of England, where agricultural wages were low, most agricultural laborers who belonged to friendly societies appear by the 1880s to have signed up for the doctor's care.[17] At mid-century perhaps 20 to 30 percent of friendly society members enjoyed contract medical care. By the century's end that proportion had increased to two-thirds, perhaps even three-fourths, of members.

13. See also Marland, *Medicine and Society in Wakefield and Huddersfield,* 188–97. The evidence assembled here and that provided by Marland is, therefore, at odds with claims that few working people could afford doctors (Horn, *Labouring Life in the Victorian Countryside,* 185) or that "on the whole the working class saw little of the members of the medical profession in the days before the National Health Insurance Act of 1911" (Schofield, *Medical Care of the Working Class,* 3).

14. E.g., Webb, 'One of the Most Useful Charities in the City,' 5; and Parry and Parry, *Rise of the Medical Profession,* 143. The most detailed source is still Hodgkinson, *Origins of the National Health Service,* who also describes other sources of medical assistance but has little to say about the friendly societies; see 195–249, 610–19.

15. Waddington, *Medical Profession,* 26.

16. Club doctors—medical men working on contract for friendly societies, trade unions, or individual employers—should be distinguished from doctors working at family clubs, which were organized by doctors themselves as a form of prepaid medical care usually for individuals who lacked access to friendly society services, such as the wives and children of friendly society members.

17. See the lists of patients attended by different club doctors of the Abthorpe Foresters in AOF, Abthorpe Court papers, ZA1605, at the back of this ledger.

At the estimate of friendly society membership given earlier (more than 50 percent of all adult males and more than 67 percent of working-class men), these figures suggest that by 1900, at a minimum, more than a third of adult males and more than 45 percent of all working-class men acquired medical attendance through friendly societies, not including medical aid associations.[18] Only a fraction of Britain's general practitioners worked full time for friendly societies and allied organizations. But most of these doctors worked under contract for friendly societies at some point in their lives, and many did so throughout an entire career.

The friendly societies also played some role in training working people in how to be patients. In 1848 the *Foresters' Miscellany* excerpted in nine rules the advice of a celebrated physician about how to summon a doctor and how to act when the doctor arrived. Send for the doctor early, before he has started his rounds, in order to let him work a visit to your house into his route in the most efficient way; state the nature of the ailment, especially when the need for attendance is urgent; call the doctor at once and in any case do not wait until the night when "darkness frightens you into alarm"; do not waste the doctor's time with polite chat; and do not consult two doctors for the same ailment.[19] This advice, especially the first rule—call the doctor early—represents the case that doctors made about why friendly societies should engage them. Too often, they said, working people waited too long to call the doctor, until he could do them no good. Friendly societies that engaged doctors on contract would relieve their members of the financial anxiety surrounding a call to the doctor. By implication, the person who called a doctor earlier rather than later would have a less severe case, recover earlier, and be less likely to die. Those were not, of course, claims that doctors could make directly. But they could be advanced indirectly.

The same magazine, which was distributed widely among AOF members, also advised about pain and its treatment, the relationship of cold weather to health, and other matters.[20] The editors saw one of its purposes as educating workingmen about formal medicine, its etiquette, advice, and treatments. In 1887 the *Miscellany* mentioned *The Family Physician* as a source of information about health.[21] Members consulting that book

18. That is, at least 67 percent of the half of adult males who belonged to friendly societies, or of the two-thirds of working-class men who belonged.
19. *Foresters' Miscellany,* Apr. 1848, 161–62.
20. *Foresters' Miscellany,* Apr. 1869, 355–56, and July 1869, 419.
21. *Foresters' Miscellany,* Sept. 1887, 272.

found a dictionary of diseases and treatments written in layman's terms, together with discussion about the signs of disease—things noticed by medical men, especially temperature, pulse, the appearance of the tongue and urine, and the facial expression. The same book advised its readers about methods of nursing, domestic surgery, and hygiene, and it provided recipes for medications in a form that could be carried to an apothecary for mixture.[22]

The friendly societies brought working-class males as a group into contact with formal medicine.[23] They also molded that contact in a certain form, providing stingily rather than generously paid care. From the beginning the friendly societies bargained with surgeons and other practitioners on terms familiar to workingmen, holding the price of medical services as low as possible, just as the members' employers held wages as low as possible. Although plentiful evidence from friendly society sources shows that working people bargained with surgeons from a position of social inferiority and that the superior social position of the surgeon mattered to both sides, the societies enjoyed considerable advantages in these negotiations, which the British Medical Association promoter Alfred Cox, when a young general practitioner, called "dutch auctions."[24] In 1871, when an alliance of friendly societies in Worcester advertised for a surgeon, they received thirty applications for a single post paying only £170 a year.[25] Market forces and the superior capacity of the societies to manipulate the market long gave them enough power to hold fees down. Doctors reacted, according to the complaints of people dissatisfied with their services, by relegating friendly society patients to an increasingly marginal position within their practices and, finally, by turning to an aggressive campaign to combat friendly society manipulation of fees with their own combinations in restraint of trade.

CONTRACT PRACTICE

Contract practice, in which a friendly society served as the intermediary between a health care provider and potential patients, existed in the latter

---

22. *Family Physician.*
23. Digby, *Pauper Palaces,* 25, 176, makes this argument for rural laborers in Norfolk, which lagged slightly behind the average across Britain.
24. Cox, *Among the Doctors,* 30. Cox reports that doctors sometimes paid bribes in order to win practices (57).
25. *Foresters' Miscellany,* Jan. 1871, 305.

years of the eighteenth century but developed rather slowly until the 1840s and 1850s.[26] In those two decades both the friendly society movement and the frequency with which societies engaged surgeons in group contracts grew rapidly. Friendly societies expanded especially because of the advent of affiliated societies, led by the Oddfellows and the Foresters, which recruited members. Their national organizations offered not only the option of transferring membership from one locale to another but also access to the expertise needed to plan secure insurance programs. Affiliated societies encouraged the engagement of doctors to certify the health of new members as well as to provide medical attendance. Electing a surgeon was sometimes the first matter of business in a new court, after the selection of officers.[27] Furthermore, the affiliated orders urged use of premium schedules for sickness and burial benefits based on experience, in place of the rule-of-thumb schedules used by many independent friendly societies.

In the early decades of the practice, most contracts between the societies and doctors provided for attendance solely on friendly society members, excluding their families. Over time, but especially from the 1840s onward, more societies contracted for medical attendance, a growing proportion of members chose to pay for contract services, and more contracts included family members. By extending the principles of insurance to medical attendance and the provision of medicines, the friendly societies made affordable services that had previously been beyond the means of most workers, or at least beyond what workers had been willing to pay. As a way of providing medical services the group contract was much older. It was the basis on which many apothecaries, surgeons, and physicians had served institutions housing the sick poor. But use of such contracts had not previously been widespread among working people. Friendly societies provided the institutional resources—a structure in which sums due under a contract could be accumulated beforehand—and the means to bargain for an agreement, the latter in the form of officers or sponsors who negotiated terms with an attending surgeon.

Although direct evidence about the motives that led late-eighteenth-century friendly societies to enter such contracts is lacking, the very contracts themselves are testimony to a change in the medical services that working people demanded. The contracts, their growth in numbers, and the rising preference among workers for friendly societies that included

26. Loudon, *Medical Care*, 254–56. Ray Earwicker, "Miners' Medical Services," 39, dates widespread provision of medical services through friendly societies only from the 1880s.
27. E.g., AOF, Court Perseverance papers, minutes, May 29, 1876–Feb. 8, 1884.

medical services among their benefits constitute an argument that working people wanted to be attended by formal practitioners. But the sources have little to say about why the working class wanted that and why, once the preference had been given expression in the initiation of contracts between some friendly societies and surgeons, for so long it developed slowly rather than rapidly.

What did surgeons offer that made contracts with them attractive? At the point when such contracts began to become common, in the 1780s or 1790s, it is difficult to distinguish surgeons from informal practitioners on grounds of either the types of services or the efficacy of the medical care they provided. Self care and informal medicine shared with the medicine of the surgeon a reliance on a humoral conception of the sources of ill health and on humoral therapies. Surgeons may have been likelier to be skilled in inoculating for smallpox that their rivals among informal practitioners, and inoculations constituted one of a few services of unambiguous efficacy. Children inoculated for smallpox contracted milder cases of the disease and died in much smaller proportions than children who contracted the disease by natural means. Moreover, the inoculation procedure mattered, since shallower incisions reduced the risk associated with this procedure. But the friendly society members who contracted for services were already adults and thus no longer at serious risk to smallpox, a disease especially dangerous for young children and young adult migrants to cities. There is no evidence to suggest that friendly society doctors inoculated the members' children. Neither inoculation nor vaccination, which began to be practiced around 1800, provides a forceful reason to explain why workingmen began to form group contracts with surgeons in the 1780s and 1790s.

Nor were economic conditions especially propitious. Food prices rose sharply in Britain during the 1790s, in general more rapidly than wages, eroding the capacity of working people to pay for medical care. Perhaps group contracts with surgeons brought a savings over what working people had paid apothecaries and informal practitioners in buying their services individually. But too little is known about the charges made by informal practitioners to say whether this is so. Certainly, the 1790s seems an unlikely period for workingmen to have introduced a new claim on family resources.

If an explanation for the timing of this shift toward working-class contracts for medical services remains elusive, there are nevertheless powerful reasons for the preference friendly society members expressed for surgeons over other potential providers. Surgeons offered the full range of services previously important to working people, and group contracts made these services available for a single small fee. Surgeons provided medications, issuing them at attendance, and, for private patients paying per attendance rather than on contract, the charge for a surgeon's services was often included in the cost of medications, or vice versa. Surgeons also provided a wide range of medical therapies, whereas informal practitioners often specialized as bonesetters, oculists, leech suppliers, midwives, or in other areas. Compared with physicians, surgeons provided affordable and unpretentious attendance.[28]

Hence, most friendly societies engaged surgeons, sometimes in association with another practitioner. In the 1830s a Lancashire lodge of Oddfellows hired both their surgeon, Arrell, and an unnamed leech supplier, the surgeon attending members and the leech supplier furnishing leeches to members and their families.[29] But more typical, especially by the 1850s, was the assignment of all responsibilities to a surgeon. Among twenty-one practitioners who attended members of the Abthorpe court of the Foresters between the 1840s and 1909 from their surgeries in Abthorpe and neighboring villages and towns, twenty were surgeons, one a physician, and none an alternative practitioner.[30] Either the friendly societies adhered to the 1858 Medical Act, which required them to appoint only qualified practitioners, or they carefully concealed the appointment of informal practitioners even in their own confidential documents.

For friendly society members, cost was an overriding concern. From the first, the leading question was this: how little is it necessary to pay to arrange medical attendance? The same parsimonious spirit guided members deliberating about what they were willing to pay for partial compensation for wages forgone during sickness and for burial insurance. Except perhaps for the annual feast, at which members indulged themselves with food and drink,[31] a spirit of economy dominated friendly society finance. Officers were paid for the services they rendered, for example keeping the ledger of members' contributions and of benefits. But they were paid fees so small as to constitute voluntary exploitation. According to rough estimates of the time needed to keep the books, to visit the sick, or to tend to

28. Peterson, *Medical Profession in Mid-Victorian London*, 10–11, 29.
29. IOOF, Duke of York Lodge papers, minutes, 1816–c.1840, e.g., Apr. 9, 1838.
30. AOF, Abthorpe Court papers, especially ZA1585–93 and ZA1759–1809.
31. Horn, *Labouring Life*, 150–52.

other business, officers received far less per hour spent on friendly society business than they did in wages from work.[32]

Nevertheless, in the early years of contract medical services, up to the 1870s, friendly society officers were sometimes paid more in a year to keep the books and fulfill their other duties than contracting surgeons were paid to attend the sick. In St. Asaph in North Wales, Court Loyal Bodelwyddan paid its secretary £3 5s. in 1869, but its surgeon, G. W. Roberts, only £3. Not until 1872 did the surgeon, attending over forty members, earn more than the secretary, who kept the books and managed court business.[33]

Until the 1870s the bargaining power of the friendly society itself, aided up to the 1860s at least by an oversupply of practitioners, was enough to hold down fees for medical attendance. Each lodge or court needed only to find a single surgeon who would accept what they proposed to pay in order to use that to bargain with other potential suppliers. Thus when members of the Bedford Oddfellows living in nearby Kempston asked to have their own surgeon appointed, their brothers in Bedford agreed as long as the Kempston surgeon would serve on the same terms as the lodge's other doctors.[34]

Even so, the stipends friendly societies paid often constituted a substantial portion of a doctor's income. An unidentified Durham doctor recorded his gross earnings in 1846–48:[35] from February 1, 1846, until January 31, 1847, he earned £126 11s., of which £27 3d., or 21.3 percent of his total income, came from friendly societies; from February 1, 1847, to January 31, 1848, he earned £167 6s., of which £57 4s. 9d., or 34.2 percent, derived from friendly society contacts. Since private patients often did not pay as reliably or as rapidly as the friendly societies did, these proportions probably overstate the friendly societies' part in this doctor's putative earnings. Nevertheless, they suggest how large a part contracts with friendly societies could play in a doctor's actual income.

Beginning in the 1860s, medical men in many communities tried to work together in order to push their fees up, thereby taking a more active hand in achieving what many practitioners had expected the Medical Act

32. See also Greenbaum, "Economic Cooperation among Urban Industrial Workers," who explores the issue of incentives for officers of such organizations.
33. AOF, Court Loyal Bodelwyddan papers, D/DM/510/2.
34. IOOF, Maiden Queen Lodge papers, OF8/2, minutes, Dec. 10, 1895.
35. Doctor's account, D/X 872/2. In 1846–47 the doctor also paid 15s. 8d. to friendly societies, so that his net income from them was slightly lower.

of 1858 to accomplish by regulating entry to the profession.[36] The long sickness of Dr. Beechey prompted members of the Kempston Friendly Society in 1873 to elect a new surgeon, Oliver C. Combs, offering him 3s. 6d. per member each year, a rate that had been raised only two years earlier from 2s. 6d. But Combs declined, explaining in a letter that the medical men of Bedford had agreed not to take any new club work for less than 5s.[37] Not all Bedford medical men had agreed, or at least not all were prepared to hold to the agreement. The surgeon Adams consented to take the work at 5s., what the Bedford medical men wanted, but also to give the society a quid pro quo. Each year thereafter the society drank the doctor's gift, a donation of 10s. that bought beer at the club's dinner. In 1883 the club ordered 13.5 gallons of beer for twenty-six members.[38]

MEDICAL AID ASSOCIATIONS

Under growing pressure from doctors to raise consulting fees, and also out of a sense of the potential of collaboration, friendly societies responded by forming cooperative organizations. They shared information and prepared a friendly society position on issues important to their members. In the Amalgamated Friendly Societies' Association, members met for discussion and debate, intending to improve their ability to speak in public. The Cambridge Victoria Friendly Societies' Asylum, formed in 1837, cared for members in old age, including men who belonged to societies that had failed.[39] The Yorkshire Foresters' Orphanage and Convalescent Home tended the orphaned children of AOF members and, for the members themselves, provided facilities for convalescence.[40] As early as the 1830s, but with increasing frequency in the 1870s and 1880s, regional groups of units in the affiliated societies, and some clusters of independent friendly societies, founded homes for old members who had no relatives and convalescent homes for men recovering from chronic sickness.

Working people with such diseases as tuberculosis, who could not af-

36. On expectations about what the Medical Act would achieve in the way of higher incomes, see Waddington, *Medical Profession*, 144, 148–49. See also Hodgkinson, *Origins of the National Health Service*, 608–10.

37. Kempston Friendly Society papers, DDX157/2, minutes, Dec. 9, 1872 ff., July 30, 1880, May 6, 1892, and in DDX157/3, minutes, May 23, 1883.

38. Ibid., DDX157/3, management committee minutes, May 4, 1883.

39. *Cambridge Victoria Friendly Societies' Asylum*, 6.

40. See a receipt for subscription to the home, AOF, Court of Three Mary's papers, TU:10/2.

ford to follow the commonplace late-nineteenth-century advice of taking the air at private clinics, gained access to such treatments in friendly society facilities where room, board, medicines, medical attendance, and nursing were provided for modest charges.[41] In the North-eastern Counties Friendly Societies' Convalescent Home, in Grange-over-Sands, members of any supporting club could spend two or three weeks recuperating from diseases not requiring constant medical attendance. During 1904, when the home marked its fourteenth anniversary, 493 men were served.[42] The home's purpose was to counteract the ill effects of climate on chronic chest diseases.

Friendly societies also took a collaborative role in promoting the effort to teach lay people how to perform simple, often life-saving medical procedures. When a surgeon addressed members of the St. John's Ambulance Association in 1888, the *Foresters' Miscellany* reported some of the examples he gave of unfortunate consequences from want of understanding that bleeding from a wound could be stopped by applying pressure. According to the surgeon, a man once burst a varicose vein and bled. His wife, eager to help, "simply placed his foot in a bucket and went and fetched the doctor. When she returned the bucket was pretty nearly full, and she placed his foot in another. . . . By the time the doctor arrived the poor man was in the next world."[43]

Within the medical economy of the working class, however, the most important thing gained from collaboration among friendly societies was the medical aid association. In place of the club contract, or in addition to it,[44] medical aid associations enrolled subscribers for medical attendance from all participating friendly societies, as well as private individuals and family members, rented a surgery, stocked it with medicines and equipment, engaged their own doctors, midwives, and apothecaries or dispensers, and appointed a lay board of governors. Like the works clubs formed in certain industries, especially mining, and like the family clubs

41. See, for example, *Foresters' Miscellany,* July 1848, 208–9, regarding the Metropolitan Benefit Societies' Asylum in Islington; and the advertisements for such facilities in National United Order of Free Gardeners, *Directory,* of which a copy may be found at West Yorkshire Archive Service, Huddersfield, KC41 23/24.

42. Independent Order of Rechabites papers, 1914–1961.

43. *Foresters' Miscellany,* Jan. 1888, 11–12.

44. Leicester Bond Street Friendly Society papers, DE1884/2, minutes, June 9, 1892. But in 1876 this society joined the local medical aid association and dismissed its surgeon (DE1884/1, minutes, Mar. 14–June 8, 1876). In short, from 1876 to 1892 medical aid association doctors attended the men in this society, but in 1892 society members gained the option of being attended by a doctor of their own choice.

that some doctors set up for working-class families,[45] medical aid associations provided an alternative to contract practice. But the friendly societies bitterly resented works clubs because employers sometimes denied their workers the option of joining a friendly society.[46] Medical aid associations, in contrast, they welcomed as a means to gain inexpensive access to medical services and as a further step toward working-class patient control over the financial relationship with doctors.

The United Friendly Societies' Medical Association in Manchester charged four shillings a year per adult (less for children) and provided surgery services at four clinics for seven days a week, mornings and afternoons, and evenings on every day but Sunday.[47] Worcester's Amalgamated Friendly Societies' Medical Association, formed when the town's doctors threatened to raise fees for club doctors to five shillings a member per year, served all friendly society members who wished to join at four shillings per year, four shillings for a wife, and one shilling per child.[48] Two features of the medical aid associations were especially appealing. First, they extended the bargaining power of friendly societies from individual clubs to all clubs within the reach of an association's facilities. Second, they regularly treated family members, whereas many individual clubs continued to provide services only for members.[49] The National Insurance Act of 1911, too, provided treatment only for the worker, not for family members. Yet medical aid associations arose not out of a tranquil extension of ongoing friendly society activities but from conflict.

In a paragraph repeated nearly verbatim for more than twenty years, the AOF directory explained the origins of the medical aid associations with a simple metahistory. In the days before conflicts arose, "kind and congenial" club doctors provided good medical care and advised the friendly societies to which they belonged, about other matters, too. "As time rolled

---

45. Earwicker, "Miners' Medical Services"; and Benson, *British Coalminers in the Nineteenth Century*, 180–82, describe works clubs; Cox, *Among the Doctors*, 35, 38, 49, mentions both works and family clubs from his experience as an apprentice dispenser and young general practitioner; and Smith, *The People's Health*, 370–71, discusses the background and practice of both.

46. E.g., Grand United Order of Oddfellows, Charity Lodge papers, S/CL/4, minutes, Mar. 26, 1898.

47. AOF, Manchester District, *Quarterly Report* (1890). See also Cambridge Friendly Societies' Medical Association, *Rules*.

48. *Foresters' Miscellany*, Jan. 1871, 305.

49. Rumsey, *Essays on State Medicine*, 159, claims that club doctors entered side deals in which, to secure votes for reelection, they agreed to attend family members without charge. Gilbert, *Evolution of National Insurance*, 309, echoes this claim, citing the testimony of a doctor. How commonplace such deals were is uncertain.

on, the connection between the Surgeon and the Society assumed a more strictly business-like aspect," the doctors demanding more compensation and the members complaining that, compared to the doctor's private patients, they got little attention and were supplied with medicines of inferior quality.[50] To settle the conflict, different friendly societies in the same town joined to form a medical aid association, regaining control over the relationship with their doctors by making them employees of the friendly societies. The point, as explained by J. Pope, president of the Friendly Societies' Medical Alliance in 1883, was to counter the "sort of Trades Unionism" by which the medical men had sought to raise their fees.[51] In Exeter, Pope had been involved in a nasty lawsuit by means of which local medical practitioners tried to close the Exeter association. His view was that the medical employees of the associations were overpaid. The nature of the conflict was evident. Rival attempts to form combinations in restraint of trade produced strong feelings on the part of doctors toward workingmen and of workingmen toward doctors.

Other proponents of the medical aid associations preferred to lay stress not on the advantage they provided working people in bargaining with doctors but on their role in making medical attendance standard for women and children who had rarely been attended, and then only in cases where death threatened. For members, their wives, and children, the associations provided medical assistance early in a case and promised thereby to save their patients from longer and more perilous sicknesses. T. Ballan Stead, long a leading figure in the AOF, claimed in 1884, "Amongst the working classes there is, perhaps, no greater source of shortened lives than want of means to call in a doctor when one is needed."[52] Working people who have made no provision for medical care turn first to "make-shift remedies" of their own design. Home remedies in great variety "are applied or given in the order in which they are recommended, and the consequence is a jumble of liquids which retard rather than assist the patient's recovery." People turn most willingly to druggists or to older women who have gained a reputation in the community for knowing what heals but who can rarely recommend useful therapies. "Fetching the doctor at the latest possible moment seems an instinctive feeling" in many working-

50. E.g., AOF, *Directory,* 1891, 559; and *Foresters' Miscellany,* Nov. 1886, 329. Such complaints were made in evidence given the Parliamentary Medical Relief Committee in 1844. See Rumsey, *Essays on State Medicine,* 158–59, 257–58.

51. *Friendly Societies' Journal,* Apr. 1883, 51.

52. Stead, "New Era in Medical Aid," 83. To the same effect "Sick Clubs," 354, presumably by the editor, Samuel Shawcross.

class families who do not belong to friendly societies. To Stead it mattered that people should be treated effectively and cured early in the course of a sickness. But it mattered also to the friendly societies, who, as Stead recognized, saved money when members recovered sooner.[53]

Stead's views were seconded by Dr. George White in comments to members of a lodge of the Loyal Order of Ancient Shepherds. White advised them "not to be long in sending for him as it caused losses to the Lodge & also to the members themselves" if they waited to seek treatment.[54]

Although medical aid associations were expected to pay their own way according to the schedule of fees adopted by their governors, who were friendly society members, the societies that formed them often had to pay in something. In 1899 the Loughborough association raised £804 18s. 6d., half in contributions from members and half from friendly societies. Its largest expenditures were £126 for a dispenser, Mr. A. Harding, and £400 for three doctors, Charles Symington and two associates.[55] By 1880 the medical aid association movement was large enough to warrant formation of the Friendly Societies' Medical Alliance, which held annual conferences in order to promote friendly society interests, to help organize new medical aid associations, and to serve as an agency for engaging doctors willing to work for such associations, against resistance from the British Medical Association, which refused to allow the medical aid associations to advertise for doctors in its publications.

The alliance also collected information from its member medical aid associations, a summary of which the AOF published in its annual directories. The first association to join the alliance was formed in Preston in 1869. It operated a dispensary employing a resident surgeon with an assistant and also engaged a consulting physician.[56] By the end of 1873 at least seven medical aid associations had been established, with 22,120 members. Collectively they spent £3,369 6s. 11d., which means that they provided a wide range of medical services—consultations at home or at the dispensary, medications, and delivery of infants—for an annual cost of slightly more than 3s. per member.[57]

53. Stead, "New Era in Medical Aid."
54. Loyal Order of Ancient Shepherds, Heatherbell Lodge papers, uncatalogued minutes, Oct. 17, 1911.
55. E.g., Loughborough Friendly Societies' Medical Aid Association papers, misc 1061\1, the annual report for 1899.
56. Ancient Noble Order of United Oddfellows papers, Grand Lodge Circular, FO/2/45, Jan. 1871, 6.
57. AOF, Directory, 1874, 284.

Table 2.1
MEDICAL AID ASSOCIATION PRACTICE IN 1874

	Bradford	Greenock	Lincoln	N'hamptn	Preston	Worcester
Members	2,889	2,897	1,763	3,445	—	3,154
Expenses	£492 3s.	£207 7s. 10d.	£308 17s. 8d.	£492 8s. 2d.	£711 16s. 5d.	£431 4s. 11d.
Cases	907			4,978	3,191	2,247
Visits at home	—	1,773	595	5,875	12,944	28,817
Contacts at dispensary		1,615	1,810	15,426	22,595	7,830
Visits and contacts	3,263	3,388	2,405	21,301	35,539	10,647
Prescriptions	6,725	2,337			13,780	
Deaths	45	13	28	46	105	28

Source: Data from AOF, Directory, 1875, 270–71.

Telling details for six of the associations operating in 1874 appear in table 2.1. Among the five reporting the number of their members, the medical aid association doctors amassed 41,004 patient contacts, a rate equal to 2.9 contacts per member. In this group the people who belonged paid just under 1s. (0.94s.) per contact. If spending on medications could be deducted, the rate would be lower still. But the point is already clear. Members of medical aid associations paid remarkably little for medical care. Whatever the quality of the medical services received, the cost of those services was low.

Historians and other commentators have sometimes expressed strong views about the quality of medical care available from club and medical aid association doctors without being able to substantiate their views. For some it seems axiomatic that working people should have had inferior medical care, and it is possible to find testimony that that was indeed the case. Judged on the basis of the price paid, that conclusion is inescapable. Working people paid less for medical care than did the elite, and so they must have received less.

But it is more difficult to reach this conclusion if the comparison is based on the efficacy of medicine. That is so not because the rich did not receive some distinctive therapies but because it is difficult to compare the outcome of therapies in controlled circumstances. Did the more expensive and numerous medicaments, and the more frequent attendances, that we suppose the rich to have received constitute better medical care in an era when many medicaments the doctor provided produced a humoral response but few improved the pace of a cure? Other scholars and commentators have judged club doctors to have given good care, usually on similar grounds: some sources provide testimony to that effect. As David Green has pointed out, the supply of doctors was large enough to put pressure on club doctors to provide services satisfactory to their working-class patients, for they were at risk of being replaced.[58] The testimony is inconclusive because it is too evenly balanced, and the arguments from logic tend to cancel one another.

Some quantitative comparisons, too, produce inconclusive results. For example, it is known that friendly society members lived longer than people of the same age and gender in Britain in general.[59] But this advan-

58. Green, *Working-Class Patients*, 70–77, reviews opinions and presents his own.
59. Compare the death rates among English and Welsh males for different periods in Mitchell, *British Historical Statistics*, 60–61; and the summary of friendly society experience in Watson, *Sickness and Mortality Experience*, 22.

tage cannot necessarily be attributed to medical care. Too little information is available to control for all of the factors influencing morbidity and mortality besides medical care. Nevertheless, quantitative evidence sheds some further light on the subject.

Among the medical aid associations represented in table 2.1 it is apparent that few cases of sickness resulted in death. For all 14,148 members in the five associations, the death rate in 1874 totaled only 11.3 per thousand, a level considerably below the crude death rate of the British population, though one close to the mortality of people aged twenty-five to forty-four, probably the dominant ages of association members.[60] More telling is the ratio of cases to deaths. In the four associations for which both the number of deaths and the number of cases is known, the case fatality rate amounted to no more than 21.6 per thousand. An overwhelming proportion—not much less than 98 percent—of sickness episodes ended in recovery or continued convalescence, at least within the year 1874. Some patients probably died later. But of course some of the deaths reported in 1874 occurred to people who had fallen sick before 1874. In any case, the important implication is that, in these medical aid associations at least, working-class men, women, and children were consulting doctors often and surviving nearly all of their sicknesses.[61] If this body of experience is taken as a measure of the quality of health care available to medical aid association patrons, the low case-fatality ratio would suggest that they were given very good care. From the two medical aid associations reporting both the number of cases and the number of prescriptions, it appears that association apothecaries and doctors liberally dosed their patients. On average each new case received slightly more than five medications.

In quantitative terms, as measured by such things as the frequency of contact between the sick and their doctors and the cost of such contacts, and perhaps also in qualitative terms, as implied by the ratio of home to dispensary visits and the case-fatality ratio, the large body of experience summarized in table 2.1 suggests that the 1870s amounted to a golden age of working-class medical care. Medical services for the sick were given frequently and inexpensively, often in the patient's home, the patients' preference for a liberal use of medications was met, and most patients survived their sicknesses. Of course, on the other side of this equation stand the high death rates of that period. Death rates for adults declined in

60. See Mitchell, *British Historical Statistics*, 60.
61. However, it is possible that the medical aid associations did not count the deaths of members being treated elsewhere, such as in hospitals.

the 1870s. Even so, if the death rate is the measure of health, it is more accurate to describe the 1870s as a rude and savage than as a golden age.

In later years the medical aid association movement grew rapidly. By 1890 the Friendly Societies' Medical Alliance counted fifty-four member associations in England and Wales with 247,417 members, but it did not include many Welsh associations. Among the thirty-six member associations reporting expenditures, the annual per capita cost of providing services had increased slightly, to 3.2s.[62] In 1903 the alliance counted fifty-nine medical aid associations with 256,362 members paying nearly 3.5s. a year for medical services.[63] The AOF directories no longer report the other interesting particulars available for 1874. It is apparent that the cost of medical services remained low, but there are no longer any indications about the quality or quantity of care.

Although the information in AOF directories is incomplete, especially in listing only a single medical aid association for Wales, it can nevertheless provide an idea of the breadth of these institutions. Map 2.1 shows the location of sixty-six associations listed at one time or another in the AOF directories, and map 2.2 the relative cost per member among associations in twenty-one English counties in 1874. Only a weak pattern is apparent. Medical aid association patients in central England, and perhaps also in counties near London, paid significantly more for medical services than did their counterparts in the north or west. The most striking point, however, is that costs varied so widely. As with wages and rents,[64] regional markets dominated in pricing medical services in this form.

THE SHROPSHIRE PROVIDENT SOCIETY

Rising tension during the 1860s between practitioners and friendly society members over costs and benefits is captured in the records of the Shropshire Provident Society, formed in 1851. From the outset the Shropshire Society provided medical attendance for members in each of the expanding number of its branches by charging a monthly fee of four pence per member and paying attending surgeons at the same rate, four shillings

62. AOF, *Directory*, 1891, 559–62.
63. AOF, *Directory*, 1904, 569–73. The information concerning costs derives from the reports of forty-five associations.
64. Hunt, *Regional Wage Variations in Britain*, 64, 82–85, passim.

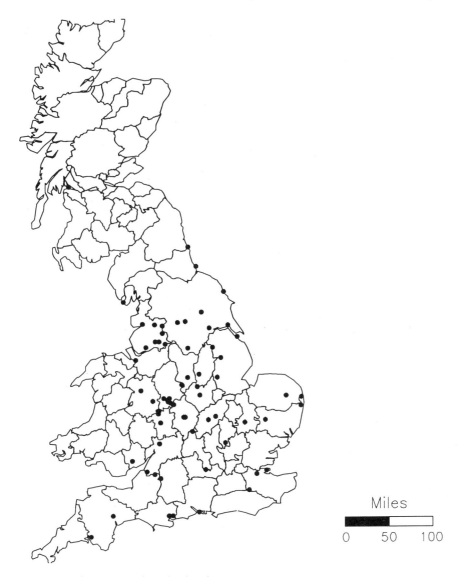

Map 2.1. Locations of Medical Aid Associations, 1874–1903
Source: AOF, *Directories,* 1875, 270–71; 1885, 472–75; 1895, 593–96; 1904, 570–73.

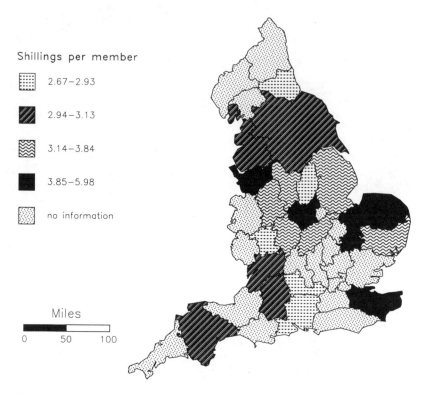

Shillings per member

2.67–2.93

2.94–3.13

3.14–3.84

3.85–5.98

no information

Miles

0   50   100

Map 2.2. Costs per Member in Medical Aid Associations in England, 1874–
1903
Source: AOF, Directories, 1875, 270–71; 1885, 472–75; 1895, 593–96; 1904,
570–73.

a year.[65] In return, its contracting surgeons provided attendance and medicines; they examined members who presented as sick, certifying their eligibility for benefits and their recovery; and gave treatment. Those fees and
payments remained unchanged from 1851 until 1869, when the surgeon
of one branch, in Longnor, managed to extract a fee of five shillings per
member per year by refusing any longer to attend members under the old
terms. But the society did not raise fees paid surgeons serving other
branches. In 1878 the management committee considered raising fees and

65. Shropshire Provident Society papers, 436/6727–28, management committee minutes,
1850–87; and 436/6730, minutes of the Shrewsbury branch subcommittee, 1851–95. Members insuring for sickness benefits initially paid four pence a month, and those insuring only
for other benefits, which did not require regular attendance during sickness episodes, one
pence per month.

payments but took no action. In April 1880 the secretary of the Madeley branch reported that their surgeon had resigned and that it had proved difficult to find a replacement for the customary payment. But the management committee decided to put off action until completing a valuation of the society's financial position.

In succeeding months the committee sought advice from its actuary, Francis G. P. Neison Jr., and in August launched an investigation into how much other friendly societies paid their surgeons. This decision is remarkable, because on previous occasions when other friendly societies had approached the Shropshire society about matters of common interest, the society had taken the view that its interests were not affected. Only when pressed by complaints from surgeons and members about medical fees did the society give up its aloof posture. The results of that inquiry are not apparent, but the management committee did not immediately approve a general increase in fees, preferring to consider each case individually.

Late in 1880 the Shrewsbury branch was allowed to raise its fees and payments. It had struggled with the problem since 1875, when the surgeon Samuel Wood resigned, after giving "skillful and willing services for an all but nominal remuneration" since 1851.[66] Wood's partner declined the appointment, as did two other surgeons, because they would not attend for the four shilling fee. As a result the branch prevailed on Wood to continue providing attendance until completing arrangements with the Salop Medical Aid Association, set up in the 1870s to give the collaborating friendly societies greater control over medical costs. As one of the friendly society leaders observed in an organizational meeting, "the doctors were getting tighter upon us"; the medical aid association would furnish "efficient medical attendance and proper medicine" on terms set by the friendly societies.[67]

Although a new practitioner approached the Shrewsbury branch in 1878 offering to attend its members, the arrangement with the Salop Medical Aid Association continued. It, too, faced pressure to raise fees, and its decision in 1880 to raise payments forced the Shrewsbury branch to increase fees and payments to five shillings a member. Not until May 1881 did the Shropshire Provident Society as a whole raise its payments to five shillings per member per year in all branches, with some of the additional payment being funded not by higher fees on members but from the soci-

66. Ibid., 436/6730, Feb. 5, 1875.
67. AOF, District Management Committee papers, 4727/1, Jan. 11, 1872.

ety's surplus assets. Neison's 1879 valuation had found a surplus of £1,478 on assets of £13,065. Nevertheless, during the 1880s the turnover of surgeons increased, presumably because those under contract remained dissatisfied with their pay.

THE BATTLE OF THE CLUBS

Two issues aggravated tension between friendly societies and doctors into what the *Lancet* referred to, in a series of spirited articles published in 1896, as the battle of the clubs. Doctors wanted to raise the fees that friendly society members paid for contract medical services, and they wanted to prevent clubs from enrolling members who could afford to pay the fees that doctors charged for private care.[68] They wanted to keep men, like sculptor Thomas Wilkinson Wallis, who earned more than £250 a year from joining a friendly society to get cut-rate medical care.[69] David Green interprets this struggle between clubs and doctors as the interplay of a free market in which, on balance, the clubs showed a willingness to go some distance toward meeting the doctors' demands for higher fees but the doctors acted in an intransigent way, trying to establish monopoly control over the provision and pricing of medical services.[70] It is more accurate to acknowledge that both sides turned to combinations in restraint of trade as a way of consolidating or improving their bargaining position. Both sought to undermine and manipulate the free market to their own advantage.

At first doctors organized locally, forming medical societies and drafting agreements intended to present a solid front in favor of higher fees and, if possible, also to exclude higher-wage earners from friendly society membership.[71] In the 1890s some among them sought to use the power of the General Medical Council to remove from the medical register doctors

68. See the 1896 *Lancet* for articles about doctors and contract practice in Australia, the United States, Hungary, Belgium, France, and Britain. Cox, *Among the Doctors,* 30, 57, 60, discusses his view of the struggle; Parry and Parry, *Rise of the Medical Profession,* 151–54, explain how the British Medical Association saw the struggle.

69. Wallis recorded his income and spending on drugs and doctors. From 1847 through 1856 he spent 1.13 percent of his income on drugs and doctors, not including what he paid to belong to the Oddfellows. In that period he earned an average of more than £250 a year. Wallis, *Autobiography,* 79–80, 113–14, 136–37.

70. Green, *Working-Class Patients,* 4, 30–32, passim; and Green, "Doctors versus Workers," i–xii.

71. Such strategies are described in articles in the *British Medical Journal.* See, e.g., Mackenzie, "Battle of the Clubs"; and Phillips, "Battle of the Clubs."

employed by medical aid associations, on a charge of professional misconduct.[72] In 1900 one doctor, "a Birmingham consultant," wrote a hectoring letter to workingmen. In his view working people paid too little for medical services, so little that doctors needed to see seventy or eighty patients a day to make a living, and all the patient could expect was "a kind word and a bottle of something which shall not injure you."[73] To get the medical advice they wanted, workingmen needed to pay half a guinea—10.5s.—a year and give up their desire to hire their own medical men. The friendly societies responded by insisting all the more intently on the inability of working people to pay such fees, by resisting the arrogance of doctors demanding to control the relationship with patients, and by bargaining all the more aggressively for medical services.

Pointedly, the British Medical Association and its members argued that they had gone along with friendly society contract practice because it served a class of persons who required lower medical fees. But the medical aid associations might admit people who did not need this advantage. By the 1890s many doctors believed they were being exploited. Their complaints became a major feature of the BMA's 1905 report on the undesirable features of contract practice.[74] Too many people who could afford to pay the fees of private practice were escaping such fees by joining friendly societies, medical aid associations, and other groups or by presenting at hospitals. The BMA wanted these groups to act like provident dispensaries, which gave discounted medical services to poorer people but put a ceiling on how much their subscribers could earn. Doctors were willing to treat working people at reduced rates, but only those whose wages the medical men deemed suitably low. For doctors, it had become an article of faith that their own incomes were too modest and, furthermore, that they were too modest because people who could afford to pay were slipping through a system that attempted to price medical services according to socioeconomic status. At the Gloucester Infirmary one investigation resulted in the finding that nearly 41 percent of patients who presented could afford to pay for treatment, either as private patients or as subscribers to the city's provident dispensary.[75]

To the doctors' laments the Friendly Societies' Medical Alliance re-

72. Green, *Working-Class Patients,* 36–47.
73. "Open Letter to the Working Men of Birmingham," 3.
74. "Investigation into the Economic Conditions of Contract Medical Practice in the United Kingdom."
75. Whitcombe, "Suggestions Founded on the Recent Enquiry." Whitcombe was a solicitor, but the complaints he made in this pamphlet were often made also by doctors.

sponded with a frank and telling argument. The old club system of contract practice was defective. True enough, it gained medical attendance for its members at a rate of three or four shillings a year each. But the club doctor usually regarded that obligation as secondary to private practice. Care of friendly society patients was often turned over to assistants, even ones inexperienced or unqualified. In South Wales and elsewhere some doctors treated large numbers of patients by hiring poorly paid and overworked assistants.[76] There and elsewhere friendly society members spent hours waiting at the surgery to be attended and were given medicines in too small quantity or obliged to have prescriptions filled by the doctor's chemist. They were treated as charity patients, with a "general want of sympathy" and with indifference. The medical aid associations had been created to redress these shortcomings, hiring doctors who would not (in most cases) engage in private practice and providing medicines without giving the contract doctor any pecuniary interest in them.[77] If the article of faith for doctors was that people who could afford private-practice medical services were paying at prices meant only for working people, the article of faith among friendly society members was that doctors working on contract provided services of poorer quality.

The Shropshire Provident Society, like other friendly societies, continued to resist paying higher fees for medical attendance, managing to supply attendance to their members at low cost. But the sick clubs' power in bargaining with medical practitioners lost force in 1911, when the National Insurance Act created a separate category for state members. Unlike the men and women who belonged to friendly societies before the act, who after 1911 were called voluntary members, the terms for medical attendance to state members were set by the government. Public authorities found themselves subject to pressure from medical interests, especially the British Medical Association, to raise fees, and the friendly societies were slow to react. Perhaps they did not immediately realize that their modest payments to doctors would be endangered by the comparatively generous fees paid on behalf of state patients, for whom the Medical Benefit Fund created by the act paid seven shillings per individual per year.[78]

76. Cox, *Among the Doctors,* 30, describes niggardly treatment of patients, but in works clubs rather than friendly society contract practices.

77. British Medical Association papers, MP337/C102.

78. IOOF, Loyal Vale of Clun Lodge papers, 1927/1, minutes for 1912 and 1913; and British Medical Association papers, MP337/C102. On the act and the friendly societies' concerns about it, see Gilbert, *Evolution of National Insurance,* 289–447. For background of the act, see Brand, *Doctors and the State;* Ritter, *Social Welfare in Germany and Britain,*

In Doncaster the medical society formed in 1911 set as its objectives providing a forum for scientific and ethical discussions and advancing the interests of the profession, specifically seeing that voluntary friendly society members paid at least 8s. 6d. per member per year for medical services.[79] The Buchan Medical Society, a small local group in Buchan, near Aberdeen, formed to promote good fellowship among medical practitioners in the community and to share case studies, held a special meeting on June 24, 1911, when the national insurance bill was pending. Although the members disagreed about the bill itself, they agreed unanimously that, should the bill pass, "none of us will agree to act for any of the friendly societies, without the consent of the members of this Society, and according to the policy of the British Medical Association." They also appointed an agent to lobby members of parliament.[80]

The practitioners in Buchan wanted not only the higher fees, 8s. 6d., proposed for the insurance act, but they also wanted that fee to exclude medicines and extras, allowing them to charge more according to the distance they traveled to see a patient and for vaccination, treating a fracture or dislocation, and other services. A key aim lay in obtaining a schedule that allowed doctors to make house calls at the ordinary fee, 2s. 6d. per visit plus mileage, only between eight and ten in the morning. The remainder of the ordinary working day, from 10 A.M. to 6 P.M., and the night would be reserved for urgent calls, charged at 9d. per mile rather than the 6d. they wished to charge for morning calls.

The BMA had long sought to promote the economic interests of its members and specifically to counter the power that friendly societies had gained by collaborating among themselves while exploiting divisions within each local medical community. In 1911 the BMA campaigned for a higher minimum contract fee and against friendly society medical aid associations. In the BMA view, these forms of contract practice exploited doctors, paying them too little and burdening them with too many patients. The Medico-Political Committee, which campaigned actively against medical aid associations, pointed to such examples as the Blaenavon Medical Aid Society, which employed one surgeon at £800 and an

esp. 131–78; and Hennock, *British Social Reform and German Precedents.* On the consequences of the act, see Green, *Working-Class Patients,* and Klein, *Complaints against Doctors,* as well as Fox, *Health Policies, Health Politics;* and Hollingsworth, Hage, and Hanneman, *State Intervention in Medical Care.*

79. Doncaster Medical Society papers, 1911, DS 22/1, minutes. The doctors' case is put by Parry and Parry, *Rise of the Medical Profession,* 151–54.

80. Buchan Medical Society papers, 1163/1/1a, minutes, June 24, 1911–May 18, 1912.

assistant at £350 a year and expected them to attend some eleven thousand patients. Together the two surgeons averaged 112 consultations a day.

But the BMA did not merely attack directly. It pitched its campaign against the medical aid associations on two matters of alleged principle. First, patients should have a free choice of doctors, in place of the medical staff of the aid associations. Without any apparent sense of irony or humor, the BMA sought to end the friendly societies' opportunity to form combinations in restraint of medical trade by creating a superior combination. Second, the medical staff should direct the associations, or at least sit on their boards. BMA leaders could not bear that control of these organizations lay with working-class appointees serving on boards; most especially they could not tolerate the practice of patients making complaints about medical service to lay officials, over the heads of the doctors.[81]

Some members of the Medico-Political Committee felt strongly enough that they were willing to compromise the health and well-being of medical aid association patients as a means of securing medical control of these organizations. In 1914 those members seriously entertained the idea of persuading the medical staff at voluntary hospitals to refuse professional recognition to doctors who worked for medical aid associations and, "except in cases of grave urgency," to refuse to treat patients sent them by medical aid associations. But the hospital campaign was not adopted in 1914, at the peak of this controversy, and medical aid associations remained a leading problem for the BMA into the 1940s.[82]

While more effective collaboration among doctors in setting fees helped erode the friendly societies' negotiating advantage, it is also true that the societies undercut their own interests. A spirit of friendly rivalry and cooperation had usually marked the relations of local units of different affiliated societies and independent sick clubs. They joined together in processions, jointly organized fund-raising campaigns for such objects as the foundation of a tuberculosis sanitarium or an insane asylum, and, most important, collaborated in forming medical associations. But in the 1890s and thereafter on a growing number of occasions, friendly rivalry gave way to undercutting. The Heatherbell Lodge of the Loyal Order of Ancient Shepherds in 1911 entertained five applications from surgeons willing to attend its members. As a condition of acceptance, however, the lodge, a

81. British Medical Association papers, MP337/C102. For other signs of the loss of lay control over doctors, see Jewson, "Disappearance of the Sick Man." Similar arguments had been made by doctors in the 1850s. Parry and Parry, *Rise of the Medical Profession*, 143–45.
82. British Medical Association papers, MP556/C211, MP807/C277, MP513/C191, and MP578/C216.

huge outfit with about eight hundred members, required that candidates agree to stop attending any other societies. In the end they elected George White, who had previously attended four lodges with a total of about four hundred members. White was delighted. He visited the lodge, where the members excused him from the initiation ceremony, "and promised that as far as his power & ability lay, *Medically* & *Socially* he would do his best for the Lodge."[83]

During the 1920s, under constant pressure from the BMA, the National Health Insurance schedule of fees paid rose sharply, from the 7s. per member per year set in 1911 to 11s. in 1926. Some friendly societies managed to hold payments down. The Whitchurch Oddfellows still paid only 4s. a year because, in the opinion of one physician, they owned their doctor's surgery and had helped him pay for his practice, and they engaged a doctor who did not belong to the BMA and, moreover, whose "standing is not high, to say the least of it."[84] Whether the judgment about standing refers to collegiality, social status, or medical skill is not apparent. Other doctors new to Shrewsbury were able to demand more, up to 12s. per member per year. All this seems to have been meant to encourage Dr. W. W. Anderson of Whitchurch, who wished to raise his fees above the 6s. the Oddfellows paid him in 1926. Anderson apparently wanted the Odd-fellows to pay the BMA-approved minima of 11s. per adult and 7s. 6d. per youth. After negotiations in which the Oddfellows combined with other friendly societies in the area, they declined to pay more than 10s. and 6s. 6d. respectively.[85] How the dispute was resolved is not apparent. But it is clear that, during the 1920s and between the two periods of economic downturn, 1920–21 and 1929–31, the friendly societies lost much of their control over what they paid for medical attendance.

Workingmen who belonged to friendly societies and working-class fam-ilies enrolled in medical aid associations set the financial terms under which they would first engage doctors. From the 1780s, when the friendly societies initially promoted contract medical services for their members, until 1912, when the National Insurance Act went into force, working people took advantage of their superior organization and an oversupply of doctors in Britain to extract medical services on their own terms. They extracted frequent and convenient services, whether or not those services

---

83. Loyal Order of Ancient Shepherds, Heatherbell Lodge, uncatalogued minutes, Sept. 5, 1911–Oct. 17, 1912.

84. Shropshire Provident Society papers, 2794/14, letter of May 17, 1926.

85. Shropshire Provident Society papers, 2794/14, letters of June 14 and Aug. 26, 1926.

were of good quality. In the least costly of all forms of contract service, the medical aid associations, the contract doctor saw working-class patients frequently, often in their own homes, and provided them with numerous medications. The very charge that working people did not get services equivalent in quality to those provided private patients—that doctors skimped on time and medications—figured in an important way in negotiations with doctors. Doctors countered that the friendly societies, and especially their medical aid associations, paid too little to expect good care. Neither contention accurately described pay or care. Instead, these characterizations were rhetorical points in a public debate in which each side maneuvered in ways calculated to improve its bargaining position.

The National Insurance Act of 1911 broke up working-class control and foreshadowed the victory of doctors in the battle of the clubs. Because medical services for state patients were compensated at higher rates, the friendly societies could retain their bargaining power only so long as they could enroll enough members to give them some control over price setting. Two developments undermined their position. First, the public purse provided some of the benefits the friendly societies had offered without assessing separate charges. That made friendly societies attractive chiefly to the men and women who had already invested too much in them to forfeit by leaving, but not to young adults and new members. Second, the purchasing power of friendly society sickness payments and burial benefits diminished. That made the friendly societies marginal rather than central sources of assistance in sickness. In sum, the heyday of the friendly societies had passed; for them to have retained the economic power they had had from the 1780s to 1912 would have called for extraordinary action to reverse political and economic trends. In the absence of such action, the BMA, which had long fought a losing contest with working people, found itself with sudden conjunctural advantages. To those it added the greater political clout it managed to exercise in negotiations for the insurance act.

But the medical men's victory remained for a long time incomplete. Many friendly societies managed for two or three decades after 1911 to retain contracts with their doctors on terms that provided them with medical services at lower costs than those paid for members of the state insurance program. Although the friendly society members were older than voluntary members and thus more prone to need medical treatment, they paid less. The members of medical aid associations, too, preserved their superior position into the 1940s, finally giving way before National Health Insurance.

CHAPTER 3

The Political Economy of Patients and Practitioners

WORKING-CLASS PEOPLE in nineteenth-century Britain often distrusted doctors,[1] and doctors felt increasingly estranged from working-class patients. Medical practitioners and friendly society members alike suspected they were being taken advantage of, or would be taken advantage of, by the other party. Unfortunately, both were right. For a long time the friendly societies, aided by an oversupply of formal practitioners, held a strong enough hand to contract for medical services at reduced fees. Doctors submitted. But it may be that the working-class patients who paid less for contract service also got less—less of the doctor's time, fewer prescriptions without side payments, less expensive medicaments, a smaller chance of being attended in their own homes at their convenience rather than in the doctor's surgery at his convenience. Perhaps working-class patients got more cursory attention from doctors who, consciously or not, budgeted their time according to what patients paid for it.

It is easier to establish the differential between what friendly society members and private patients paid for medical care than it is to compare what they received in the way of care. To judge the level of care provided to friendly society members requires information about three things: the terms of care for friendly society members, the terms of care for private patients, and the terms of trade between doctors and working-class patients. The fees working people paid and those doctors received are instructive by themselves. They acquire additional meaning when considered in terms of the political economy, meaning in this instance the trend of earnings in each group: which group improved its position relative to the

1. Wood, *Poverty and the Workhouse*, 32.

75

other? Unfortunately, there is no firm point of comparison to use in establishing whether patients or doctors were getting more. The question is a tricky one. But it is an appropriate question to ask, for two reasons. First, doctors and club members fretted about which side was getting the better of the contact. Second, doctors and working-class patients set the terms of their relationship in the nineteenth century, especially in its second half. Hence, the latter decades of that century constitute a base period against which more recent experience should be compared. In the long run, which group has gained more advantage?

CONTRACT PRACTICE

The contracts between friendly societies and doctors, whether negotiated by individual clubs or by groups of clubs organized as a medical aid association, imply by their very existence that workingmen got a bargain, paying less for medical care equivalent to or better than what they would otherwise have received. Initially, in the late eighteenth century, the workingmen's advantage may have consisted of nothing more than substituting licensed medical men, usually surgeons, for informal practitioners, with an implied but still uncertain gain in the quality of care. As early as the 1840s club members were bargaining among surgeons, often in circumstances in which nearly every surgeon in a community vied to be the club doctor. Many features of that situation remained in place in the early twentieth century for medical aid associations that were large enough to pay an attractive annual stipend. In 1905, for example, twenty-two medical men applied for the post of second medical officer to the Lincoln Oddfellows medical aid association, a position that paid £240 a year.[2]

If friendly society members gained more medical care in the process, they gained it at once over other surgeons, who could plausibly expect to provide contract services; other physicians, who rarely deigned to become candidates; and informal practitioners, who did not offer the same range of services that surgeon-apothecaries could provide but who, until the Medical Act of 1858, were eligible to serve as friendly society doctors. In such circumstances, questions about the quality of care revolve around whether friendly societies consistently hired less skillful surgeons, engaging men who would practice for lower fees under contract because they could not get higher fees from private patients, as well as around the issue

2. Lincoln Oddfellows Medical Committee papers, Misc. Dep. 96/2, minutes.

of whether the surgeons they did hire provided lower-quality care to friendly society patients than to private patients.

From the surgeon's point of view group contracts with friendly societies, like those with poor law authorities, brought a certain income in return for an uncertain scale of responsibilities. How many men would fall sick during the year, and how often would they need to be attended? Surgeons' ledgers fail to reveal the scale of responsibilities. Because of the contract payment, the surgeon and his accountant did not need to record each contact and each medication, as they did for other patients. Fortunately, court records sometimes permit reconstruction of these matters.

Attending practitioners provided three key services to the friendly societies. First, they examined individuals applying for membership to decide whether their health was satisfactory. For life insurers and for some friendly societies, such examinations earned separate and sometimes generous fees. The Shropshire Provident Society paid ten shillings for a medical exam. But most friendly societies expected examinations to be covered by the annual contract payments they made. Second, doctors attended friendly society members when they were sick, distinguishing sickness from wellness, providing therapy, and filling in forms certifying eligibility for benefits. The societies expected their doctors to fill those forms— reporting name, date, opinion about sickness status, and, rarely, a diagnosis—without charge and grumbled vigorously when the doctors wanted compensation for the service. One lodge described such a proposed charge as extortion.[3] Third, the doctors provided medicines, but not always the bottles in which liquid medicines were dispensed. They did not furnish appliances, such as trusses, and, as a rule, they performed only procedures that were already commonplace in their practice.[4]

AOF Court Equity in Cambridge paid its surgeon about 3s. 6d. per member per year for medical attendance in 1879, in the midst of a period during which some additional evidence is available about what court members got for their money.[5] In return, the surgeon worked court members into his private practice. The additional data derive from 1877 and 1882, when the average membership of the court totaled 274 men, and the surgeon's pay, assuming that the 1879 rate obtained, fell just short of £48.

3. Loyal Vale of Clun Lodge papers, 1927/1, minutes, Nov. 8, 1912.
4. E.g., Shropshire Providence Society papers, 436/6728, minutes, Mar. 29, 1884.
5. AOF, Court Equity papers, R78/70. This figure is estimated on the basis of the sum paid the surgeon for the half year ending June 30, 1879, plus the number of members at the beginning of the year, entrants, and exits. Various ways of computing the number of men at risk indicate the surgeon was paid between 3s. 4d. and 3s. 7d. per member per year.

On average in those two years, sixty-six members fell sick, and their sicknesses lasted a total of 3,644 days.

The key point, however, is how often the members were attended, which can be estimated for 1877. From the surgeon's certificates that survive it is apparent that the court's surgeon had to recertify a sickness every one or two weeks. Taking the rate at a consultation every two weeks, which will produce a lower total, Court Equity's surgeon had a minimum of 262 contacts with sick members during 1877, an average of 4.5 contacts per sick member. This is certainly an understatement, for it refers only to the certification process. Members visited the surgeon, or called for him to visit them, as needed by their sickness rather than merely to serve the administrative need for certifying their sicknesses. What is more, twenty-one men joined Court Equity in 1877, raising the number of contacts to at least 283.[6] That figure, albeit a minimum, suggests that Court Equity's doctor attended members less often than once a day through the year. The demand on this doctor's time does not seem to have been heavy.

In 1883 the Cambridge Oddfellows, the Foresters, and members of other sick clubs jointly formed the Cambridge Friendly Societies' Medical Association (CFSMA), which provided medical attendance and medicines for members and their families. The CFSMA engaged a surgeon as full-time medical officer and a dispenser to serve a rapidly increasing number of subscribers. Table 3.1 shows the CFSMA's record from 1883 through 1897. On a daily basis, assuming a medical officer was available seven days a week, the burden grew from 12.2 contacts per day in 1884 to 45.1 in 1890. A second surgeon was appointed in 1891. Even so, in 1897 Dr. Stinson attended on 18,937 occasions—51.9 a day—and Dr. Campbell on 10,028 occasions—27.5 a day. The cost per attendance dropped from 9.7d. per visit in 1884 to 3.8d. in 1897, and the cost per prescription from 3.1d. in 1887 to 2.6d. in 1897.[7] The CFSMA was a highly efficient supplier of medical services.

Doctors working at the Northampton Friendly Societies' Medical Institute in 1873–74 attended 3,445 men, women, and children. On average for those two years each member had 1.13 incidents of sickness and saw the institute's doctors 4.35 times. Thus, each sickness involved an average

6. No evidence is available about how often or in what quantities the surgeon provided medications.

7. Respectively, dividing expenditures on medical officers by the annual total of visits and payments to dispensers plus the cost of drugs by the number of prescriptions filled. Thus, both estimates disregard overheads—administration, rent, heat, and light—but the things left out do not affect the trends reported and have only a small effect on the rates.

Table 3.1
CFSMA Activities, 1883–1897

	1883[a]	1884	1885[a]	1886	1887	1888	1889	1890	1891	1892	1893	1894	1895	1896	1897
Society members	1,567	1,711	1,811	1,911	2,046	2,133	2,312	2,458	2,713	2,812	2,944	3,105	3,253	3,373	3,411
Family members	173	266	315	495	731	876	996	1,130	1,182	1,215	1,313	1,393	1,631	1,969	2,320
Total	1,740	1,977	2,126	2,406	2,777	3,009	3,308	3,588	3,895	4,027	4,257	4,498	4,884	5,342	5,731
Home visits	—	1,263	743	1,663	1,985	2,132	2,595	3,367	4,829	4,037	4,221	5,992	6,303	7,508	7,470
Surgery visits	—	3,179	2,914	7,042	7,722	8,539	10,586	13,104	13,810	12,862	14,463	17,134	20,208	21,439	21,495
Total	2,521	4,442	3,657	8,705	9,707	10,671	13,181	16,471	18,639	16,899	18,684	23,126	26,511	28,947	28,965
Prescriptions dispensed	—	—	—	4,950[b]	10,433	12,808	14,099	19,472	18,121	15,919	19,333	20,744	27,921	30,918	33,150
Candidates for Entrance															
Passed	91	238	110	188	243	227	342	354	486	409	367	395	419	420	409
Rejected	7	4	2	—	—	—	11	26	35	22	6	12	35	36	27
Sick certificates granted															
On	354	469	252	528	493	482	487	863	692	736	847	707	996	935	903
Off	147	375	205	464	464	456	446	794	650	721	761	731	927	870	879
Confinements	13	21	10	37	38	43	48	36	52	35	46	48	37	88	88
Deaths	4	18	5	37	21	29	20	33	27	34	41	32	50	44	43

Source: Data from Cambridge Friendly Societies' Medical Association papers, 1897 annual report.
[a]Membership for 12 months; visits for 6 months only.
[b]Membership for 8 months only.

of 3.85 consultations, three-quarters at the Institute's clinic and the remainder at the member's home.[8] In this medical aid association as in these associations in general, working people consulted their doctors freely, perhaps as often as every other day when sick. Certainly, the Northampton Institute's members saw their doctors far more often than was required by friendly society rules about the certification of sickness.

Individual sick clubs contracted with doctors in two ways. Some courts, especially in the early nineteenth century, paid a flat retainer, the size of which did not change as the court gained or lost members. Others set fees at a per member rate, which provides an easier basis for comparison. Figure 3.1 shows the average per member payment for medical services in thirty societies distributed widely across Britain in both cities and rural areas.[9] These data show a clear trend toward higher fees, in three stages. From the 1840s to the 1870s most courts and lodges paid their doctors about 3s. per member per year. In the early 1870s, fees jumped up toward 4s., where they remained into the 1890s. Then the average jumped again to 4s. 6d. In the late eighteenth and early nineteenth centuries, friendly societies had paid between 1s. and 2s. 6d. per member for contract services. In the 1920s they paid sharply rising fees, reaching as much as 13s. 6d. in 1927.[10] Considering only the fees themselves, without adjusting for price change or for changes in the demand for medical services, the evidence from friendly society accounts seems to support Ian Waddington's conclusion that the limitation of access to the ranks of qualified practitioners, promoted by the Medical Act of 1858, and a deterioration in the ratio of doctors to the population during the period 1861–81 led to higher incomes for doctors.[11]

Individual lodges often paid for medical services at the same rate for lengthy periods, a practice that promoted the tendency evident in figure 3.1 for doctors' fees to remain at the same level and then to rise abruptly. Sometimes the fees a lodge paid were fixed in its rules. Raising them required not merely a special meeting where rule changes might be adopted but also the printing and distribution of new sets of rules to members. This sticky pattern suggests that pressure for higher fees had to

8. *Foresters' Miscellany,* Apr. 1875, 373.

9. Green, *Working-Class Patients,* 15–17, provides additional instances of fees.

10. Loyal Fane Friendly Society papers, Loyal Fane II/2, minutes, Nov. 20, 1927.

11. Waddington, *Medical Profession in the Industrial Revolution,* 148–52. On the crowded profession early in the nineteenth century, see Loudon, *Medical Care and the General Practitioner,* 7–8, 208–27, 309.

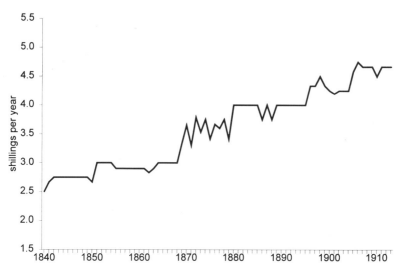

Fig. 3.1. Average Payments for Medical Services, 1840–1913
Source: Data from AOF, Abthorpe Court papers, rules, ZA1692; AOF, Court
Loyal Bodelwyddan papers, minutes, D/DM/510/2–3; AOF, Court Loggerheads
papers, cashbook, D/DM/217/9; Dr. Edwards' papers, ledger, D/DM/63/33;
Shropshire Provident Society papers, minutes, 436/6728; Leicester Bond Street
Friendly Society papers, minutes, DE1884/1; Lytham Sick Club papers, minutes,
RCLy/2/1; IOOF, Pleasant Retreat Lodge papers, minutes, DDX433/2; IOOF,
Loyal Queen Adelaide Lodge of Chipping papers, DDX814/2/1; AOF, Court
Equity papers, balance sheets, R78/70; Kempston Friendly Society papers,
minutes, DDX157/1; Melchbourne Club papers, minutes, P73/28/1–2;
Eversholt Friendly Society papers, minutes, X783/1/1; IOOF, Idris Lodge
papers, minutes, 8476D; IOOF, Temple of Love Lodge papers, 3545C; Great
Northern Railway Locomotive Friendly Society papers, minutes, DS9/1/1–2;
IOOF, Loyal Star of the North Lodge papers, minutes, D/IOO/1–3; High
Pavement Chapel Provident Friendly Society papers, minutes, HiF 2; AOF,
Court Ancient City papers, minutes, 37203; IOOF, Loyal Steam Plough Lodge
papers, minutes, 1898–1913; AOF, Court Conqueror papers, rules, KC40
8/1/1; AOF, Court of Three Mary's papers, minutes, bills and accounts,
TU:10/2, TU:97/1; Royal Berkshire Friendly Society papers, rules, D/EBy/Q34;
Neave Collection, rules of AOF courts 634 and 719 and H. H. Cranswich
Foresters' Friendly Society, DFR/17; IOOF, St. Peter's Lodge papers, minutes,
DFR/13; IOOF, Farmers Refuge Lodge papers, minutes, DFR/12; and Sudbury
Friendly Society, surgeon's book, GF505/5/2.

build up, so that the administrative manner in which fees were set added
to tensions between friendly societies and doctors.

Calculated on a per member basis, fees rose over time. So, too, did the
average age of friendly society members. Because the risk of being sick
increases with age, additional fees did not necessarily mean additional

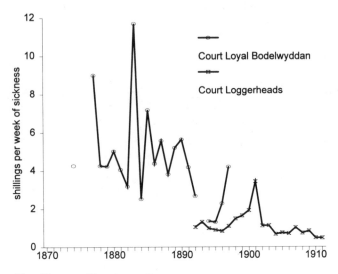

Fig. 3.2. Two Contract Practices, 1870–1911
Source: Data from AOF, Court Loyal Bodelwyddan papers, minutes,
D/DM/510/2–3; and AOF, Court Loggerheads papers, cashbook,
D/DM/217/9.

income, measured by the time doctors devoted to the health complaints of
friendly society patients. Moreover, the average amount of sickness time
was rising, at least in the period 1872–1910, after taking age into account.
Thus, it is possible that the net fees doctors received, gauged in terms of
friendly society demands on them for services, may have diminished. Figure 3.2 provides information pertinent to these issues from two units of the
AOF located in North Wales, Court Loyal Bodelwyddan in St. Asaph and
Court Loggerheads in Llanferes, showing how much the doctor for each
court was paid for each week of sickness. Under neither contract service
nor private practice were patients charged in this way. But the measure of
shillings per week of sickness can serve as a gauge of the demand on a
doctor's time.

Each curve should be examined separately, for the courts paid their
doctors at different rates. Court Loyal Bodelwyddan paid a comparatively
generous average of 4.6s. per week of sickness, but Court Loggerheads
paid its doctor much less, an average of only 1.1s. per week of sickness.
Each curve shows a trend decline in payments. Members' sickness time
increased more than did payments to their doctors, and doctors' compensation shrank. By the early years of the twentieth century the Llanferes
court paid its doctor less than 1s. a week to treat sick members. These

declining rates of compensation per week of sickness meant also that the friendly societies did not shoulder the medical costs of rising sickness time. They had to pay benefits for longer periods, but their doctors bore the burden of longer periods of treatment.

In 1905 the BMA presented results from a survey of doctors engaged chiefly in contract practice, attempting to speak to the issue of pay for service. Most respondents indicated that contract practice required work equal to or less than that required by private practice.[12] Among doctors who supplied more detailed information, the anonymous authors of the report tried to estimate cost per consultation, but their assumptions patently overstate the rate of contacts.[13] The best-substantiated conclusion of the report was that contract doctors thought themselves underpaid. No analogous investigation of the attitudes of working people toward their pay exists, but it seems safe to infer that working people, too, thought themselves underpaid.

PRIVATE PRACTICE

Doctors whose ledgers have survived did not as a rule record individual contacts with friendly society members, entering only the revenue from the contract.[14] They often did enter such information about contacts with private patients. Sometimes they identified their patients by occupation, which makes it possible to examine ledgers to discover whether private patients and members of friendly societies in the same occupations paid equal amounts for medical services.

In the 1860s, 1870s, and 1880s, a period for which comparatively plentiful information is available, doctors sometimes charged separately for consultations and the medicines they supplied at consultation, but more often they combined the two services. Thus although their ledgers

12. Arthur Newsholme recalled working in private practice for five years during the 1880s, when he served as medical officer for an Oddfellows lodge. He welcomed the extra income and found that the members were not demanding. Newsholme, *Fifty Years in Public Health*, 130.

13. "Investigation into the Economic Conditions of Contract Medical Practice," 14. When they lacked information on the number of consultations from a respondent, the authors assumed a rate of one consultation for one medication. But doctors' ledgers and other sources regularly show that this assumption produces an inflated estimate, because doctors usually provided significantly more than one medication per consultation. See below, this chapter.

14. Sometimes ledgers also indicate additional charges doctors could make to friendly society members who lived outside the boundaries of the area where the doctor's services were considered to be prepaid.

show some elements of a fee schedule, the schedule was not always followed. It is especially likely that charges made for a consultation at the doctor's surgery were included within the cost of medications.

Moreover, doctors sometimes charged different fees for what appear from ledger entries to be identical services. Often the rich paid more, either in higher charges for the same medications or services or in more numerous services and more plentiful medications. If those caveats are kept in mind, a selection of ledgers from sites in Wales, Scotland, and England indicates that surgeons levied similar fees across Britain. Typically they charged 1s. or 1s. 6d. for a consultation at their surgery and 2s. 6d. for a consultation at a patient's home close to the doctor's residence, usually within a mile, a fee sometimes collected via the sale of medications rather than as a specific charge for consultation. For traveling greater distances they charged more, often at a rate of 1s. a mile.[15] Almost all consultations led to a sale of medications, so that ordinary patients, including people working in agriculture and manufacturing or in retail trades, paid at least 1s. 6d. to 2s. to visit a doctor and obtain medicines.[16] On average they paid considerably more. One sample, from the ledgers of an unidentified doctor practicing in Oxfordshire, shows that in the period 1869–70 patients were charged an average of slightly more than 4s. 6d. per contact day.[17]

Frederick Hall, a surgeon practicing in Wragby, Lincolnshire, accumulated 12,504 contacts in 1876–78 with private patients, an average of 11.4 a day during his seven-day workweek. In addition, his contract-patient contacts can be estimated at 1.5 a day, so that his total load reached nearly thirteen contacts a day.[18] Hall charged his private patients an average of 5.56s. per contact day, of which he collected 4.70s.[19] He had a lucrative

15. Inferred from the charges made by the Wragby surgeon Frederick Hall, from doctor's ledger, Misc. Don. 477/1.

16. Doctor's ledger, D/DM/301/3, 1855–1860; Buchan Medical Society papers, 1163/2/1/1a, minutes, Aug. 2, 1864, for the society's schedule of fees; Buchan Medical Society papers, 1163/2/7/10, the schedule of fees of the Garioch and Northern Medical Association, 1863; Dr. William Noot ledger, 1876, 12540D; doctor's ledger, Misc. Sq. III/1 and IV/1, the ledgers of an unidentified doctor for the period 1869–1873; and John Stephen Taylor Collection, D/597, ledger from 1888–1919.

17. Doctor's ledger, Misc. Sq. IV/1, a sample consisting of all patient contacts and charges from ledger, 100–119. A contact day includes charges for medications as well as examination.

18. Doctor's ledger, Misc Don. 477/1, covering the period 1875–85.

19. These averages are based on transactions charged and payments received in 1877 and 1878. Some of what Hall received each year was paid for services rendered one or, rarely, two years earlier. Hence the charges for 1877 might be associated with revenues for 1878. Even

practice, with gross charges averaging £1,159.66 a year and collections of £979.71. In 1877 and 1878 Hall's private practice accounted for 91.4 percent of all his charges.[20]

Hall served private patients in Wragby, paupers on medical relief in several poor law unions in the vicinity, and several friendly societies. He was unusual in being, for a few years, the only medical practitioner living in Wragby. In most British communities the size of Wragby, two or three doctors would have split these various responsibilities. Hall recorded receipts from the poor law unions but not the number of his patient contacts. Another source from the region indicates that medical men treating patients for the Boston Provident Dispensary in 1855 earned 2.23s. per case, although the records do not show how often cases were attended.[21] According to a sample, Hall saw private patients an average of 5.7 times per episode of sickness. Taking that as an upper-bound estimate of the number of contacts per case, Boston Provident Dispensary doctors may have earned as little as 4.7d. per contact or, at the other extreme, assuming one contact per case, as much as 2.23s. In any event, these two samples suggest that medical care was delivered in nineteenth-century Britain at sharply lower cost for charitable cases than for private patients. That comes as no surprise, and it is affirmed by other sources.[22]

No typical or average rate of payments in private practice can be extracted from this sketchy information. Nevertheless, it is apparent that, at a per member rate of 3s. to 4s. a year, the friendly societies paid an amount that would, in private practice, have brought not quite a single contact for each member with a doctor, including medications provided by the doctor. In short, doctors charged friendly societies at a rate that indicates they expected to make less than one visit per year per member. The evidence shows that they saw members more often than that and that, therefore, friendly society members got cut-rate services. The friendly societies paid doctors more than the private dispensaries and poor law unions did but less than private patients.

Since at least some doctors charged their patients different amounts

---

so, the averages would be so nearly the same as not to matter. (These quantities are based on preliminary results of an analysis of Hall's practice.)

20. That is, he billed £2,319 6s. 5d. for all services in those two years, including those provided friendly societies and poor law unions. Digby, *Making a Medical Market*, 142–48, provides extensive information about the advertised income from practices. Hall was doing very well for a country doctor.

21. Thompson, *History and Antiquities of Boston*, 294–95. Mark James kindly supplied this information and reference.

22. Hodgkinson, *Origins of the National Health Service*, 26–45, 297, and passim.

according to their social position or wealth, it may be more telling to compare what friendly society members paid with what was paid by private patients in similar occupations. Hall charged his wealthier patients slightly more for some medications. For the most common medication he provided, the family members and servants alike in two landowning households, the Turners and Heneages, paid 3s. 6d., whereas working people paid only 3s. But he levied the same charges to rich and working poor alike for journeys, deliveries, implements, and some other goods and services. Hall got more from the rich in one way. He provided them with more medications and services, in one sample charging for an average of 2.64 items per contact day compared to 1.69 items for working-class and lower-middle-class family members. But he appears to have gotten less from the rich in another way. Working people—grocers, wheelwrights, postmen, laborers, gardeners, and the like—paid him more promptly, and they also paid him a larger proportion of what he charged them than did people in his practice in general or the rich in particular.

Hall could discount the cost of his services in setting fees for friendly societies because he knew that in private practice he would collect less than he charged. As the quantities given above indicate, he collected 84.5 percent of the charges made in 1877 and 1878. Moreover, the friendly societies paid promptly for medical services, giving the doctor a slight advantage if he thought about the present value of current and future receipts. On those grounds it was appropriate to charge contract patients less than private patients. But for Hall and many other doctors, friendly society patients paid much less still.[23]

POOR LAW MEDICAL RELIEF

The poor law provided medical relief to people deemed to be both destitute and sick in a system in which national policy attempted unsuccessfully to regulate local action. Each administrative unit, the poor law union, engaged one or more medical officers, and most also appointed relieving officers whose task it was to judge the economic and medical eligibility of applicants for assistance. The 1834 law sought to provide relief on terms niggardly enough to discourage people from relying on it, and it suc-

23. In "Investigation into the Economic Conditions of Contract Medical Practice," 15, one respondent acknowledged that he charged less in contract than in private practice but that he also had fewer bad debts. Other respondents overlooked the issue of bad debts. In general, respondents to the BMA survey believed they were being paid too little.

ceeded. Nearly every observer concluded that poverty was far more wide-spread than pauperism, that being the specific condition required for assis-tance. Whereas a quarter to a third of the population lived in poverty, only 4.3 percent received poor law relief in 1860. That proportion declined across the second half of the century. In its medical relief the poor law was meant to concentrate aid on the treatment of people who could recover. Thus, most unions limited assistance to a matter of weeks, or at the most a few months, without anticipating the need for aid to people undergoing lengthier convalescence or facing prolonged disability. With that intended effect came also unintended limitations. By appointing lay relieving offi-cers and by stigmatizing relief, designating the sick poor as paupers and thus using the same term for people the union doctor treated at his surgery or in their own homes as it did for people in the workhouse, most poor law unions discouraged people from seeking treatment in the earliest stages of sickness.[24]

Thus three schemes of assistance for the sick poor existed in England and Wales in the nineteenth century. The poor law assisted paupers, in-cluding people out of work and those reduced to destitution by their sicknesses. Charitable agencies, especially the voluntary hospitals and public dispensaries, helped the urban poor. The friendly societies and medical aid associations arranged contract medical services for most people in the working class. Each system had a target population. In practice the groups they served overlapped at the edges. For example, the friendly society member whose club did not engage a contract doctor, or did not engage one for his wife and children, must often have turned to the public dispensary or voluntary hospital, if one was available.

Although the working-class ethic fiercely resisted the appellation of pauper, the friendly society member who lost his job and whose member-ship lapsed before sickness set in must often have applied for relief. But it is important to notice that the friendly societies, rather than the poor law unions, provided best for long-term sickness. The man or woman who was sick for three months or longer could expect very little from the union without entering the workhouse but could count on continuing benefits from the friendly society. Two categories of destitution can, therefore, be distinguished. In one, the disabled, the lunatic, the blind who were not

24. Hodgkinson, *Origins of the National Health Service,* 295–96, 693; Digby, *Pauper Palaces,* 12, 84; and Flinn, "Medical Services under the New Poor Law." Digby, *Making a Medical Market,* 244, argues that medical care under the new poor law was worse than under the old law.

friendly society members entered and remained in a workhouse, not to work but because the workhouse was also an infirmary and increasingly a hospital. In the other, those who were members lived on their own receiving half or quarter benefits from their sick club.

All three schemes draw attention to the possibility that their clients received inferior medical services. Doctors working for poor law unions also regarded themselves as underpaid. They complained far more often in public about their inadequate pay than their patients complained formally about the quality of the medical care they received. Almost nothing is known about private and informal complaints. Therefore, the evidence consists chiefly of what doctors and poor law administrators wrote. Not surprisingly, they found many faults with the system but maintained that paupers received not just adequate but good medical care. Workhouse infirmaries were overcrowded; too many patients came for treatment too late in the course of their sicknesses. But the doctors were good.[25]

Whether or not the testimony of doctors and officials is to be believed, poor law medical relief implies some things about the medical care that friendly society members received. First, poor law authorities set out to avoid providing medical care attractive enough to draw patients from the ranks of the provident poor. They aimed to serve as few people as possible rather than to assist the sick in general.[26] Second, friendly societies were visibly more successful than poor law unions at stimulating rivalry among the doctors of a community for the medical posts they offered. They paid more, they paid reliably, and they demanded less in one crucial aspect: a doctor working for the poor law union was expected to treat paupers scattered across the entire territory of the union or the part of it that he served, an area often larger and costlier in time to serve than the area in which the members of a friendly society lived. Frederick Hall, the Wragby doctor, spent much of each day traveling to patients who required home treatment. He charged the rich for travel and sometimes also for waiting time. But neither the poor nor working people could afford the added charge, so Hall and other doctors tried to save time by reducing the extent of their horseback travel.

Poor law medical relief, in which the doctors themselves believed they provided good care, stands as a floor of medical care in nineteenth-century Britain. If it was indeed good, then, because of the important advantages of

25. Hodgkinson, *Origins of the National Health Service*, 17, 23–26, 65, 133, 277, 351–52, passim.
26. Ibid., 8.

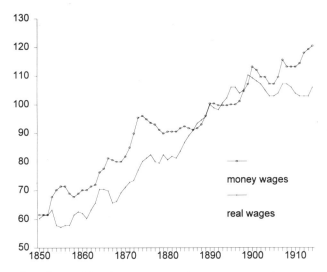

Fig. 3.3. Index of Wage Trends, 1850–1914 (1890–94 = 100)
Source: Data from Mitchell, *British Historical Statistics,* 149–50.

friendly society over poor law care, that emerges as an argument that friendly society medical care was better.

THE RELATIVE COST OF MEDICAL SERVICES

Data about medical fees take on additional meaning when interpreted in the light of price and wage trends.[27] Figure 3.3 depicts the course of wages in the second half of the nineteenth century, considered in four dimensions. The first curve follows changes in average wages taken at current values, and the second curve adjusts these for price change, showing how the purchasing power of wages shifted over the period 1850–1914. Between 1850 and 1900, real wages increased by about 75 percent, but for the next fifteen years they failed to increase further. Until 1900, working people enjoyed real and substantial gains in income.

The extent to which working people understood that wages were rising more rapidly than prices is uncertain. Clearly, they lived these price and wage changes. From limited testimony in AOF sources, they seem to have

27. Mitchell, *British Historical Statistics,* 149–51, 163, 170, drawing on the work of others, most notably G. H. Wood and A. L. Bowley. Wood and Bowley supply separate but overlapping indices, which have been spliced here at 1894–95 and adjusted to a base period of 1890–94.

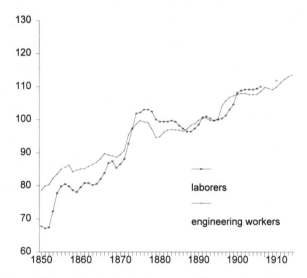

Fig. 3.4. Index of Wage Trends for Laborers and Engineering Workers, 1850–1914 (1890–94 = 100)
Source: Data from Mitchell, *British Historical Statistics,* 149–50.

felt that the two things were rising at more or less the same pace and that, in any case, they were no better off.[28] If this is an accurate view of their perception, then it follows that friendly society members would have been eager to prevent any sharper increase in what they paid for medical services than the increase of their wages.

Figure 3.4 tracks the wages at current values of ordinary laborers and those of skilled engineering workers, groups at more or less opposite extremes in the spectrum of wages earned by working-class men. Both curves closely follow changes in wages in general. But they suggest further that less-skilled workers benefited relatively more from the great upward momentum of wages in this period than did highly skilled workers. The wages of ordinary laborers rose along a steeper gradient than did those of skilled engineering workers, though the latter continued to earn much more. Hence, in the last decades of the nineteenth century, the relative cost of medical care diminished more for working people with fewer skills.

It is against this background that medical fees can be examined further. Figure 3.5 reproduces the curve of average wages in current prices and compares it with medical fees, which appear here as index numbers rather

28. See a brief discussion of this point embedded in a wandering essay of moral advice in "Circumstances and Self Not Synonymous," 286.

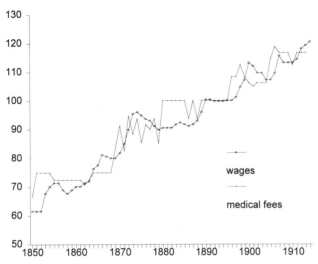

Fig. 3.5. Index of Wages and Medical Fees, 1850–1914 (1890–94 = 100)
Source: Data from AOF, Abthorpe Court papers, rules, ZA1692; AOF, Court
Loyal Bodelwyddan papers, minutes, D/DM/510/2–3; AOF, Court Loggerheads
papers, cashbook, D/DM/217/9; Dr. Edwards' papers, ledger, D/DM/63/33;
Shropshire Provident Society papers, minutes, 436/6728; Leicester Bond Street
Friendly Society papers, minutes, DE1884/1; Lytham Sick Club papers, minutes,
RCLy/2/1; IOOF, Pleasant Retreat Lodge papers, minutes, DDX433/2; IOOF,
Loyal Queen Adelaide Lodge of Chipping papers, DDX814/2/1; AOF, Court
Equity papers, balance sheets, R78/70; Kempston Friendly Society papers,
minutes, DDX157/1; Melchbourne Club papers, minutes, P73/28/1–2;
Eversholt Friendly Society papers, minutes, X783/1/1; IOOF, Idris Lodge
papers, minutes, 8476D; IOOF, Temple of Love papers, 3545C; Great Northern
Railway Locomotive Friendly Society papers, minutes, DS9/1/1–2; IOOF, Loyal
Star of the North Lodge papers, minutes, D/IOO/1–3; High Pavement Chapel
Provident Friendly Society papers, minutes, HiF 2; AOF, Court Ancient City
papers, minutes, 37203; IOOF, Loyal Steam Plough Lodge papers, minutes,
1898–1913; AOF Court Conqueror papers, rules, KC40 8/1/1; AOF, Court of
Three Mary's papers, bills and accounts, TU:10/2 and TU:97/1; Royal Berkshire
Friendly Society papers, rules, D/EBy/Q34; Neave Collection, rules of AOF
Courts 634 and 719 and H. H. Cranswich Foresters' Friendly Society, DFR/17;
IOOF, St. Peter's Lodge papers, minutes, DFR/13; IOOF, Farmers Refuge Lodge
papers, minutes, DFR/12; Sudbury Friendly Society, surgeon's book,
GF505/5/2; and Mitchell, *British Historical Statistics,* 149–50.

than amounts. Although medical fees were sticky, tending to remain at the
same level for years at a time, their upward course closely tracked the
growth of wages. Fees may have been slightly higher, in relative terms, in
the 1850s and slightly lower in the last years before 1914. Like wages,
medical fees increased more rapidly than did the price of food and other

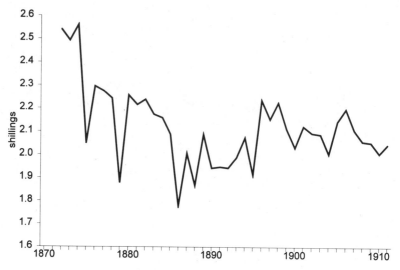

Fig. 3.6. Medical Fees per Week of Sickness, 1870–1911
Source: Data from AOF, Abthorpe Court papers, rules, ZA1692; AOF, Court
Loyal Bodelwyddan papers, minutes, D/DM/510/2–3; AOF, Court Loggerheads
papers, cashbook, D/DM/217/9; Dr. Edwards' papers, ledger, D/DM/63/33;
Shropshire Provident Society papers, minutes, 436/6728; Leicester Bond Street
Friendly Society papers, minutes, DE1884/1; Lytham Sick Club papers, minutes,
RCLy/2/1; IOOF, Pleasant Retreat Lodge papers, minutes, DDX433/2; IOOF,
Loyal Queen Adelaide Lodge of Chipping papers, DDX814/2/1; AOF, Court
Equity papers, balance sheets, R78/70; Kempston Friendly Society papers,
minutes, DDX157/1; Melchbourne Club papers, minutes, P73/28/1–2;
Eversholt Friendly Society papers, minutes, X783/1/1; IOOF, Idris Lodge
papers, minutes, 8476D; IOOF, Temple of Love papers, 3545C; Great Northern
Railway Locomotive Friendly Society papers, minutes, DS9/1/1–2; IOOF, Loyal
Star of the North Lodge papers, minutes, D/IOO/1–3; High Pavement Chapel
Provident Friendly Society papers, minutes, HiF 2; AOF, Court Ancient City
papers, minutes, 37203; IOOF, Loyal Steam Plough Lodge papers, minutes,
1898–1913; AOF Court Conqueror papers, rules, KC40 8/1/1; AOF, Court of
Three Mary's papers, bills and accounts, TU:10/2 and TU:97/1; Royal Berkshire
Friendly Society papers, rules, D/EBy/Q34; Neave Collection, rules of AOF
courts 634 and 719, and H. H. Cranswich Foresters' Friendly Society, DFR/17;
IOOF, St. Peter's Lodge papers, minutes, DFR/13; IOOF, Farmers Refuge Lodge
papers, minutes, DFR/12; and Sudbury Friendly Society, surgeon's book,
GF505/5/2.

consumer goods. But there was no marked change over that period in the
capacity of wage earners to pay for medical services on the terms provided
to friendly society members.

In terms, therefore, of the costs of contract services, it is difficult to argue
that doctors or friendly society members gained much of an advantage,

unless doctors actually gave services of deteriorating quality as time passed. Adjusting for price change alone removes the appearance that the incomes of doctors gained across the second half of the nineteenth century, insofar at least as that may be judged on the basis of what friendly society members paid for medical services. Doctors' incomes may have risen because more working people were hiring formal practitioners than had done so earlier in the century, but they did not rise because working people were paying more for medical services. In short, if medical incomes improved, this evidence would suggest they did so because doctors worked harder, seeing more patients, rather than because in real values the fees they received from individual working-class patients rose.

Figure 3.6 alters the terms of the analysis by comparing the average fees that friendly society members paid for contract medical services per week of sickness among AOF members in the period 1872–1911, holding age constant.[29] This approach seeks to adjust for changes in the characteristics of the working people using contract medical services, specifically in age and aggregate sickness time. It is inexact, however, in that too little evidence is available about how often sick men saw their doctors and thus about the degree to which an increase in sickness time promoted an increase in the number of consultations per episode. Sick men saw their doctors at least as often as every week or two. But that rate concerns certification of sickness rather than attendance, and it fails to show how consultation patterns changed during the course of prolonged sicknesses or over time.

At one extreme, sicknesses became more protracted, but workingmen may not have continued to consult their doctors at the same frequency throughout the course of long episodes. At the other extreme, men may have seen their doctors with some regularity—once a week or even more often—throughout the course of an episode, because their contract allowed them to call the doctor when they needed him. Without more evidence it is not possible to decide whether the lengthening of episodes observed in the years 1872–1911 added to the number of contacts patients had with doctors.

Per week of sickness, the cost of medical attendance dropped sharply from the early 1870s to the late 1880s, then rose for about a decade before declining once more in the early years of the twentieth century. Across the period as a whole, working people clearly gained, according to this gauge.

29. Construction of the sickness rates used in this figure is explained in chapter 7.

Sickness time increased much more rapidly than did medical fees, especially from the 1870s to the 1890s. Working people not only negotiated advantageous terms for medical treatment, they also preserved and enhanced those terms across a period during which they were sick more of the time and therefore needed more medical attention.

Throughout the period up to 1910 the portion of their income that working people spent on contract medical care remained small. Ordinary laborers, those who earned the least among their peers, had to pay an average of only 0.57 percent of their annual wages to obtain the medical services provided through friendly societies.[30] Skilled workers paid less still. Compared to the family budgets reconstructed by A. L. Bowley and E. H. Hunt, medical care contracted through the friendly societies represented one of the smallest items of expenditure.[31] At less than 1d. a week, medical costs amounted to roughly a quarter of what farm laborers spent on sugar or tea. In fact, workingmen spent somewhat more than that on medical services. The contracts that friendly societies arranged with a doctor covered only services from that practitioner. The man who needed to see a specialist, to enter a hospital or an asylum, or even to consult another practitioner had to pay for those services over and above what he had paid for the court doctor, though individual friendly societies sometimes contributed something toward additional costs.[32] For the member himself the costs of medical care were still modest, compared to wages. But when these provisions excluded care for family members, that care cost more. For example, in female friendly societies the women who belonged

30. I.e., an average medical fee in the period 1850–1909, 3.78s., divided by the annualized cash wages of 668.74s. Digby, *Making a Medical Market*, 47, reports that Board of Trade returns yield an estimate that 1 to 2 percent of the workingman's income went toward medical attendance. That figure includes premiums for regular friendly society benefits.

31. Bowley, *Wages and Income in the United Kingdom*, 36; Hunt, *Regional Wage Variations in Britain*, 77–105. Bowley attempted to adjust his estimates to include other family earnings, but he does not appear to have considered income from secondary occupations. See Benson, *Penny Capitalists*, who deals with secondary economic activity as well as working-class capitalism. If secondary activity was widespread, wage estimates would more substantially understate earnings, because they assume only employment in primary jobs.

32. E.g., on five occasions between 1900 and 1908, the Loyal Steam Plough Lodge of the Oddfellows in Kirton in Holland (Lincolnshire) considered requests for help in paying outside medical bills. Thrice they agreed, contributing 7s. 6d. in 1900 for a minor operation that one member needed, £5 in 1906 toward what another member owed an outside practitioner, and £1 in 1907 for the cost of anesthetics used in a finger amputation for a member's son. Twice they refused, declining in 1908 to buy a cork leg for a member or to help another member who had consulted someone other than the lodge doctor. IOOF, Loyal Steam Plough Lodge papers, minutes, May 22, 1900, June 26, 1906, Mar. 5, 1907, Mar. 3, 1908, and Nov. 10, 1908.

usually received benefits for childbirth, but the wives of men in male friendly societies did not.

The Dundee stonemason with gravel, James Smith, left a record of what he paid for doctor's and nursing services in nine years during which he also recorded his earnings. His accounts provide a point of comparison for judging how much in doctor's fees could be saved by joining a friendly society. For the nine years, all between 1838 and 1851, Smith paid out a total of £17 8s. 7.5d., which may exclude what he spent on medicines, from earnings of £522 14s. 6d. Thus, he spent at least 3.3 percent of his earnings on medical care.[33] Smith's expenses were unusually heavy. He was incapacitated in 1849, so that his earnings fell and his medical expenses rose. He also had a large family, though for his wife and children he rarely called doctors except for grave sicknesses, like the illness of his first wife in 1846, which resulted in her death, and the bout his son George had with water in the head, also fatal.[34]

Taking the friendly society evidence at face value, figure 3.5 suggests that working-class wages increased as rapidly as, perhaps a little more rapidly than, medical fees paid by friendly societies for contract care. Figure 3.6 shows that as friendly society members, and perhaps working-men in general, suffered increasingly protracted sicknesses they paid less for medical services. By 1899 tension between the two parties, the doctors represented by the British Medical Association and friendly societies by the National Conference of Friendly Societies, reached such a level that a conciliation board was set up to arbitrate disputes. It appears to have done nothing to solve the problem. Men in friendly societies struck a hard bargain for medical services, negotiating effectively to hold costs down, even though their demand for care, as measured by sickness time, was rising. In the prewar era they got the better of the bargain in terms of cost.

In the postwar period, wages continued to increase, but medical fees rose more rapidly still. In the late 1920s current wages averaged an index of 234, but medical fees, at 11s. per adult male friendly society member, jumped to an index of 275 without a corresponding increase in sickness

---

33. Memoirs of James Smith, 108 ff, for 1838–41 and 1847–51. Smith's entries for "sundries" may include purchases of medications.

34. However, Smith and his second wife did arrange an expensive course of treatment for one son, Richard, who stammered. Richard was sent to Edinburgh to be attended for four weeks by a Mr. Bell at a cost of £7 16s. 5d.

See also chapter 4 for further discussion of the costs of medical services for people who did not belong to friendly societies.

time. Although the evidence assembled here deals only with the fees paid by working people for medical care, it suggests that doctors in Britain did not begin to enjoy higher incomes until the 1920s. After that their incomes, compared to those of workingmen, rose rapidly.[35]

Within the friendly societies, medical care for the British working class was a remarkable bargain. Measured in the real price of what friendly society members paid, the cost of care increased along with real wages across the period 1850–1914. Working people paid more for medical services at the end of the period than at its beginning, but as a proportion of their wages the cost of medical services remained stable. Sickness time increased. Hence, assuming no deterioration in attendance rates, working people gained the advantage. Over time they paid somewhat less, as a proportion of their income, for medical services for each week of sickness. In the intermediate run the terms of trade shifted in their favor. Since the initial bargains that workingmen in friendly societies struck with doctors made medical care available to them at cut-rate prices, it is clear that workingmen held the advantage in the nineteenth century. Over time they added slightly to that advantage.

The National Insurance Act of 1911 undermined the capacity of friendly societies to organize on their own in restraint of trade and thus to hold medical fees down, without placing the same limits on doctors' organizations. The result was that the friendly societies lost the battle of the clubs. Thereafter, the wages of working people continued to increase. But the incomes of doctors rose much more rapidly, and the terms of trade shifted decisively in favor of doctors.

This and the previous chapter add new evidence about the quality of medical care in the form of quantitative indices: how many visits, how many medications. The friendly societies extracted not just cheap medical care but also medical care to their own specifications. The men and women who belonged were often treated by the same doctors who treated the rich and the destitute. They seem to have gotten fewer medications than did the rich; perhaps they also got less of the doctor's time. But they seem to have gotten better care than people receiving poor law medical relief. The charge that friendly society members sometimes made, that their doctors gave them less than they gave their private patients, is not to be taken at face value. It was a rhetorical point intended to undermine the doctors'

35. Digby and Bosanquet, "Doctors and Patients," 75–76.

efforts to elevate their fees rather than an assessment of the medical care working people received. Friendly society members could grumble throughout a long sickness about the attention their doctor paid them, but the many who subscribed for medical care were attended on their own terms by licensed practitioners, no matter how long their sicknesses lasted.

CHAPTER 4

The Friendly Societies' Moral Economy

INDIVIDUAL DOCTORS who treated working people seem to have been confident about the utility and efficacy of their services, at least in their public mien, even though few of the treatments they provided seem likely, by present standards, to have had curative properties. It is not clear how doctors sustained their confidence. Perhaps the question arises in this form only because, a century later, doctors and patients alike have so much more confidence in the power of doctors to cure. Nineteenth-century working-class patients, in contrast, wanted doctors to provide medications that produced a physical effect, even if only so modest an effect as the foul taste of a cough syrup. They wanted, no doubt, to become well; but there is very little indication that they truly expected doctors to do something that would make them well.

What should doctors expect from patients and patients from doctors? This question seems to raise the issue of health: doctors expect to treat patients who are sick, trying to ease their discomfort or even to make them well; patients expect doctors to provide therapies that they cannot provide for themselves and to assist the healing course of Nature. It may be that workingmen in Britain took these expectations to doctors who greeted them in kind. But the evidence of that does not appear in friendly society sources. There, the manifest expectations of doctors and patients revolve not around relief or cure but instead around cost, as we have seen, and the degree of attentiveness on the doctor's part.

Workingmen and their doctors came together in the doctors' surgeries and the men's homes but also in club meetings. Doctors visited in order to reassure the men of their commitment to the men's health, but awkwardly, in a gathering of unequals. Doctors visited also to confront charges and, when challenged, to explain why they should be kept on as club surgeon.

At some other meetings, when the doctor was not present, members aired their grievances about unfaithful medical attendance. Sometimes the death of a fellow member prompted a critical review of the medical care he had received, and that, in turn, led to a general scrutiny of the club doctor. Doctors treated members of the sick clubs, but they were also drawn into a complex system the friendly societies had erected to keep the sick under surveillance and to discourage malingering. In that system doctors, too, were under observation.

Until the 1890s the men in friendly societies regularly asserted their capacity to make decisions for themselves. They could decide whether the care a doctor had given sufficed as easily as they could determine whether the actuary's advice about club finances needed to be taken. Suddenly, in the 1890s, as club minutes testify, workingmen lost their nerve.

SURVEILLANCE OF THE SICK

A threshold separates wellness from sickness, but it lacks an objective or readily specified character. Individuals know when they are sick and when they are well, when they suspect that sickness is coming on and also when they feel they are getting well. Although we tend to be confident in our own judgment, we tend also to be suspicious of others, in a way suggested by a small event that occurred during the preparation of files for this book. One of the student employees, who had just returned from a week off and had given an unconvincing description of the health problems that had caused her absence, questioned the merit of a diagnosis given for a Scots railway employee's absence from work in the early twentieth century. The railway worker seemed to her to have stopped work for insufficient reason.

Suspicions about the merit of claims arise in friendly society records. They make up the most common medical item discussed in the minutes of local meetings. Friendly society officials and members alike suspected that some fellow members might impose on them by claiming to be sick when they were well or by claiming still to be sick after they had recovered. To guard against that possibility, some clubs scrutinized each claim separately.[1] But most transferred that responsibility initially to a sick steward and later, as club doctors were appointed, jointly to the steward and the doctor. By the 1870s most clubs had for some time employed general practitioners and divided the responsibilities for record keeping and visit-

---

1. Loyal Order of Ancient Shepherds, Lorne Lodge papers, minutes, Aug. 13, 1890.

ing the sick. Sometimes the steward visited sick members within a certain radius of the club's meeting site, two or three miles, while members living further afield had to produce a surgeon's certificate.[2] But the trend was clearly toward dual examination and visitation of all claimants.

The doctor's primary responsibilities were to certify sickness and to provide medical attendance, the specifics of which were, until the late nineteenth century, usually left unstated, to be determined by the surgeon and friendly society officials. When in 1841 the Lund Oddfellows engaged one of their members as lodge surgeon, they drew up a formal contract but stated the surgeon's duties in only a few words: the doctor was "to find medicines and attend professionally as need requires on each and every sick or lame member."[3] Increasingly in the 1870s and thereafter, partly because the informal arrangements had led to misunderstandings, these terms were made more specific. The Abthorpe Foresters, typical of many others, spelled out these duties in their rules: Surgeons registered under the Medical Act are elected and continue at the pleasure of the court. They must examine all candidates, attend all members living within five miles of the New Inn (a public house where the court met), and provide "proper and sufficient medical and surgical attendance and medicines," each doing "his utmost to restore the health of the afflicted brother." If a member can walk to the surgeon's residence, he should attend the surgeon; if he cannot, the surgeon should attend him in his home. When the surgeon is away he is responsible for naming another surgeon to attend his patients. In the Abthorpe Court, three or four surgeons at any given time attended members scattered in neighboring villages and Abthorpe itself, temporarily a place much larger than other villages in the area.[4]

Friendly society doctors were also charged with certifying a member's sickness and recovery. Thus, each court's attending doctor decided, in negotiations with the member presenting as sick, whether the individual was unable to work because of sickness. These responsibilities the doctor carried as part of the burden of his post and usually fulfilled without extra charge. Each sickness therefore required at least two contacts with the attending doctor, more if it lasted long enough to mandate a series of

2. E. g., Rochdale Lower Place Sick and Burial Society papers, DDX261, minutes, Feb. 3, 1862; and IOOF, Loyal Queen Adelaide Lodge of Chipping papers, DDX814/2/1, resolutions, June 26, 1886.
3. Neave Collection, DFR 13, minutes of the Lund Oddfellows, Mar. 27, 1841.
4. AOF, Abthorpe Court papers, ZA1692, 1884 rules, quotes from 9.

weekly or fortnightly certifications of continuing sickness.[5] So far as the minutes reveal, even disputes over certification were left to doctors to decide. Dr. Sleigh, one of two medical men serving an AOF court in Suffolk, refused in 1909 to provide a sickness certificate to H. Quantrell, who thereupon obtained one from Dr. Carey. But the court secretary refused to pay him benefits, calling on the two doctors to try to reach agreement with one another. When they could not, the case was referred to another doctor. In the end, Quantrell was paid when all the doctors involved agreed that he was disabled, though they continued to disagree about some features of his case.[6]

Sick stewards visited members on benefit each week or fortnight, bringing the benefits in cash. In many courts they reported regularly at meetings on the extent to which members were complying with rules, the names of the sick and their condition, and other matters.[7] As officers earning a salary, albeit small, they had an obligation not merely to see the sick but also to attend court meetings, and they might be fined for failure to perform either task.[8] Sick visitors served two functions. On one hand, in today's jargon, they provided social support, showing the sick member that his brethren were anxious about his condition and preserving the community for sick members, who could not attend meetings.[9] During the fatal sickness of E. W. Walford, a member of the Bedford Oddfellows, the sick visitor stopped by each week from June until September 1931, jotting notes about his visits. Until late August, Walford was "about the same," but then his condition deteriorated. In the last week of September he was "very ill."[10]

On the other hand, the sick visitor was also a spy. It was his duty to decide whether the member on benefit was indeed sick and to report to the

5. See, e.g., Leicester Bond Street Friendly Society papers, DE1884/1, minutes, May 31, 1852, requiring weekly certifications from the surgeon, Mr. Moore; and Loyal Order of Ancient Shepherds, Robbie Burns Lodge papers, minutes (uncatalogued), Feb. 10, 1894.

6. AOF, Court Flower of Suffolk papers, minutes, Feb. 6–Mar. 21, 1909.

7. See, e.g., the reports of John Quin to Court Powis, in Welshpool, at AOF, Court Powis papers, minutes, 1884–1900; and those of the Court Cock Royal Woodwards in AOF, Court Cock Royal papers, D/125/4, minutes. *Foresters' Miscellany,* July 1869, 405, relates the importance of visiting during sickness in the eyes of the wife of a Forester.

8. See, e.g., IOOF, Temple of Love Lodge papers, Resolution Book, MS 3547C, May 28, 1895.

9. "Sick Clubs." Sick and convalescent members were expected and required to remain indoors after eight or so in the evening, which means they could neither attend court meetings nor, more important as a part of community activity, socialize by going to a tavern.

10. IOOF, Maiden Queen Lodge papers, OF/19/1.

court on occasions when he suspected a man on benefits was well enough to work or when signs in the member's behavior—such as absence from home when the visitor called—suggested he had begun to behave as though he were well and, hence, that he was merely feigning sickness. Members who returned to work while still receiving claims were cautioned, fined, or even expelled, as were members deemed to have pretended to be sick. Men also faced a fine or even expulsion if they defied the doctor's orders. In Welshpool, Edward Garner was punished because he went back to work when the court doctor considered him still at risk to falling because of his illness and even though he had notified the court secretary that he intended to resume work.[11] Ernest Ambrose describes sick visitors in his club walking "miles to visit a sick member on the club to make sure he was genuine. Woe betide him if he was found carrying a pail of water or digging a root of potatoes in his garden."[12]

Stewards also spied on the doctor. It was their duty to ask whether the club doctor was attending as often as needed and providing proper medicines and to report back to the club any complaints from a sick member.[13] In the last quarter of 1888 the sick visitors for the Bedford Oddfellows twice prompted the lodge to complain about Dr. Chillingworth's attendance.[14] When they found medical services wanting, they instructed their officers to write the medical men seeking an explanation or to provide a warning, or they arranged a confrontation at the lodge, where the surgeon had to explain his behavior. Moreover, the visitor's intimate knowledge of each sick member's complaint allowed him to second guess the doctor. Sick stewards were not medical practitioners, formal or informal. But they did assume a stance of medical knowledgeability. They represented the working-class layman's claim to know the difference between sickness and wellness.

Part of a court's meeting time was taken up by hearing reports from its sick visitor and deciding what action to take in cases where rules appeared to have been violated or expectations left unsatisfied. Court officers confronted members accused of making fraudulent sickness claims, asking for

11. AOF, Court Powis papers, minutes, Sept. 27–Nov. 22, 1884. The *Quarterly Report* of the AOF shows, however, that members were rarely expelled. AOF, *Quarterly Reports of the Executive Council,* minutes for 1875–89.

12. Ambrose, *Melford Memories,* 114.

13. "Sick Clubs." Thus, the sick stewards carried the same responsibility of surveillance of the sick and their doctors that relieving officers under the New Poor Law bore. But the stewards did not authorize visits to the club doctor.

14. See above, this chapter.

an explanation. Many times a member was let off with only a fine and a caution. For example, Robert Bleazard Sr. was allowed to travel on the advice of the Chipping Oddfellows' surgeon as an aid to recovery. But on his trip he was seen in a public house at 9:15 P.M. by members of the No Danger Lodge in Longridge, who reported him. Bleazard was fined 5s.[15] A Bedford Oddfellow was expelled in 1902 for having tampered with the doctor's certificate, altering the closing date of an episode to change June 21 into June 26 in order to collect 6s. 8d. more in benefits.[16] He lost the small sum fraudulently claimed, a week's benefits he was owed, his investment in future sickness and burial coverage, and the community of his peers.[17]

One of the means friendly societies used to encourage members to return to work as soon as they recovered was the rule prohibiting men on benefits from visiting public houses or drinking alcoholic beverages in public. For many workingmen the pub was an important center of social life, which had to be forgone during sickness. The temptation to go out for a drink, or more than one, was nevertheless strong. The most common charge brought against men on benefit was not that they had returned to work without declaring themselves off benefits but that they had been seen in a tavern. For a first charge most men admitted their offense, pleaded an extenuating circumstance, such as the social pressure involved in an invitation from a friend to visit a pub, and begged for leniency. In such circumstances most clubs were satisfied to fine the miscreant. But repeated offenses led to expulsion.[18]

Internal evidence could be made to reveal areas of abuse. After F. Harrison and two other members were found away from home when visited, Bedford Oddfellows compared the sickness patterns of county members, who were certified by the medical officer but not regularly visited by the sick visitor, with that of city members, who submitted to certification and visits. The county members made more claims. Hence, the lodge resolved to appoint a sick visitor for the county.[19]

In short, the friendly societies erected safeguards against fraud and took

15. IOOF, Loyal Queen Adelaide of Chipping Lodge papers, DDX814/2/1, Sept.–Nov. 1886.

16. IOOF, Maiden Queen Lodge papers, OF8/3, minutes, July 21, 1902.

17. However, for a similar offense in a Leicester friendly society, in which not the sick member but the secretary was judged at fault, the punishment was merely a fine. Leicester Bond Street Friendly Society papers, minutes, DE1884/1, Feb. 13, 1855.

18. See, e.g., AOF, Court Powis papers, minutes, Aug. 1, 1895, the case of John Allen.

19. IOOF, Maiden Queen Lodge papers, OF8/1, minutes, Mar. 9, 1888.

upon themselves the task of settling the disputes occasioned by their surveillance. But the important point is absent from the minutes and other
sources: friendly society members did not disagree among themselves
about their ability, aided by doctors and sick visitors, to distinguish sickness from wellness. Their agents could be trusted to tell the difference.
When questionable cases arose and the brethren asked whether a member
was really sick and unable to work, when they wrote the doctor for more
information or asked the sick visitor or the secretary to make a special
visit, they were satisfied with the answer. Rarely did they pursue a case any
further. In the friendly societies the seemingly natural suspicion that people
feel about their capacity to rely on the judgments of others concerning
sickness and wellness was quieted by confidence in these intermediaries.

Nor in these societies, which existed in order to serve needs potentially
trapped in contentions about the reality of sickness or wellness, was contentiousness commonplace. In the Abthorpe Court of the Foresters, minutes survive for the period from 1893 through 1911. In those years benefits
were paid for 1,127 new sickness episodes and more than 111,700 days of
sickness.[20] Yet the minutes indicate that only on six occasions were questions raised about whether claims were warranted. In other societies and
local units, too, the rate of complaints and investigations was low. Though
they stood at the center of potential contentions, the friendly societies
paradoxically had less to fret about concerning the validity of sickness
claims than they did from many other features of their business, which
would seem at first glance to have been less contentious issues.

DOCTORS AND WORKINGMEN

Many doctors who attended friendly society members belonged to the
societies, more as a means of gaining access to clients than because they
needed the sickness and burial benefits the societies provided or wanted
fellowship with workingmen. Doctors attended meetings rarely, and, in
the accounts examined, they seldom drew benefits for sickness or burial.
Since most lodges and courts allowed both honorary and benefit members,
the doctors may have joined mostly as honorary members, though that

20. See AOF, Abthorpe Court papers, chiefly ZA1581–ZA1604, but these data have also
been checked and expanded from other parts of this large collection. New episodes are
distinguished as periods of sickness occurring fourteen days or more after a previous episode.
The Abthorpe Court did not count Sundays, but here the number of days has been augmented
to seven days per week.

cannot be decided without explicit evidence, such as from contribution ledgers. In any case, the minutes and other sources report cordial meetings as well as confrontations. W. J. Tubbs, who practiced in Upwell, joined an Oddfellows lodge at its formation, served as lodge surgeon, and regularly attended annual dinners. In 1864, replying to a toast to the health of the lodge surgeons, he jollied his fellows with good humor: should the men drink too much he promised to attend them the next morning, if they came early; over the life of the lodge he had seen it prosper like bees in a hive, "but he hoped they would not sting each other."[21] Yet Tubbs did not attend ordinary lodge meetings, he said, because he could not stand the tobacco smoke. He was a member, but not on the same terms as the workingmen who belonged.

Dr. Jabez Carter, one of the surgeons attending the Bedford Oddfellows, visited the lodge in February 1907 and was asked to speak. He touched all the right chords, saying that, as lodge surgeon, "he had always respected the various calls made upon him and looked upon our members as being very respectable[,] well looked after[,] and possessing good livers."[22] The Oddfellows must have wanted to hear that they were respectable men who got good medical services and could drink like fish. Whether any of that was true mattered little at the moment. What mattered was that the doctor honored lodge members by being present, even if he honored them in a condescending manner, speaking not as a man who shared their lives and their concerns but as a social superior whose burden was to humor them.

In April 1892 the surgeon West visited the Loyal Fane Friendly Society in Fulbeck. According to the secretary who kept the minutes, West

> spent a verry comfortable and social Evening with the Members & there expressed his great desire to become acquainted with the Loyal Fane Lodge[.] [H]e decided to accept us as a body of Members under his Medical Care at the same rate as our Late Dr. Barton received & said it should be his great study to do his utmost to promote our welfare by using his best skill to Keep all our Members in good health.[23]

What is noteworthy is how painfully this and the remainder of the secretary's entry stands out from other entries in the minutes. Ordinarily reserved and laconic, at Dr. West's visit the secretary was voluble; typically businesslike, on this evening he wrote about sentiment and feelings. West's

21. Greer, *Tubbs: A Nineteenth-Century G. P.,* 57.
22. IOOF, Maiden Queen Lodge papers, OF8/3, minutes, Feb. 11, 1907.
23. Loyal Fane Friendly Society papers, Loyal Fane II/1, minutes, Apr. 19, 1892.

visit was a special occasion, one that evidently made the members feel awkward.

Carter's visit to the Oddfellows and West's to the Loyal Fane club illustrate one mode of behavior of friendly society members toward their doctors revealed by the minutes. In polite meetings both parties behaved correctly. The members showed that they were honored to receive attention from their doctors; the doctors offered reassurance about their interest in the members' health and an attitude of friendly condescension. Everyone seems to have been uncomfortable, but the discomfort was the familiar one of an encounter of people from different social classes. The interests of the two parties were at odds, but in polite meetings no one had the ill grace to raise that matter.

Rarely was a meeting of the club doctor and the club members free of strain. On September 3, 1891, the members of Robin Hood Lodge of Oddfellows invited John Johnston, a surgeon practicing in Bolton who had served them for twelve years, to their lodge meeting. They gave Johnston an illuminated address. Several men praised Johnston, who responded in suitably humble fashion. The Oddfellows were pleased with Johnston's long service, but more especially they were pleased that, though many of them had fallen sick in the 1890–91 influenza epidemic, all had recovered, which they attributed to Johnston's "kindness of heart and faithful attention." Johnston recorded his impressions of the event in his diary. He was proud of the honor and moved by the sentiments expressed by the workingmen Oddfellows. More especially, he was struck by the uniqueness of the event: "it is a most unusual thing for a Dr to receive a testimonial from one of his clubs. Nay more[,] it is the first time I have ever heard of it[,] for the relations of clubs & their Drs are seldom so friendly as to suggest such a thing."[24]

More commonplace in the minutes is the record of a second mode of behavior. In the privacy of their meeting hall, in meetings where the doctor was not present, friendly society members sometimes spoke harshly of their doctors. Prompted by what they saw as a failing on the doctor's part, usually his neglect to visit sick members often enough, the members challenged their doctor. Although nineteenth-century doctors sometimes wrote or spoke disparagingly about the skills of fellow practitioners, friendly society members rarely challenged their doctor's skill. Indeed, the

24. Johnston Papers, ZJO/1/14. The first quote is from the *Bolton Evening News,* Sept. 8, 1891, a clipping of which Johnston pasted in his diary, and the second from the diary itself.

charge that a doctor did not attend often enough can be taken as testimony to the efficacy that workingmen associated with medical attendance. Instead, friendly society men challenged their doctor's commitment to their good health. The doctor who did not attend members often enough seemed to disdain them as a class of patients. Though exact words are seldom detailed, the minutes leave no doubt that on such occasions harsh words were often spoken. After one member complained, others often remembered earlier signs of inattention in their own experience and retailed stories they had heard from men not present. A single incident often quickly became described as a pattern of neglect. Members expected to be slighted, and they readily became heated about slights. Emboldened by the secrecy and solidarity of club meetings, members challenged their doctors in a way they did not do face to face.[25]

Much of the aggrievement on the part of friendly society members and their doctors sprang from fundamental disagreement over what medical services were worth. Regularly and repeatedly medical men sought to inflate the value of their services, and just as regularly workingmen and their agents undervalued medical services. Another side of this conflict, discussed above, is illustrated by an exchange in the *Foresters' Miscellany* in 1884 between the AOF official T. Ballan Stead and the long-winded J. Maunsell, a physician and fellow Forester.[26] Stead acknowledged this fundamental difference of opinion about the value of medical services and addressed himself not to resolving it but to finding additional ways for the friendly societies to economize on the cost of medical services. Could drugs be obtained more cheaply if the clubs bought in bulk by forming medical aid associations, which would employ a doctor and stock a dispensary? Could such associations economize further on other overheads? In any case, the medical aid associations constituted only one means by which working people might, through collaboration, assist themselves. Stead urged the formation of friendly society convalescent homes and proposed a vague plan for friendly society collaboration in providing nursing services.

Maunsell countered that the friendly society medical aid associations wanted too much for too little. They wanted "to get the [medical] work

---

25. However, some stories of insolent or aggressive behavior of workingmen to their doctors, especially when inebriated, appear in nineteenth-century memoirs. See, e.g., Mullin, *Story of a Toiler's Life,* 148–49, describing how working people treated a Welsh doctor for whom Mullin served briefly as locum tenens.

26. Stead, "New Era in Medical Aid"; Maunsell, "New Era of Medical Aid."

done too cheaply," to include subscribers who could afford to pay as private patients, and to bind doctors in ways that undermined ambition and good care. Before the medical aid associations existed, Maunsell claimed, the doctors of a community could expect payments averaging one pound per person per year from the people who subsequently joined the associations. Once in the associations, however, they got only a fraction of that. Moreover, the associations expected their medical men to attend too many patients. No one could, in Maunsell's view, attend the sick among more than three thousand people, and then only if the three thousand lived within a radius of three miles. Since the medical aid associations demanded more than was reasonable, doctors would have to react in some way. Perhaps, Maunsell suggested slyly, they would deny medical aid association subscribers services at the hospitals the doctors controlled, though of course the "traditions of the medical profession do not permit" such steps.[27]

No number of exchanges could resolve the question of the proper value of medical services. In addition, neither doctors nor friendly societies were willing to allow the competitive forces of the market to settle the issue, as they both showed by forming combinations in restraint of trade.

COMPLAINTS ABOUT DOCTORS

Only a few sickness claims prompted disputes about their validity. Even fewer claims led to questions about the quality of medical service rendered. At first glance, nineteenth-century workingmen, like their twentieth-century counterparts in the populace at large and like the nineteenth-century recipients of poor law medical relief,[28] seem to have been content with the medical services they gained by belonging to friendly societies, as workingmen seem also to have been content with the medical attendance they received in other circumstances.

One gauge of apparent approval derives from the patients comment book kept at the Ashton District Infirmary in Ashton-under-Lyne between October 21, 1906, and August 14, 1909. Most Ashton patients entered because of injuries, and most stayed four weeks or longer. At their depar-

27. See also Elizabeth Edwards's discussion of tension in Cambridge after formation of a medical aid association, in *Friendly Societies*, 481–82.
28. Klein, *Complaints against Doctors*, esp. 106; Hodgkinson, *Origins of the National Health Service*, 133–36.

ture infirmary authorities recorded patients' names with diagnoses and their response to two questions: "Were you satisfied with the Treatment? Have you any Complaints to make?"

The answers must have been gratifying. Of 1,830 responses to the first question, only four patients indicated they were dissatisfied. Although nothing can be said about the opinions of patients who died, those who recovered or left to convalesce believed that the physicians, surgeons, and other practitioners of the Ashton Infirmary almost never provided unsatisfactory treatments. Their expressed rate of dissatisfaction was higher than the rate of formal complaints under the National Health Service around 1970, at nine complaints per million patients. But both are remarkable for the degree to which they suggest that patients were content with the medical services they received early in the century and have remained content.[29]

A higher proportion of Ashton Infirmary patients had some complaint, however. Of 1,817 responses to the second question, thirty patients voiced complaints, and a further forty-two said that they had no complaints but then mentioned something that had troubled them. If only the thirty are counted, the rate of complaints comes to 1.7 percent; if the forty-two are added, the rate is nearly 4 percent. Male patients did most of the complaining, and they complained chiefly about the nurses and the food. Arthur Beaumont said he had no complaints to make but added, in the words of the person who kept the register, that "some of the Nurses could be very haughty & unless men were most deferential they were often neglected. Several times he had known patients ask for the bed pan or bottle twenty or thirty minutes before it was given to them & often they wd. be in distress." Harry Brown believed the meals "short of butter," and Thomas Brown found the potatoes "quite cold 2 or 3 times" and was "short of bread once or twice, [but there was] plenty of butter." Nurse Worthington annoyed several patients. Thomas Hyde believed she wanted "to do too much 'ordering'," Anne Lees found her "too sarcastic," and Sarah Madden thought her "too 'snappy' & overbearing." Like the doctors, the nurses gave satisfactory medical care. But sometimes they were impatient. A few patients also complained that they were being released too early or

29. See Klein, *Complaints against Doctors,* 32, 104–6, showing that formal complaints have never been numerous under the NHS. However, Klein estimates the rate as a proportion of patients on doctors' lists, whereas the Ashton Infirmary rate is based on complaints per patients treated.

had, for personal reasons, to leave before they had recovered fully. Others remarked that they wished they had entered the infirmary earlier.[30]

In the friendly society records, too, complaints about the quality of medical care were seldom made.[31] To all appearances working people rarely told their doctors that they were unhappy with their medical skills. Other doctors may have shared the reservations about practice that J. A. N. Longley recorded in his diary. In 1902 Longley wrote of his dispensary practice, "the poor do not interest me very much." He fretted about "losing one's interest in cases, not taking the trouble to make a diagnosis, but just giving a 'bottle.'" Later entries in his diary suggest that Longley gave in to his lack of interest in treatment, for they consist chiefly of a record of his interests outside medicine.[32] The public record about how working-class people felt about the medical attention they received suggests that they were either unaware of or untroubled by such reservations.

However, in the privacy of their lodge meetings, as we have seen, friendly society members complained more often and more freely. Sufficiently roused, they appointed one of their officers, or a committee, to get in touch with the doctor by writing or visit, confronting him with the stories and charges against him.[33] Fairness required that the doctor be given a chance to explain or to defend himself. On January 6, 1892, three members of a Foresters court in St. Andrews complained of their treatment at the hands of the court surgeon, D. Hamilton Thyle. The members resolved to have the secretary write Thyle setting forth the complaints. At the next meeting, on January 20, Thyle responded, asking to present his side of the matter and stating that he was not aware of having given any cause for complaint. Now calmer and more timid, the members instructed the secretary to write again to the effect that the court had reviewed the complaints, would take no further action, and regretted having troubled him. In future, they hoped, the surgeon would attend members at any hour, insofar as possible.[34]

In most cases the confrontation was enough, and later minutes imply

30. Ashton District Infirmary Archives, patients' comment book, DDH/1/133.
31. In Klein's study of the NHS, formal complaints are dwarfed by informal complaints, as estimated by the clerks of executive councils. However, that rate, too, is modest. See Klein, *Complaints against Doctors*, 106.
32. Longley papers, 35694/1–8.
33. See, e. g., AOF, Court of Three Mary's papers, minutes, TU:97/1, July 9–Sept. 29, 1860; High Pavement Chapel Provident Friendly Society papers, HiF 2, minutes, passim, 1872 ff.
34. AOF, Court Ancient City papers, 37,204, minutes, Jan. 6, 1892–Jan. 20, 1892.

that it usually occurred after the heat of the accusatory meeting had passed. On May 10, 1881, when the members of Loyal Fane Lodge suspected that their treasurer had converted money owed the doctor to his own use, they called a special meeting on the same day. But clubs accusing doctors of being inattentive or of other failings regularly let days or weeks pass between the accusations and the confrontation.[35] In most cases doctors accused of neglect in the meeting hall continued in service, although sometimes it is not clear whether that was because members were persuaded by the doctor's response or because they preferred not to press the matter. If on the financial side the friendly societies long had bargaining power over their doctors, on the social and rhetorical sides they were at a disadvantage. The doctor's knowledge of medicine outweighed, in the scale of their values, their own occupational expertise, and the doctor's superior social standing required a timid and usually submissive respect for him.[36]

As employers the friendly societies could not behave toward their doctors as abruptly as the poor law guardians often did. Nor did they exact terms as niggardly as those paid for poor law medical relief. Perhaps the inferior social status of the club members aided the doctor in negotiating his pay, compared at least with what transpired between doctors and guardians. But it seems more likely that the clubs paid more for medical care per case and per week of sickness because they wanted to distinguish themselves from paupers and because they could afford to do so.

Doctors may have complained as often about their patients as patients did about doctors, but the comparison cannot be made on the same terms because of the want of sources analogous to friendly society minutes. The Bolton general practitioner John Johnston, nevertheless, recorded two stories that show how patients, and fellow doctors, peeved him. In one, the patient's error was impatience. Mrs. C. fell getting out of bed and believed she had broken her leg. Away when the call came, Johnston was represented by his locum tenens, who decided that her leg was not broken. Rather than wait for Johnston and call him again, Mrs. C. summoned another doctor, who declared the leg broken and ordered a course of treatment that lasted fifteen weeks. During that treatment Mrs C. decided

35. Loyal Fane Friendly Society papers, Loyal Fane II/1, minutes, May 10, 1881.
36. On the social pretensions of medical men and their efforts to improve their social standing, see Peterson, *Medical Profession in Mid-Victorian London*, esp. 194–206. Whereas Peterson emphasizes the inferior position of medical men compared to elites, friendly society sources emphasize their superior status compared to working people.

the leg had not actually been broken, blamed her substitute doctor for the leg ulcer that had formed under her bandages, and refused to pay his bill.[37]

In another story the patient's error was duplicity. A patient under another doctor's care summoned Johnston after assuring him that the other doctor had been told not to call again. Johnston treated the patient up to his or her death, after which he learned that he and the other doctor had both been attending. Johnston was upset, perhaps because the patient had lied to him or because he feared invidious comparisons between the two programs of treatment but more probably because he regarded consulting two doctors as a breach of medical ethics.

Friendly societies elected their doctors, meaning literally that they held votes among competing aspirants. Repeatedly in the 1860s and 1870s one lodge of Lancashire Oddfellows changed surgeons, voting each six months and choosing among as many as four candidates, even though the lodge paid no more than two shillings a member per year for attendance.[38] When their current surgeon died or resigned, Oddfellows in Durham voted in 1882 among five aspirants, and in 1909 among six.[39] Other lodges and courts used a more complicated system of election, in which members voted both for and against candidates. In 1869 the Kempston Friendly Society elected Frederick Beechey as surgeon. Beechey won by gaining forty-two positive votes to twenty-four negative, whereas his opponent, Robinson, had twenty-seven positive votes and forty-one negative.[40] Doctors submitted to demands for rebates, the scrutiny of their services by friendly society officers, the complaints of members disappointed either by the doctor's failure to attend or to cure, the scrutiny of their medical judgments by laypeople, and to much more.

The surgeon Griffith Roberts rushed to join the St. Asaph Foresters in North Wales in 1862, evidently hoping to be named court surgeon and to earn the £3 10s. a year the court paid for medical attendance. But his brothers elected Llewelyn Lodge.[41] Lodge soon wanted more money, and the court refused, accepting his resignation and electing Brother Roberts, who served until 1876. The minutes do not reveal what was said about Dr. Lodge at the meeting on June 25, 1864. Whatever was said so troubled the

37. Johnston Papers, ZJO/3/4.
38. IOOF, Pleasant Retreat Lodge papers, DDX433\2, minutes, 1856–76.
39. IOOF, Loyal Star of the North Lodge papers, D/IOO/1, Nov. 13, 1882, and D/IOO/3, Dec. 30, 1909.
40. Kempston Friendly Society papers, DDX157/1, minutes, Apr. 16, 1869.
41. AOF, Court Loyal Bodelwyddan papers, D/DM/510/2, Jan. 20, 1862, and following entries.

members that they required everyone present to sign a statement agreeing not to tell Dr. Lodge what had been said about him. Lodge's complaint is not difficult to understand. He and his successor earned an annual sum equivalent to 2s. 6d. per member.

Roberts moved to Denbigh in 1875 but continued to hold surgery hours in St. Asaph. The St. Asaph Foresters considered replacing him but were satisfied when Roberts joined them at a meeting and promised both to attend members in St. Asaph two days a week and, at his own expense, to find a practitioner to attend members in cases of emergency. Nevertheless, a year's trial persuaded court members to ask for Roberts's resignation, on grounds that he could not attend them satisfactorily at such a distance. A proposal to reelect Lodge lost, and the court chose Dr. Browne, who served for four years, until late 1880, when he moved out of the neighborhood. The court then voted on whether to rehire Lodge or Roberts, thirteen members voting for Roberts, eleven for Lodge, and two declining to vote. The winner, Roberts, resumed attending members on regular visits to St. Asaph but by 1884 decided that he no longer wished to pay for renting a consulting room there, proposing instead that members write to him to arrange a visit or, in emergencies, send a telegram or take the train to Denbigh. That further deterioration in service persuaded the St. Asaph Foresters to dismiss Roberts again in 1885 and, after twenty-three years, to amend their rules to allow payment of more than 2s. 6d. a member per year.

The surgeons Lodge, Browne, and Roberts did not wish either to give up the friendly society business or to submit to the financial terms the Foresters (and other societies) required. Their lack of independence is as apparent in their long submission to the Foresters' ceiling fee as it is also in the extra steps they took to persuade the Foresters to retain their services. Court officials did not have to call on the surgeon; he came to their meetings in order to make his case. But at the same time, the court refused to pay enough to secure the kind of attendance wanted. Most of the members wanted Roberts, but Roberts evidently could not make enough money in St. Asaph, so the Foresters had to be content with a part-time and absentee doctor and, ultimately, with appointments arranged by postcard. Llewelyn Lodge remained available to them in St. Asaph, but most members preferred part-time attendance by Roberts. Even at the niggardly fees they paid for medical attendance, St. Asaph Foresters could be choosy about the doctor they engaged.

Members of the Leicester Bond Street Friendly Society complained in

1876 that their surgeon, Mr. Clarke, had shortchanged them in medicines and attendance. Even though Clarke was an officer in the club and not merely its employee, a committee of investigation was appointed, and Clarke was asked to explain himself. The committee found his explanation unsatisfactory and proposed to raise the issue at the annual meeting, which would be attended by most members. The minutes fail to show the outcome of this dispute, but they do reveal that this club joined a medical aid association later in 1876. Apparently Clarke was not dismissed but was instead replaced by the doctors working for the medical aid association.[42]

In June 1887 the widow of Thomas Merridale met with her late husband's friendly society colleagues in Eversholt to tell them that the club's doctor, Hawkins, had not attended her husband once in the six weeks' illness preceding his death, although he was repeatedly asked to visit. The members adopted a unanimous resolution of astonishment, called a special meeting for the following week to consider dismissing Hawkins, and entertained a suggestion that Dr. Lucas of Woburn be appointed Hawkins's successor. At the special meeting the members voted to dismiss Hawkins and to notify him that he was being let go because he would not visit the members at their homes. Among three contenders to succeed him, the club chose Dr. Lucas of Woburn, who accepted on the same terms as his predecessor: 5s. per member per year, the doctor visiting all members unable to go to his surgery.[43]

In January 1885, G. M. Crackwell complained to his brethren in a Cambridgeshire Oddfellows lodge about the care their surgeon, R. Ceeley, was giving R. Brett. Brett needed to be visited more than once a week, and lodge members asked their delegate to the surgeon to speak to Ceeley. The same complaint was repeated in February, when Ceeley was accused of neglect. Nine days had passed between visits. Brett wanted to report Ceeley to the lodge's Medical Aid Committee. Though asked to visit Brett, long sick and recently worse off, twice a week, Ceeley did not do so. He wrote to the lodge informing them that his visits did not need to be more frequent as, in the wording of the minutes, "he could not do him any good."[44] Brett died on March 7. To his friends and lodge brothers, it must have seemed that more attentive care from Dr. Ceeley would have pro-

42. Leicester Bond Street Friendly Society papers, DE1884/1, minutes, Mar. 14–June 8, 1876.
43. Eversholt Friendly Society papers, X783/1/1, minutes, June 6–June 27, 1887. For a similar case, although with fewer details, see IOOF, Loyal Star of the North Lodge papers, D/IOO/1, minutes, Oct. 5–Dec. 21, 1875.
44. IOOF, Loyal Merton Hall Lodge papers, R78/70, minutes, Jan. 5–Mar. 16, 1885.

longed Brett's life or at least made him more comfortable in his last sickness. But the lodge lacked either the moral or the contractual authority to compel its surgeon to attend on terms set by a member.

The lodge meeting was a place to relieve frustrations about the real and imagined failures of club doctors. There, members spoke freely, even daringly, using private language they would not use in meetings where the doctor was present or in conversations with and letters to their doctors. But in the final analysis, their complaints do not appear to amount to anything approaching an indictment of doctors for poor treatment. Friendly society members were concerned at least as often about the intractable nature of bad health as they were about such specific failings on the part of their doctors as infrequent attendance or inadequate medication. Their anger and anguish subsided without leading to action against a doctor who could not make sick men well. When complaints can be studied in proportion to the number of sickness episodes, it is apparent that very few men thought themselves badly served by their doctors, or at least few thought so to the point of making an issue of the medical services they received.

If workingmen did not charge their medical men with poor treatment, still all was not well in their relationship with doctors. Friendly society sources, especially the minutes of private meetings, suggest not that workingmen believed they were receiving bad medical care but that they were sensitive to the possibility. They regarded medical men as capable of treating them as inferiors by giving less attention, weaker medications, or too little medicine. They were capable of being aggrieved. For a long time they were also capable of taking any strong sense of aggrievement out on the doctor, who was at once a social superior and an employee.

A LOSS OF NERVE

Two Bedford surgeons, Carter and Chillingworth, formed a partnership in 1884 and attended at least two friendly societies.[45] Carter beguiled the Bedford Oddfellows, playing up to their view of themselves,[46] but Chillingworth acted quite differently. Already in 1886 the men in one club instructed their secretary to reprimand him for his neglect of some mem-

45. IOOF, Maiden Queen Lodge papers, OF8/1, minutes, Oct. 23, 1888; IOOF, Kempston Friendly Society papers, DDX157/2, minutes, Apr. 13, 1883–May 7, 1886.
46. See above, this chapter.

bers and for the second time adopted a resolution requiring medical certification of sickness at least every two weeks. Nevertheless, in 1887 they reelected Carter and Chillingworth as medical officers. In 1888 the Bedford Oddfellows demanded an explanation of unspecified misconduct by Chillingworth and entertained a complaint of neglect. The Kempston club found cause again in 1889 to be dissatisfied, the surgeons having failed to visit a member during his recent sickness. But their earlier aggressiveness had disappeared. In place of a reprimand they settled for a timid letter calling the surgeons' attention to this case.

In the last decade of the nineteenth century, friendly society sources show, the spirit of independence that had for so long characterized sick clubs in their dealings with social superiors collapsed.[47] Independence gave way to failing nerve and an unwillingness any longer to challenge superiors. Standish Meacham argues that, around 1890, strife replaced cooperation and harmony in the relations of the working class to the larger society.[48] Membership in labor unions rose sharply in the first decade of the twentieth century, a period in which real wages briefly declined, and strikes became more numerous. But the testimony from friendly society minutes, in which working people describe their contacts with social superiors, suggests the opposite course. It relates a shift away from the self-confident assertiveness of mid-century toward timidity. The minutes show another aspect of the submissiveness that Stephen Yeo noticed in studying the comments of friendly society leaders and the interpretation of those comments by historians. As Yeo remarked, the societies seemed to stand for the independence and commitment to self-help of working people when the future held a growing assumption of welfare responsibilities by the state.[49] The minutes, a source for grassroots sentiment, show not a last stand in favor of self-help, which friendly society leaders made in negotiations over the National Insurance Act of 1911, but a loss of nerve before superior authority that began two decades earlier. The members were prescient.

Previously, friendly society members had defied surgeons who failed to provide attendance they deemed satisfactory as readily as they had stood up to government officials who sought to direct local friendly society activities, national officers and actuaries who wished to give them advice,

47. See especially Tholfsen, *Working-Class Radicalism*, 246–57, 288–305, for an elaboration of working-class subculture and the friendly societies' part in its expression.
48. Meacham, *A Life Apart*, passim, esp. 213–17.
49. Yeo, "Working-Class Association, Private Capital, Welfare, and the State."

or members who violated club rules and wanted to escape punishment.[50] Across Britain clubs summoned their doctors to defend themselves against charges that they had failed to carry out their duties and dismissed doctors whose services they deemed inadequate. Doctors were the social superiors of most friendly society members, and they knew things the brothers did not.[51] Even so, they were still tradesmen, capable of giving inadequate service and subject to dismissal for that. At the end of the century much of this defiant spirit, this insistence not only on remaining in charge of their own affairs but also of appraising those outsiders who sought to advise or direct them, disappeared.

Kempston Friendly Society members long refused to submit the club's accounts for valuation by an actuary. In 1855 they rejected a warning from John Tidd Pratt, Registrar General of Friendly Societies, that their club was in deficit, refusing by a vote of forty-six to sixteen either to reduce benefits or to raise premiums. Later, they increased benefits against the advice of Vicar Williams, who served as treasurer, even defying Williams and forcing him to resign in 1875 when he threatened to appeal to the law courts in order to force the members to accept his advice.[52] The members were mostly agricultural laborers; many could not sign their own names. But they had enough confidence in their own judgment to stand up to their so-called betters. By the 1890s much of that confidence had been lost.

Kempston Friendly Society members finally gave in on the controversial matter of the valuation of their assets in 1896 and reduced benefits for older members when the valuation showed a deficit of £2,601. As recently as 1887 they had allowed another treasurer to resign rather than lower benefits. In 1901 they were told that, despite excessive recent sickness claims and inadequate changes in their benefit rules, their deficit amounted to no more than £372. Even so they did not reverse their earlier decision or reassert their obviously accurate sense that the actuaries had misstated the magnitude of their problem.[53] In 1892, the nearby Abthorpe Foresters submitted to their actuary's advice, suspending benefits for members who had been sick for lengthy periods.

During the 1890s, to a greater degree than at any previous time, friendly

50. On independence among members of friendly societies in Kentish London, see Crossick, *Artisan Elite,* 192–98.

51. In explaining the rising prestige of medical men, Peterson, *Medical Profession,* 3–4 and passim, stresses social factors over the efficacy of medicine.

52. Kempston Friendly Society papers, DDX157/1, minutes, May 28 and Dec. 13, 1855, Dec. 8, 1875.

53. Ibid., DDX157/2, May 1, 1896, and Sept. 27, 1901.

society actuaries claimed control over finance. In place of the defiant attitude so often evident in earlier years, when societies had rejected the advice
of their actuaries and refused to listen to explanations about how assets
were valued, appeared a submissive attitude. As late as 1893 members of
the Leicester Bond Street Friendly Society refused to allow actuaries to
value its assets. But repeatedly in the years that followed they submitted
to the opinion of the actuaries, turning back proposals from members to
share out surplus assets or to elevate benefits.[54] Paradoxically, when the
societies had most often lacked the assets required to meet their commit-
ments, in the mid-nineteenth century, they had been the most inclined to
reject advice. But when their positions were more secure, as they were by
the 1890s, they were the likeliest to accept the cautious advice of their
actuaries. As explained below,[55] the quality of the advice the actuaries
gave remained flawed throughout, judged with the advantage of hindsight.
They regularly undervalued assets by adopting estimates of future earnings and claims that were too pessimistic.

The experience of Court Powis, in Welshpool, illustrates this loss of
nerve. In a conflict with the AOF executive council about what was necessary to gain financial stability, court members at first openly defied their
national officers. When that failed they turned to subterfuge, and then to
submission. Until the 1890s this court insisted on collecting flat premiums
rather than premiums graduated according to the member's age at entry,
which would have led to higher payments for sick benefits and which many
other courts had adopted as early as the 1850s. AOF officials warned that
practices of this sort were responsible for the court's poor financial position, revealed at regular valuations by actuaries, and urged the court to
alter its rules. A long discussion of these issues at a meeting on December
15, 1895, produced no decision. Unruly members disrupted the meeting,
preventing a vote being taken. A few months later, when the court's actuary suggested he would be willing to travel to Welshpool to explain how
the financial position could be improved, members asked him instead to
write and thereby save them the cost of his journey.

Their later actions reveal that it was not just a spirit of economy but also
a desire to evade the issue that motivated them. In July 1897 the court's
management committee, charged with a preliminary review of business,
agreed to submit to the wishes of the AOF executive council and recom-

54. E. g., Leicester Bond Street Friendly Society papers, DE1884/2, minutes, Feb. 10,
1921.
55. See chapter 5.

mended that action to the entire court. In a meeting at the month's end the court appeared to agree, adopting by unanimous vote the council's appeal to implement a schedule of graduated premiums. But the vote concealed the court's real action, for a graduated schedule was not implemented. The AOF suspended Court Powis in 1898. For another year court members tried to temporize, pleading that they did not understand the executive council's reasoning and arguing that their own financial position had improved to the point at which, according to their actuary, assets totaled nearly 96 percent of liabilities. But in 1899 the court gave in, asking the actuary to draw up a schedule of graduated premiums and adopting new rules. Whereas in earlier decades AOF courts had often defied the executive council, even to the point of breaking off from the order, by the end of the century they had grown timid.[56]

Complaints about neglect by medical officers continue to appear in the minutes of friendly society meetings in the 1890s and thereafter. But they were much less likely to be followed by action, even to the extent of passing the complaint along to the attending doctor. In 1882 the Kempston club secretary wrote to Dr. Adams about complaints from members and got a reply: Adams wrote that he was not aware of any negligence on his part, but he also admitted to occasional oversights. Again in 1883 they charged Adams and Carter with failing to visit a sick member, James Keep, even though Adams had been in the neighborhood, and they threatened to engage another doctor. Carter then met with the club and explained to the members' satisfaction why he and his partner had not attended Keep.[57]

But two decades later attitudes had changed. In May 1903, Arthur Ashpole reported that the surgeon had failed to attend his children when sent for, and other members at the meeting added their own complaints. The club's management committee investigated and discovered that the surgeon's duties were nowhere specified. Rather than complain about neglect, as they had done so willingly in the past, members asked the surgeons to state what services they were prepared to offer for the five shillings that members and family members wanting medical attendance paid each year. The surgeons answered that they would see patients able to attend the dispensary in Kempston on Tuesday and Friday mornings at 11:45 or in Bedford any weekday from 9 to 10 A.M. Patients too ill to attend should send their dispensary cards to the Kempston surgery before

56. AOF, Court Powis papers, minutes, Dec. 15, 1894–Sept. 21, 1899.
57. Kempston Friendly Society papers, DDX157/3, management committee minutes, May 17, 1882, June 29, 1883.

11:45 on Tuesday and Fridays or otherwise to Bedford. The management committee accepted this minimal specification as sufficient and did not pursue the members' complaints.

The friendly societies retained enough of a bargaining advantage to hold medical costs down. But they had lost their moral advantage, which had allowed them to hold medical practitioners to their own sense of the services the doctors would furnish. Increasingly, attending doctors scaled down their services, limiting contacts to visits to their surgeries by erecting rules about contact in the patient's home that were unrealistic, given either the difficulty many of the seriously sick would have in making their way to a surgery or the conflict between emergency medical problems, which might arise at any point, and the limited hours of service in the surgery. Members of an Oddfellows lodge in Lincolnshire seemed both surprised and delighted when their surgeon agreed in 1907 to back down from an attempt to charge separately for anesthesia in operations.[58] In 1905, when Joseph Hewison, of the Loyal Steam Plough Lodge of the Oddfellows in Lincolnshire, complained that the lodge surgeon had refused to attend him or to give him medicines, the lodge answered by refunding Hewison what he had paid in for medical attendance.[59]

In earlier years it is possible to find in the minutes examples of generosity of spirit on the part of doctors attending friendly society members, the poor compensation they received notwithstanding. But from the 1890s forward such actions are rare; they had given way to officiousness, the attitude the doctors adopted when asked to describe their responsibilities, and, on the part of the friendly society members and local officers, to frustration concealed behind timidity.[60]

Until the 1890s the working people who belonged to friendly societies adopted an independent and sometimes insolent attitude toward their social betters. They cultivated an ideology of self-help that made them independent both of the threat of poverty and poor relief and of elites. The surest measure of this independent spirit lies in the frequency with which sick club members disregarded or rejected advice given to them by social lions, professionals, and experts, even by the leaders of the friendly society

58. IOOF, Loyal Steam Plough Lodge papers, minutes, Feb. 5–Mar. 5, 1907.
59. Ibid., Nov. 14, 1905.
60. But see AOF, Beaminster Branch papers, minutes, PC/BE:5/3, Jan. 26, 1897, a note of thanks from Dr. Spurr for the sympathetic manner of the toast to his health at the court's annual dinner, and Oct. 26, 1898, when court members gave Dr. Spurr a present on his marriage.

movement. But in the 1890s they lost their nerve. Long before the National Insurance Act of 1911, which has so often been identified as the first serious blow to self-help and to the friendly societies, the men who belonged to sick clubs began to yield to advice and direction they had formerly resisted. Why they did this the minutes and other sources do not reveal. What these sources do show is that, with comparative suddenness, workingmen began to submit. Thus, the minutes stand at odds with other sources in what they reveal. Relying on evidence given chiefly by the people honored, or by their peers, Geoffrey Crossick has shown that clergymen, doctors, and lawyers were honored community leaders.[61] That is undoubtedly true. Their status and position were acknowledged by working people. But the friendly society minutes suggest that, within their own part of the community, working people did not dwell on the honor or importance of social elites. Until the 1890s, but much less so thereafter, they dwelt instead on their own capacity to handle their affairs.

One aspect is common in all these manifestations of the loss of nerve. Friendly society members bowed in the 1890s and thereafter before people who possessed specialized and arcane knowledge, especially the knowledge of medicine and actuarial science. What may have changed was not their view of their social superiors but their appreciation of the power of specialized knowledge. Anne Digby emphasizes the real gains doctors made in the last part of the century in the efficacy of their drugs and therapies and in the authority they commanded.[62] In the 1870s and 1880s actuaries drew more and more clubs into regular quinquennial valuations, arcane demonstrations of their putative skill at forecasting future financial demands on a club. But these things were under way for two decades before friendly society members changed their posture, so that they are partial explanations at best.

Nor is an explanation apparent in the characteristics of the clubs themselves. In their rate of growth, the occupational composition of their members, and other respects, the clubs maintained during the 1890s trends that had been under way earlier. It is true that they withdrew more into themselves. They organized fewer public processions in the last years of the nineteenth century. They also found the members less eager to attend annual banquets and club meetings. The fraternal qualities of the friendly society movement lost some force. Decades earlier the men and women

61. Crossick, *Artisan Elite*, 88–104.
62. Digby, *Making a Medical Market*, 100.

who belonged to sick clubs had shed initiation rites and cultivated their spirit of community in meetings, banquets, and processions. In the 1890s those things too were withering, so that there was less enthusiasm for the community and the movement, although still as much for its insurance. The societies continued to gain members into the new century. But in the 1890s they became more introspective. The loss of nerve evident in friendly society dealings with doctors, actuaries, and others may signal waning confidence in the capacity of working people to make secure judgments. But it may also signal merely that the regulars and officers in local clubs no longer had behind them the support, or even the active participation, of the members, so that the officers felt obliged to behave more timidly.

The issue of the quality of medical care has come up in each of the last three chapters, and this is a good point to draw together the strong hints and suggestions that emerge from medical and friendly society sources. For doctors, and sometimes also for historians, the issue of quality is taken to focus on the choice of doctors rather than on the number of medical contacts, medications, or other quantitative indicators. Friendly society members did not fret about choice, except as regards cost. Choice first emerged as a key issue in the case doctors made about how the new system of national insurance should be structured rather than in demands from patients. The club members were willing to use every doctor in a community successively, or all at any given time to attend only a single doctor chosen by majority vote, as long as the price was right. Perhaps friendly society members were unable to judge doctors on the quality of care they gave. Or perhaps nineteenth-century doctors only imagined that substantial differences existed among them in the quality of care they gave. Until some evidence can be produced that bears directly on the question whether, in the main, some doctors were much better than others, it will not be possible to decide who was deceived.

Working people suspected doctors would shortchange them, and in the friendly societies and medical aid associations they stood watch against this threat. Doctors desperately wanted higher incomes, consonant with the social status to which they aspired. But they were too numerous in nineteenth-century Britain to be able to negotiate better pay. They were, however, willing to imply that the care they gave might be inferior. Like working people, they tried to use the rhetoric of inferior care.

In friendly societies and medical aid associations, working people set the terms not only of payment but also of attendance. Doctors had to see their contract patients often, even in the patients' own homes, and furnish the large number of medicaments that these patients wanted. However tempting it was to shortchange these patients, doctors could not afford to do so because the friendly societies maintained an effective system of surveillance. In the end, therefore, the way that workingmen used the threat of inferior care trumped the doctors' use of it, because, in relative terms, patients were in shorter supply than doctors.

Further evidence about whether friendly society members received good medical care will emerge in part 2. There it will be shown that, to an increasing degree, these men survived their sicknesses for longer periods of time. And there the case will be made that access to doctors, which friendly society members increasingly enjoyed, made a difference not in the prevention of sickness but in its management. Perhaps doctors did give better care to their private patients. But the care they gave friendly society contract patients was good enough to improve their health.

PART TWO

Sickness and Its Trends and Determinants

CHAPTER 5

Sickness: The Friendly
Society Definition

BEING SICK, as everyone can agree, is not the same thing as being well. But where is the line to be drawn? This is not a question that can be answered in unequivocal terms.[1] The friendly societies gave a succinct answer in their rules, but they gave the matter detailed consideration. A definition of sickness or wellness is, of course, a complex thing to provide, the more so when the issue of health is confounded by the question of insurance. Even so, the friendly society definition is not uncommonly complex. Any threshold, even one as simple as the line dividing the decision to complain about one's health to a loved one from the decision not to complain, is also complex because it bears on so many aspects of health and on so many issues that have little or nothing to do with health.

In the friendly societies sickness was any health condition that rendered a person unable to work. Wellness, therefore, was the ability to work. That, at least, is the explicit resolution of the problem, a resolution remarkable because it gave the friendly societies so few problems. In the minutes of meetings, where members deliberated about conflicts, there is scarcely any mention of disagreement about the definition of sickness or suggestion that this functional definition created problems. The men and women who belonged and the people who advised them, including doctors, felt confident about their ability to distinguish sickness from wellness, not because they had failed to notice that this was a problem but because they dealt with this issue so often that they saw its resolution clearly.

The confidence of friendly society members in their capacity to differentiate good health from poor health existed in part because, to an increasing

---

1. See the discussions at Johansson, "Health Transition"; Riley, "From a High Mortality Regime to a High Morbidity Regime"; and Johansson, "Measuring the Cultural Inflation of Morbidity."

degree as time passed, clubs turned the problem over to doctors. Members who deemed themselves sick called on the club doctor for confirmation. If the doctor agreed, he signed the club's certification form, giving a name and a date but, until the late nineteenth century, rarely a diagnosis.[2] No one could be considered sick without certification, but it was possible to be under treatment without missing work.

As Charles Hardwick pointed out in 1859, the friendly society definition of sickness did not coincide with the medical definition, because it contained the provision about inability to work.[3] Just as modern respondents to health surveys in Britain and elsewhere often distinguish between disease (the presence of biological disturbance) and illness (disease plus inability to function),[4] friendly society members distinguished between the person who needed medical care and the person who also needed time off from work. Thus, one could be sick but not sick enough to take time off from work, or one could be sick and unable to work, but one could not be considered sick without a third party's certification. Either the doctor, who made the decision in most local clubs, or the steward, or more typically both, had to agree that sickness existed.

Friendly society members pioneered a distinction made in modern sociology. Sickness existed when it was acknowledged by others rather than only by the sick person.[5] This specification of sickness anticipated many elements of the description that Talcott Parsons gave in inaugurating the modern effort to understand sickness behavior. Parsons portrayed illness as partly biological and partly social in definition. Like most friendly society members, he believed also that physicians legitimize illness, which is therefore a type of behavior rather than a biological condition, and,

2. No evidence was uncovered about the proportion of men who presented as sick but failed to obtain the doctor's certification.

3. Hardwick, *History, Present Position, and Social Importance of Friendly Societies,* 70–71.

4. Calnan, *Health and Illness,* 134. More often, medical sociologists distinguish three categories: disease is a biological or physiological malfunction, illness is an individual's awareness of malfunction, and sickness is the social role appropriate to malfunction. See Susser, Watson, and Hopper, *Sociology in Medicine,* 16. In those terms, the use of the term *sickness* by friendly society members was quite appropriate. Some sociologists continue this discussion by emphasizing the ambiguity of ill health, defined in these various ways. For example, Turner, *Medical Power and Social Knowledge,* 11, 14–15, points to repetitive-strain injury and anorexia nervosa as cases of malfunctions that are difficult to pin down. Most examples of sickness ambiguity focus on conditions such as these, which defy ready medical specification, rather than on the commonplace ailments within the experience of friendly society members.

5. Twaddle, *Sickness Behavior and the Sick Role,* 18, gives the sociological point of view.

further, that the sick, in order to get well, need to seek competent help and to cooperate with the helper.[6]

In further anticipation of Parsons and modern social theory, the friendly societies promoted a functional definition of sickness as opposed both to a medical definition, which stresses the presence of disease, and to what is often called an experiential definition. Like working people in the second half of the twentieth century, who usually define sickness as the inability to function as usual,[7] sick club members focused neither on the physiological aspects of poor health (the medical model) nor on aspects related to their individual development (the experiential model). As proletarians standing at the epicenter of industrial capitalism, how could nineteenth-century working people have avoided a definition that stressed the individual's ability to fulfill economic tasks set by employers and, in the larger frame, serve the needs of a capitalist society? But friendly society functionalism emerged before industrial capitalism. Inability to work was the definition given to sickness in the eighteenth century, when the friendly society movement first flourished in Britain. That is not proof of working-class independence, much less of a community of interest between workers and employers in the preindustrial world. Instead, it is a further sign, along with the very existence of insurance against wages lost to sickness, of the workers' keen focus on *wage* labor and the maintenance of its income stream.

In this form, friendly society functionalism allows working people to be seen to have anticipated many of the needs of the modern business firm well in advance of the emergence of such firms. Working-class householders organized their own risk sharing in mutual insurance at a time when the only widespread form of insurance already in existence covered shipping losses. They used mutual insurance to guard themselves against interruptions in their flow of income long before any other organized institutions in society had found a similar means of protecting themselves. Thus, the friendly society definition of sickness points up another way in which this movement represented a singular, original, and intricate working-class solution to working-class problems.

Friendly societies also created a group culture which, on the surface, was a culture of fraternity and mutual aid. In reality, that system of beliefs and practices had as much to do with formulating rules about sickness and

6. Parsons, *Social System*, 431, 436–37.
7. Calnan, *Health and Illness*, 27.

wellness as with promoting brotherhood or working-class solidarity. Men, and later women and children, who joined friendly societies learned new friendly society rules about distinguishing sickness from wellness. The aim here is to reconstruct those rules, examining them in the light of how they may be supposed to have made friendly society members act differently from other people.

By drafting rules to specify sickness and wellness, the friendly societies made obvious the need to consider the various possible meanings of sickness and the deceptions, witting and unwitting, in which people may engage. Their close scrutiny of this issue provides evidence where it is usually lacking about the complex aspects of definition and differentiation. The friendly societies tried with some considerable success to understand how their own definitions differed from those applied by other people, especially doctors. In the process, they call attention to the modest degree to which we who experience and study sickness have managed to understand the way in which that experience is differentiated by the many groups that detect it. How do doctors decide when a patient is sick, and thereby worth attention and valid medicaments rather than placebos? How do family members decide? neighbors? employers and colleagues at work? How do nurses decide about degrees of sickness and deservedness of care among their patients? These are not questions that will be addressed here, but they are questions that acquire more specific form in the examination that the friendly societies gave sickness.

Two sources—rules and logic—have dominated previous reconstructions of differences between friendly society members and other people. The rules of friendly societies describe how they intended to operate, often in great detail.[8] Historians have turned to logic to interpret these intentions. For example, the rules show that doctors were employees of the friendly societies rather than of the individual members. Doctors were likely, therefore, to have been encouraged to favor the interests of the society, which benefited from an early return to work that reduced the drain on resources of a more protracted sickness.[9] In fact, the doctor's status depended on the friendly society. In the works clubs run by employers, the employer hired a doctor. Works club doctors may have followed the employer's wishes in deciding when men had recovered, and they are likely to have let medical judgments be influenced by the employer's view

8. See, e.g., *Rules of the Independent Order of Oddfellows.*
9. See, e.g., Hamilton, *Healers,* 226.

of work efficiency. In the two largest affiliated societies, the Foresters and the Oddfellows, the local clubs elected their doctors. Doctors were neither employees of individual members nor dependent on the national or even the local officers. Their tenure in the job depended on the goodwill of the members. As we have seen, the minutes of club meetings in which doctors were elected or discharged and where the terms of their service were discussed indicate that the members' view of a doctor was driven by concern about the attentiveness and cost of care rather than about the doctor's rigor or leniency in deciding when a member could return to work.[10]

INSURANCE AND SICKNESS

Costs and benefits affect how often people believe that their sicknesses warrant taking time off from work. In the Netherlands, for example, sickness absence rates have been much higher in recent years than in neighboring Belgium or Germany, at least in part because the Belgians and Germans require medical certification and enforce a waiting period before claims begin, whereas the Dutch do not.[11] As Rienk Prins shows in comparing absenteeism in the three countries, different rules about compensation result in different practices in making sickness claims. Hence no two bodies of information about sickness absence and claims should be compared without taking rules about compensation into account. In the present case, that has two implications. First, sickness absence rates from AOF members should not be compared with those of other groups in other times without a careful attempt to see how differences in rules affect practice. Second, AOF rates over time can be compared on the same terms to the degree that a similar system of costs and benefits remained in place.

Any community, even one unencumbered by insurance against wages lost during sickness, has in place rules that govern discrimination between wellness and sickness. In the workplace, it is often observed, people violate those rules, claiming to be sick when they need a good excuse to miss work. Such practices show up in heavy absenteeism on Mondays; the nineteenth-

---

10. See chapter 4. Appendix 1 reports the results of a test of the association between a court's assets and its sickness claims, which stand in for the doctor's certifications. Members entered slightly fewer claims as reserves accumulated—that is, reserves accumulated faster in courts with fewer claims. Doctors did not certify, and members did not make, more claims when the court was more prosperous. Neither members nor doctors give any appearance of allowing the court's financial well-being to influence their claims and certifications.

11. Prins, *Sickness Absence,* 201.

century British miners' notorious St. Monday, the first Monday after pay-day;[12] or the Mondays and Fridays that London schoolteachers missed early in the twentieth century.[13] The friendly societies avoided such claims by two means: they did not pay for only one or two days of sickness and they required certification of sickness, by a doctor or a club official. It is also true that sickness does not necessarily translate into days missed from work. Recent surveys show that even where comparatively generous bene-fits and easy access exist for sickness claims, such as in the Netherlands, people regard themselves as sick more of the time than they take off from work.[14] That, too, must have been true in the past, only more so because the benefits were not generous and the access not easy. Since both the scale of benefits and the ease of access to them affect the number of claims people will make, what matters here is to explore the terms of benefits and access and how those changed in the period under study. These issues are treated at length in appendix 1 in order that they may be summarized here.

For most working people, joining a friendly society meant gaining ac-cess for the first time to a formal system of benefits. This friendly society system was up and working decades before the Foresters began to publish statistics about sickness time in each court. Within the AOF, rules govern-ing ease of access to insurance benefits remained much the same across time, although as time passed more sick clubs specified that they meant to include mental ailments as well as injuries and diseases. Until the second decade of the twentieth century the benefits the societies paid kept pace with changes in wages, remaining close to 40 percent of wages at the lower end of the wage scale. In these and others ways, too, the friendly societies maintained a consistent set of standards, which means that the inducement to report sick remained much the same across the period under study. It was not altered in a major way until 1912, when the National Insurance Act went into effect. Until that year rates of sickness incidence and time responded to factors other than changes in the insurance scheme.

The friendly society system tended to discourage claims, compared to its modern counterparts. Not only were benefits rarely paid for short spells of sickness, but also they were typically cut in half after six months and reduced further after a year. New members also had to wait six months or a year before they became eligible for benefits. Everyone making a claim had to submit to the scrutiny of the club's sick steward or its doctor—usually

12. Benson, *British Coalminers in the Nineteenth Century,* 58.
13. Hart, "Investigation of Sickness Data," 361.
14. Prins, *Sickness Absence,* 188–89.

both. By these means—classical insurance techniques for discouraging claims—the men who set friendly society rules reduced the number and cost of claims the societies would otherwise have had to pay. Since the societies were owned and run by their members, the reason for adopting such a cautious system can be said to lie with the cost of insurance to the worker rather than the stinginess of employers.

Behavioral changes in making claims can confidently be associated with changes in inducements to make claims. Once a system of compensation is in place, further changes will be slight. Officials in the AOF and any other friendly society could expect members to behave differently from people who did not belong to friendly societies. But they had no reason to expect that people who joined would continue to modify their sickness behavior in ways that would have a substantial effect on sickness rates. Thus the AOF, like other friendly societies, confidently investigated past patterns of sickness among its members as a guide to future experience. Although the past was not an entirely accurate gauge of the future, it was accurate enough to allow the friendly societies to set premiums at rates that let them meet their quite substantial financial responsibilities.

THE SICK ROLE

Illness or sickness, that compound of disease or injury plus inability to work, authorized the friendly society member to behave differently. When the male member was well, he went to work, went out at night, visited the tavern and drank with his friends, attended club meetings, and in many other ways carried on ordinary activities. Sickness required another mode of behavior. In sickness, certainly in all but its convalescent stages, the same man was confined to his bed or at least to his house. Throughout the episode's course he did not go to work, nor did he find alternate work, tend his garden, or perform other physical tasks. He also did not socialize outside his house. Fellow members visited him at home, but there they did not drink with him, as they would have done meeting at a tavern when their colleague was well. He called on the club doctor or called the doctor to his home, heard the doctor's advice, and accepted the medications the doctor provided or prescribed.

These distinctive modes of behavior exhibit a twofold response to health problems. One part is medical. Rest, treatment by a doctor, and medications all promised recovery. Doctors and working people alike stressed the importance of early treatment, suggesting that they believed that the medical features of adopting a sick role had real efficacy for health. The other part represents a style of behavior devised by workingmen themselves. Its most obvious feature, already remarked, is the provision about staying away from taverns. When you were sick you did not see your friends at work or in the evenings, unless they called. You could not socialize or drink, which must have been a strong incentive to recover. Equally, sickness meant not merely staying away from work, which might be interpreted as blessing or punishment, but also forced and housebound inactivity.

All the manifest signs of sickness and wellness behavior among friendly society members deal with the situation after a sick role had been adopted. How the working man or woman decided that he or she was sick, and the stages through which these people passed between the first concern and the final decision to declare sickness, remain obscure. Although hospital records sometimes indicate that people deliberated before seeking admission to a hospital, there is nothing in the sick club sources consulted to suggest that working people waited to declare themselves sick. Their key decision was whether to stay away from work, or leave work, the first day. By the time friendly society support kicked in, usually, in the AOF, on the third day, the decision had already been made. In any case, it does not seem to have been problematic. In the minutes of club meetings examined, no member ever challenged another's decision to declare himself sick, although they did sometimes challenge the timing of recovery.

CLASS AND SICKNESS

Members of British elites in the nineteenth century sometimes viewed working people as shirkers, disinclined to work and unable to decide their own destiny in a reliable way. Lord Albemarle took the trouble at mid-century to advise friendly societies not to pay benefits during old age and to criticize members for meeting in public houses, drinking, and behaving boisterously.[15] In his eyes, giving shiftless people any incentive to miss work, such as sickness insurance or poor relief, provided them with all the more reason to do what they were prone to do in any case. This point of view promoted the more restrictive provisions of the New Poor Law of

15. Independent Order of Odd Fellows Manchester Unity, *Attack by Lord Albemarle*, 3-4.

1834, which aimed to correct a perceived tendency in the old law to reward unemployment.[16] It is also a main theme of elite criticism of the friendly societies and, therefore, a rhetorical point in class debate.

The working-class view of its own motives contradicts these characterizations. Nineteenth-century friendly society leaders and members alike took pride in the degree to which membership in the societies meant shouldering rather than shirking responsibilities by working men and women. Members paid for their own sicknesses and their own medical care, precisely so they would not have to fall back on poor relief or on charity in other forms. The contrast in attitudes is apparent in the interviews Jocelyn Cornwell conducted with working people living in East London about their perceptions and recollections of the meaning of health and illness early in the twentieth century. Cornwell's informants wanted to avoid being seen as people who dwelt on their sicknesses. They saw themselves as people who "worked through" their sicknesses, carrying on with the daily routine whenever they could. They tended to recall fewer sicknesses than they had in fact experienced. They regarded illness as a discreditable state and good health as a morally worthy state. For them the ability to work was of central importance. Moreover, they adopted a narrow definition of sickness, excluding from the realm of "real" illnesses those health problems associated with aging but not composed of new maladies.[17]

Although average sickness time rose in the period 1872–1910, what is surprising about the statistical evidence is how little, rather than how much, sickness was claimed. The average workingman who belonged to the AOF spent most of his adult life at work, behaving in ways much closer to the working-class depiction of itself than to Lord Albemarle's characterizations.

RULES OF SICKNESS

Behavior

Friendly societies tried to promote good behavior and, as a rule, prohibited payment of claims to members whose sickness resulted from immoral acts, injuries sustained in fights that the member initiated, and excessive drink. Most clubs adopted rules concerning behavior but wrote them

16. Boyer, *Economic History of the English Poor Law*, examines whether the argument had merit.
17. Cornwell, *Hard-Earned Lives*, esp. 117–45.

vaguely, a policy that might allow a broad attempt to monitor, as easily as a general disregard of, behavioral issues. The important point is to discover how far behavioral standards may have reduced the friendly societies' liabilities—that is, how much sickness time went uncompensated.

Some friendly societies, led by the Independent Order of Rechabites, tried to limit their members to people who had not ever or no longer did drink alcoholic beverages. Their expectation was that sickness and death rates would thereby be reduced, apparently on grounds that several studies had shown a strong association between high mortality and heavy drinking and high death rates for tavern keepers and other individuals whose occupations put them in touch with beer, wine, or spirits.[18] For them the important point was not merely to avoid drunkenness but to avoid drink. For friendly societies as a whole, however, conviviality added to the appeal of membership. Some clubs had been begun by tavern keepers, who saw a way to increase their business by drawing men into regular meetings on their premises, and even at the end of the nineteenth century, when some clubs had built their own meeting halls, others continued to assemble at public houses. The thirst of workingmen earned the condemnation of some elite observers, who believed that friendly societies encouraged men to waste money on drink. Despite this disapproval, the clubs continued to meet in taverns and the members continued to drink at meetings. Since financial records often survive it is possible to reconstruct what the men did spend on drink through their sick clubs. They ate and drank prodigiously at the annual club feast, but at meetings and funerals they typically bought only one or two rounds of beer.

The clubs encouraged social drinking. Their male members thought well of men who could "hold their liquor" and saw harm only in drunkenness. In a story retold in the *Foresters' Miscellany*, a Scot who pled to the magistrate that he "had had too little" to drink claimed "that a man might

18. William Farr, assistant registrar general, remarks on the association in 1851 in Great Britain, Registrar General of Births, Deaths, and Marriages, *Fourteenth Annual Report* (1855), xv–xxiii. For an example of friendly society awareness of this association, see *Foresters' Miscellany*, Jan. 1875, 310–11. The Rechabites published some statistics intended to prove their point, e.g. *Friendly Societies' Journal* June 1883, 80, showing that their sickness claims were lower than those in other friendly societies. But that comparison is flawed, because it does not take age into account and because the societies paying more claims had been founded earlier and had older members. More systematic comparisons were made later. See Neison, *Rates of Mortality and Sickness, 1878–1887*, and Wells-Smith, *Rate of Mortality and Sickness*. But they fail to settle the issue of whether the putative temperance of Rechabites led to superior health.

be justly held sober as long as he could speak."[19] That story was meant to be funny. It is difficult to find clear guidance from the friendly societies about the point at which someone could be said to be drunk or to drink too much. Members who suffered accidents while drinking were sometimes refused benefits. But alcoholism, although employed by the registrar general as a cause of death in the category of dietetic diseases, does not appear as a cause of sickness in the available sources.[20] Men who suffered from alcoholism evidently did not claim benefits, or they claimed them indirectly, by pleading another sickness. There is also little evidence to indicate that members were expelled for drunkenness. Samuel Leak was kicked out of a Shrewsbury court in 1863 for being seen drinking while receiving benefits. But the District Committee that reviewed the case overruled the court, deciding instead to fine Leak ten shillings and to pay him the sick pay due, which probably amounted to the same sum.[21]

Drink figures most prominently in the minutes as a means of distinguishing the member who had recovered from the man still convalescing.[22] The standard friendly society rule that members receiving benefits could not visit taverns served as a powerful stimulus to declare off benefits as soon as possible, as well as a test of a man's adherence to the rules. The tavern was a public place, likely to be visited by other members. Bad behavior there—fighting, or merely visiting while on benefits—could hardly escape notice. Indeed, the most common accusation leading to the suspension of benefits was the charge that a member had been seen drinking while on benefits. Even so, the key point is not that such charges provided the most common grounds for discontinuing benefits. It is, instead, that few claims were denied because of such behavior. From cases discussed in the minutes, it seems that qualifications of the definition of sickness based on rules about drinking had an insignificant effect on sickness rates.

In 1842 the AOF permanent secretary, Mr. D. Redfearn, was forced out of office because he ran away to America with another man's wife.[23] He was also denied future benefits. But his was not really a punishment inflicted by the AOF; Redfearn left his office and his investment behind in a preemptive action. Harry Worrall, a member of the Kempston Friendly

19. *Foresters' Miscellany*, Oct. 1876, 199.
20. See chapter 7.
21. AOF, District Management Committee papers, 4727/1, minutes, Nov. 20, 1863.
22. E.g., Winslow, "A Doctor's Opinion."
23. AOF, *Directory*, 1903, xx.

Society, was suspected in 1895 of having fallen ill because of intemperance and immoral conduct, and the club's officers investigated. The surgeon reported that while Worrall's case might be affected by excessive drinking earlier in life, he knew of no immoral conduct or recent excess. What troubled the surgeon was Worrall's uncleanness. The members decided not to withhold benefits. Nor, the same day, did they wish to expel John Pateman, who had been imprisoned for housebreaking.[24]

A member of the High Pavement Chapel Provident Friendly Society complained in April 1878 that the club doctor had refused to certify his sickness. When questioned, the doctor replied that the man's disease, which the club secretary called "cyciflus," had been "brought on by an immoral act," and the club upheld the doctor.[25] The remarkable thing is not that a friendly society associated with a chapel once denied a member benefits for a venereal disease but that venereal diseases figure so infrequently either in diagnoses of sicknesses or as points of contention in minutes. Probably friendly society members concealed such diseases or treated them at their own expense rather than allowing them to come to the attention of the community, as almost certainly would have happened had the club doctor and the sick steward become involved. Carruthers Corfield, author of *A Handbook of Medical Terms* for friendly society officials, claimed that members concealed only venereal disease and cirrhosis of the liver under other diagnoses.[26]

On August 13, 1835, Thomas Arnold, a member of the Duke of York lodge of the Oddfellows in Preston, caught a fellow member, P. G. Lewty, "on the room floor with his Trowsers below his knee . . . & her laying by his side." As fellow members testified in an emphatic but laconic group of statements: "she is a Women fit to be believed." Lewty seems to have been on the point of forcing a woman, who goes unnamed, to have intercourse. But the parties to the dispute, who described to a lodge committee what they knew and had heard about the incident, also reported that both Lewty and the woman had tried to get them to alter their stories about the event. One P. S. Crook tried to persuade Arnold to say that Lewty's trousers had not been down and that his behavior had not been out of the ordinary. In addition, the woman asked a friend, whose identity is not clear, "to say that I heard her Shriek out," which the friend refused to do on grounds that

24. Kempston Friendly Society papers, DDX157/2, minutes, Mar. 8, 1895.
25. High Pavement Chapel Provident Friendly Society papers, HiF2, minutes, Apr. 29, 1878.
26. Corfield, *Handbook of Medical Terms,* 54–55.

he or she had heard no cry. In the end, the committee of inquiry decided Lewty was innocent of the charge brought against him, a charge never formally identified. Regarding the episode as a misunderstanding, it recommended that the parties involved find a way "to live amicably."[27] Lewty escaped punishment or censure even though, by any strict interpretation of lodge rules, he must have been guilty, if not of a criminal act then at least of improper conduct.

Still, accounts of sexual misconduct or immorality in other forms are rare in friendly society sources. Most clubs claimed the right to refuse benefits when immorality had occurred, but they rarely did so. They also infrequently expelled members for immoral conduct. Although the friendly societies might have been agencies of moralistic surveillance, they did not develop in that direction. Their moral attitude seems to have been tolerance.

Court secretaries received premiums and paid benefits, a responsibility that made embezzlement too tempting for some of them. Frederick Johnson allegedly took £283 from his Wokingham court in 1888; he was charged and convicted on one count involving £12 and was sent to hard labor for a year, despite his advanced age and testimony to the effect that he suffered a condition called severe brain congestion.[28] Apparently, he sacrificed future benefits, although that did not necessarily follow. Legal action against him was undertaken without malice but as a matter of necessity. T. Jacques, treasurer of a club in Fulbeck, kept for himself certain money due the club's doctor. A motion to expel him lost, and Jacques was allowed to repay the money.[29] Stories with both outcomes could be repeated without producing any other conclusion than that friendly societies preferred to decide each case individually.[30] While they typically insisted on restitution or punishment, the societies took no strong ethical stand. They were not, in cases of financial malfeasance any more than in instances of moral failure, stern guardians of public order; more often they seem to have been led by the thought: There but for the grace of God go I.

Nevertheless, British friendly societies were capable of taking a costly

27. IOOF, Duke of York Lodge papers, DDX433/1, minutes, June 13, 1835. See also Leicester Bond Street Friendly Society papers, DE1884/1, Sept. 9, 1845, in which a charge of immorality was brought against one William Wormill and deemed proven; but Wormill was allowed to remain a member in hopes that he would regain the path of virtue.

28. "In the Law Courts."

29. Loyal Fane Friendly Society papers, Loyal Fane II/1, minutes, May 10, 1881.

30. E.g., AOF, District Managing Committee papers, 4727/1, minutes, Aug. 30, 1865; IOOF, Sir William Harpur Lodge papers, OF36/1, minutes, Mar. 5, 1860.

stand on principle. The AOF High Court resolved in 1888 to suspend all courts operating in the U. S. subsidiary of the order for their refusal to admit African American members.[31] They took that action even though the Foresters were engaged in a contest with the Oddfellows in which each sought to claim the largest membership. In short, the Foresters took the exclusion of African Americans by American courts as a serious matter.

Insanity

In the early years of the AOF, the 1830s, courts rarely stated in clear terms whether they intended to pay benefits for lunacy, an umbrella term then used to describe emotional disorders severe enough to make a person unable to live in society. Instances in which benefits were paid for emotional disorders can be cited, but so can cases where club rules prohibited such payments, and it is not apparent what the balance between them was.[32] In later decades AOF courts and other friendly societies adopted more detailed rules, often specifically including or excluding lunacy as sickness. Before mid-century the designation of madness was modified in a way meant to express more enlightened attitudes toward its victims. *Insanity* replaced *lunacy* as a characterization, acquired gradations, and was identified as a disease.[33]

As a disease, insanity could be linked to a part of the anatomy, in place of the association between lunacy and a person's spirit or soul. These characteristics were explained to Foresters by J. W. Northey in a long essay in the April 1873 number of the *Foresters' Miscellany*. Northey claimed that insanity occurs as a result of brain injuries and diseases, as well as of malformations, and speculated that its putative increase in his day could be attributed to indigestion among sedentary people, "those who yield to the seductive pleasures of . . . modern civilization" by overeating, suffering "dyspeptic morbid nervous irritability."[34] His argument implied that insanity was a consequence of physical ill health, a malady like apoplexy in its gradual and inapparent development. Madness, he argued, is preceded by such signs as nervous irritability, intolerance of the views of others, and

31. AOF, *Directory,* 1903, xxxiii–xxxv. A new subsidiary without restrictive rules was later created on the west coast.

32. See, e.g., the quarterly report dated May 25, 1844, Royal Foresters, Court Stone of Ezel papers, quarterly report dated May 25, 1844, concerning benefits paid Samuel Stocks, then in the Lunatic Asylum at Derby.

33. Scull, *Most Solitary of Afflictions,* 216–31.

34. Northey, "Sane or Insane?" the quotes from 432 and 433, respectively. Starvation, too, he held to promote insanity.

bigotry. Like physical ailments, it is a matter of degree. Just as physical conditions involving only "occasional or slight discomfort" are regarded as good health, so too madness excludes mere eccentricity, indeed every emotional state short of the "ungovernable."[35] Like people with physical diseases, the mad could recover, perhaps most effectively by self-discipline.

Behind the quaint peculiarity Northey's argument has for modern ears lies a substantive argument of considerable power. In 1873 the AOF High Court, the governing body of the order, adopted a resolution instructing individual courts not already counting insanity as sickness to do so, seeking to resolve an old dispute.[36] Northey's essay appeared in the *Miscellany* no doubt as a way of preparing delegates to the national meeting. Northey and the speakers at the 1873 meeting persuaded delegates to adopt the view that insanity was, insofar as concerned the friendly societies, who included only individuals who appeared to be sane when they joined, entirely analogous to physical disease or injury. It could, therefore, be treated as sickness, a practice the Oddfellows had already adopted.[37]

For AOF officials a settled policy about mental disorders was therefore in effect from close to the beginning of the period in which AOF experience is reconstructed here. Every court did not follow the policy of the national organization. Some began to pay benefits for insanity only later, which means that sickness time tended to rise across the entire nineteenth century and into the early twentieth century, because more and more courts enlarged the definition of sickness to include mental disorders. Nor did the inclusion of insanity as sickness resolve problems of definition and threshold. What is known about the specific maladies for which AOF courts paid benefits shows, however, that insanity seldom qualified.[38] Although cases of insanity tended to be prolonged, they were too few in number or scale to exert more than a minor influence on sickness rates or the sickness trend.

On one hand, AOF records, and those of other friendly societies too, are likely to understate the incidence and prevalence of mental illness, even

35. Ibid., 437.
36. AOF, *Directory,* 1903, xxxi. According to "Is Insanity Sickness?" J. Tidd Pratt, registrar of Friendly Societies, had confused the issue by citing Poor Law Act precedents to suggest that friendly societies were not liable to pay benefits for insanity. The AOF Executive Council warned courts that this ruling was faulty and urged them to pay benefits in such cases unless their rules specifically prohibited such payments. But the Executive Council also warned that courts might suffer financially from the often prolonged duration of spells of insanity, to the point that they might want either to adopt a special rule excluding benefits for insanity or to charge additional premiums for them. This advice was overturned in 1873.
37. [Ratcliffe], *Independent Order of Odd-Fellows,* 28.
38. See chapter 7.

though they attempted to include such maladies by assigning them physical causes. On the other hand, the importance assigned, by nineteenth-century physicians and laypeople alike, to symptoms and the difficulty of ruling out biological causes for diseases described by indefinite symptoms imply that many psychosomatic maladies were benefited. If it is true, as Edward Shorter argues, that the profile of symptoms of that period was much like the profile of the twentieth century, when, Shorter claims, more is understood about how to distinguish psychosomatic and somatic maladies,[39] then it seems inescapable that many psychosomatic ailments must have passed for somatic ailments to patients and doctors alike. In that case, what is at issue in the realm of mental illness is not the medicalization of conditions previously regarded as wellness into the category of sickness but merely the relabeling of maladies, and that in a culture perhaps becoming less rather than more tolerant of male mental problems.[40] Even so, it is likely that the friendly society record excludes much mental sickness for the simple reason that, even in today's society, which is believed to be hypochondriacally sensitive to emotional health, psychosomatic illnesses so often do not lead to work absence.[41] Those sicknesses go unnoticed not because they are outside the realm of things recognized as a departure from health but because, then and now, they are so often outside the realm of things deemed to warrant taking time off from work.

ECONOMIC TERMS OF SICKNESS

Unemployment and Sickness

Friendly society members and observers worried about the pressure that higher unemployment exerted on sickness rates.[42] As they noticed, claims rose when many people were out of work. Noel Whiteside's examination of the association between unemployment and sickness claims during 1920–39, when separate sickness and unemployment benefits were available in Britain, suggests both that workers who lost jobs were likelier to enter spurious claims of sickness and that the unemployed were most likely to become sick.[43]

39. Shorter, *From Paralysis to Fatigue*, 12, 295.
40. Oppenheim, *Shattered Nerves*, 152. Oppenheim argues further that mental disorders were characterized not through a process of medicalization but through negotiations between patients and doctors.
41. See the case studies discussed in Barsky, *Worried Sick*, 3–5, passim.
42. E.g., Neison, *Rates of Mortality and Sickness, 1871–1875*, 49.
43. Whiteside, "Counting the Cost."

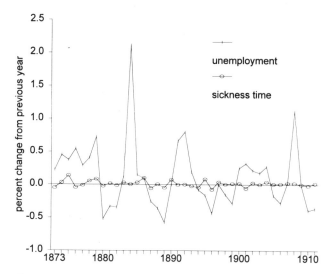

Fig. 5.1. Change in AOF Sickness Time and Unemployment, 1873–1911
Source: Data from AOF , *Directories,* 1873–1911; and Feinstein, *Statistical Tables,* T125.

During 1872–1910, when separate relief for unemployment was unavailable to most workers, sickness claims rose during economic depressions, and AOF sickness claims exhibit a statistically significant but small association with unemployment in those few trades where such data were collected.[44] Figure 5.1 shows the marked volatility in unemployment from year to year, in contrast with small year-to-year changes in sickness time. In 1879 both rose, and in 1887 both declined. But in most years they moved independently from one another. Unemployment is a bad predictor of sickness, and the reverse is also true.

Job Demands and the Sickness Threshold

Many physically demanding occupations in nineteenth-century Britain were filled chiefly by young adults. As they grew older, men and women shifted to less taxing work, adjusting the work they did to their strength and energy. When a young person was sick the work tasks that he or she could not perform often differed from the tasks an older sick person could not perform. The threshold distinguishing sickness from wellness did not remain the same across the adult life course. Men and women who could

---

44. The statistical association between sickness and various indicators of economic conditions is discussed further in chapter 6 and appendix 3.

not perform physically demanding tasks at age thirty might nevertheless have been able to perform less taxing work and might therefore have missed less work because of sickness if they had had the same jobs as their fifty-year-old counterparts. Since for working people retirement was uncommon until after 1909, when the Pension Act of 1908 went into effect, this process of adjustment continued into higher ages.[45]

It might occur, too, for a member who was unable to resume a former trade but could take lighter work. As A. H. Bailey observed in 1905, a man with rheumatism cannot carry bricks up a ladder, but he can perform a sedentary job.[46] On a case-by-case basis friendly societies considered appeals from members who wished to continue receiving benefits at a reduced level but to be allowed to work part time or to learn a less demanding trade. In 1867 the Shropshire Provident Society allowed Thomas Jones, who had been on reduced benefits of five shillings a month for many years, to learn tailoring and agreed to continue to pay him benefits for six months more.[47] Indeed, it was possible to "recover" from sickness by changing jobs. In 1889 a Kempston man, William Slater, found a job involving light work, and his club doctor refused any longer to certify his sickness.[48]

For these reasons comparisons across time may be misleading if the composition of jobs has changed in ways that add or subtract significantly from the physical demands associated with labor. Between the late nineteenth and the late twentieth centuries, the proportion of jobs that are physically taxing has diminished, as can be seen in a general way by comparing the occupations listed in censuses. That transition away from physical labor was under way in the period 1872–1910, although it is difficult to detect in so crude an index as a list of occupations. Nevertheless, there was a background shift toward a less demanding standard for distinguishing sickness from wellness and toward a standard in which the difference between what young adults and older adults could do would be less easily detected. The advent of retirement added further to this effect by removing from the workforce many old people, who formerly judged themselves sick or well according to their ability to work. In the long run,

45. On the effects of the pension act on retirement, see Johnson, "Employment and Retirement of Older Men," esp. 123.
46. Brabrook, "On the Progress of Friendly Societies," 344, in comments by A. H. Bailey on Brabrook's paper.
47. Shropshire Provident Society papers, 436/6728, minutes, Dec. 28, 1867. Also Kempston Friendly Society papers, DDX157/2, minutes, May 4, 1894.
48. Kempston Friendly Society papers, DDX157/3, minutes, Mar. 29, 1889.

the shift toward less physically taxing jobs and the generalization of retirement within the working class tended to raise the threshold between sickness and wellness. As time passed friendly society members were considered sick somewhat less often, because their work was less taxing and because they withdrew from the workforce at an age when it became more difficult to find jobs suited to their strength and energy.

Superannuation

Are old people who cannot work sick, or are they old? Until the gradual introduction of publicly funded pension benefits, which began in 1909, many people worked as long as they were physically able. Only a few managed to retire, withdrawing from the labor force while they were still able to work.[49] For example, among Foresters living in or near Ipswich who died in 1902 or 1903, most were active in their occupations at the time of their death, even at the highest ages:[50]

Age	Percent inactive
through 55	0
56–64	12
65–74	20
75+	21

Some friendly societies provided separate benefits for superannuated members.[51] Most both excluded superannuation from benefit and made no separate provision for payments to members in old age except sickness benefits, paid still when an individual could not work.

Beginning in the 1870s friendly society advisers fretted about whether unscrupulous older members would take advantage of their age to claim reduced pay in place of pensions and about how to distinguish sickness from old age itself.[52] Were the assets of the societies sufficient to support these putative claims, the scale of which no one knew? In 1878 the actuary most often employed by the AOF issued a report warning of the problem. From that time forward the superannuation issue appeared repeatedly in

49. See Quadagno, *Aging in Early Industrial Society,* 150–52; Hannah, *Inventing Retirement,* 7 ff; and Johnson, "Employment and Retirement of Older Men."

50. AOF, Ipswich District, *Half-Yearly Balance Sheets,* 1903, 1904.

51. E.g., the Morcott Friendly Society papers, beginning in 1774, rules, DE1702/4.

52. John Tidd Pratt argued in his 1853 investigation of patterns of sickness that friendly societies should pay benefits only for sicknesses lasting less than twenty-six weeks, in effect eliminating payments for chronic sickness. See Neison, *Contributions to Vital Statistics,* xxiii. This advice was rejected.

AOF deliberations at the national level and as a point of conflict between courts and the order. The courts were confident that they could distinguish between sickness and old age, but the order's officials worried that the costs of paying benefits to old members might outrun resources.[53]

Official anxiety can be traced not so much to the problem itself as to the age of the AOF. When it was organized, in 1834, most of its courts were only a few years old, having broken away from the Royal Foresters. Most members were young men in their twenties and thirties. By the 1870s, however, the young members of the 1830s had reached their sixties and seventies. For the first time the AOF could count large numbers of members at every adult age and a large proportion of old men, and for the first time it had to worry legitimately about the heavy costs associated with the high sickness rates of the aged. To individual members and to local courts, however, what officials seemed to be urging was the adoption of a hard-hearted attitude toward old members, perhaps even the denial of benefits legitimately contracted.

No solution to the problem of distinguishing sickness from old age appeared.[54] Old members suffered more diseases than their younger counterparts, but they also suffered "failing energy."[55] Some people could not work at their former jobs, or perhaps they could not work at all, not because of a specific ailment but because of age and its assorted ailments, such as debility and dyspepsia. Friendly society officials often argued that benefits should be denied in such cases, even though a member might thereby be forced onto poor relief. But members themselves typically resisted, pointing to both fraternal obligation and the difficulty of showing that sickness was not present. Rheumatism, for example, rarely posed any risk to life. Many old members who could not persuade their doctors that they were sick from another disease or injury could nevertheless accurately claim to have rheumatism. Some friendly societies tried to rule out payments in such cases but found themselves on weak legal ground. In 1871 an Oddfellows lodge refused to pay an aged member's claim for chronic rheumatism. The member took them to court, and the judge ordered payment.[56]

53. E.g., AOF, *Third Quarterly Report of the Fifty-Fourth Executive Council*, 8–9. The views of AOF officers were aired repeatedly in articles titled "Superannuation" in the *Foresters' Miscellany*, e.g., Oct. 1882, 201–8; Jan. 1883, 273–76; and May 1889, 196–200.
54. E.g., the sporadic deliberations of Maiden Queen Lodge, in IOOF, Maiden Queen Lodge papers, OF8/1, minutes, Feb. 19, 1884, July 7, 1885, and passim.
55. This phrase appears in a letter to the editor, *Foresters' Miscellany*, Apr. 1888, 192.
56. Ancient Noble Order of United Oddfellows papers, Bolton Unity, FO/2/45.

Old age and the general absence, before 1909, of pensions must have added to the friendly society ledgers some sickness time that would more accurately be attributed to age. Two features of friendly societies' experience argue, however, that these additions were modest rather than large. First, many men did not make claims, even at very advanced ages. At ages seventy to seventy-four, AOF members in the period 1871–75 claimed benefits for 23.1 percent of the time at risk. Their sickness rates were much higher than those of younger men, but the older members were still well more than three-quarters of the time.[57] Second, the advent of state-funded pensions, which diminished the appeal of using friendly society benefits as a source of pension income, had no perceptible effect on the rising trend of sickness time,[58] even though it would be expected to have reduced the likelihood that old members would enter claims.

Valuation

Early in the nineteenth century, when affiliated friendly societies were formed, the method of calculating what premiums had to be charged for a certain level of benefits had been worked out, but only hypothetical estimates were available about patterns of sickness. Thus individual clubs, which set their own premium schedules and paid their own benefits, adopted schedules according to rule-of-thumb conventions. Between the 1820s and the 1850s evidence accumulated about patterns of sickness and claims, and that evidence suggested that most clubs had fixed premiums at too low a level or benefits at too high a level. The single most contentious issue in the AOF, as in other friendly societies, during the second half of the nineteenth century arose from the effort of national officials and well-meaning observers to persuade individual clubs to adopt more cautious premium-benefit ratios.

Because there were so many friendly societies needing their services, the second half of the nineteenth century was the golden age of the actuary, who understood the arcane matter of valuation. At any moment a club faced a certain set of liabilities, the cost of which could be projected using prior patterns of sickness and mortality to supply estimates of future mortality and morbidity among individual members. Using that experi-

57. Neison, *Rates of Mortality and Sickness, 1871–1875*, 36 (62,222.17 weeks of sickness compared to 5,185.5 years at risk). Even at ages eighty-five to eighty-nine, members claimed benefits for only 40.5 percent of the time at risk.
58. See figure 6.5.

ence, actuaries estimated how much money would be paid out for sickness and burial benefits, allowing for interest that would be earned on accumulated income. Their estimates, which were defective in several respects, suggested that individual clubs were often in deficit to a degree serious enough to require them to raise premiums or reduce benefits.

Already in the 1850s AOF officers led a campaign against the custom of charging equal premiums for all members, pointing out that an individual's risk of sickness and death was influenced by his or her age. Premiums should be graduated by age, or members above a certain age should be obliged to pay higher premiums. In sum, actuaries promoted the idea of basing premiums on the leading individual risk factor, age, rather than on the principle of insurance, according to which it might have been argued that all members should pay the same premium, even if at a higher rate. The laments of actuaries about the putative financial weakness of individual clubs also helped foster the idea, held widely in the ruling class of late-nineteenth-century Britain and, since then, among historians, that the friendly societies were financially unsound and growing weaker.[59]

It is tempting to assume that the clubs that disappeared from view failed because they did not charge high enough premiums to pay the benefits they promised, and there is sufficient evidence to show that sometimes this occurred. But many clubs were absorbed by the affiliated societies, and others closed down at a moment when they still had substantial assets. William Hart, a London cooper, remarked that the first friendly society he belonged to, the Coopers' Club, dissolved in 1799, paying out its assets to members. Hart received £2 4s. 2d.[60] Although the impression of financial frailty has some validity, especially for local sick clubs, it is also true that the financial position of AOF courts, Oddfellows lodges, and friendly societies in general improved toward the end of the century and thereafter.[61] The time of financial trouble for friendly societies had been the

59. E.g., Gilbert, *Evolution of National Insurance,* 170–74. While Gilbert cites Alfred Watson's 1903 study of patterns of sickness and mortality in the Oddfellows *(Sickness and Mortality Experience),* he claims that, before World War I, the friendly societies lacked an understanding of the relation between patterns of sickness and mortality, which is what Watson's book helped supply.

60. Hudson and Hunter, "Autobiography of William Hart," 154. Hart (ibid., 155) also mentioned that he joined a second society in 1799, paying only 1s. 4d. a month for benefits of £1 a week, a ratio so generous that the club was unlikely to have lasted. But it did not dissolve until 1847. Hart does not say why it broke up.

61. See, e.g., Independent Order of Odd Fellows Manchester Unity, *Report,* xiv, which shows the history of the surplus/deficit position of the IOOF into the 1960s. The result is favorable, even though the actuaries applied strict and cautious standards. See also the comments by a well-informed insider, Wilkinson, *Friendly Society Movement,* 2–3, passim.

middle of the nineteenth century, when many local sick clubs went bust because they had not collected enough in premiums or because they had not saved enough of what they had collected.[62]

Why the actuaries erred in believing that the friendly societies were financially unsound and were growing weaker rather than stronger can be explained by the assumptions they made about the future. Those assumptions were defective in four key aspects. First, actuaries assumed that past death rates would prevail in the future. Death rates, in fact, declined, reducing the liabilities of friendly societies for paying burial benefits. Second, actuaries assumed that past rates of sickness time would prevail. But sickness time rose, increasing liabilities. However, it rose in a certain form, which was less costly. The rate of new sickness episodes actually declined over time, while the average length of sickness episodes expanded at a pace great enough to cause sickness time to rise. As actuarial valuations of individual courts show repeatedly, the largest increase came in the form of more extended sickness. Since the friendly societies regularly paid reduced benefits when sicknesses were prolonged, the added costs were minimized. Sickness time increased more than did sickness payments.

Third, actuaries assumed that the low rates of interest that had prevailed in the past should be used to appraise future earnings on friendly society assets, but in fact interest rates and earnings rose. Fourth, actuaries assumed that future price changes would cancel each other out. In fact, especially after 1900, prices rose, undercutting the value of friendly society assets and benefits and eroding their liabilities.

Projections about the future are regularly based on the past and are often inaccurate. British actuaries can be faulted for their high caution but not for their assumptions, which were plausible enough when they were made. What is important, in the final analysis, is not that the actuaries made so many bad guesses but that their worries about the financial integrity of the friendly societies proved to be unfounded. Some clubs, it is true, failed, and others had to reduce benefits or increase premiums. The Abthorpe Foresters cut the benefits they paid in 1892. Other clubs within affiliated societies obtained assistance from the national organization.[63] But one of the features of the affiliated societies was that members of one unit could transfer to another, so that few of their members need have been

---

62. Hardy, "Friendly Societies," 255. Also Gosden, *Self-Help*, 17–23.
63. AOF, *Third Quarterly Report of the Fifty-Fourth Executive Council*, 22–36, details appeals from fourteen courts that were helped in one year.

disappointed by the failure of the sick club they first joined.[64] People leaving one court in the AOF and other affiliated orders acquired "clearance" to join other courts.[65] Unless the move was temporary, the new court reported on sickness and burial, so that a member's health statistics moved with him or her. Failure was a more serious problem for the members of unaffiliated clubs, especially those too old to join another club.

In the intermediate run, stretching to the last years of the nineteenth century, the financial position of the friendly societies improved rather than deteriorated. The fears that had troubled financial advisers in the mid-nineteenth century receded as larger and larger proportions of clubs satisfied the actuaries' strict and conservative interpretation of how much was needed in the way of assets to achieve solvency. In the long run, all the anguish over whether premiums and assets were adequate, and all the conflicts between officials who warned that they had to charge more and local clubs that resisted, led to the creation of assets that were consumed not so much by paying benefits as by inflation. In the 1920s the friendly societies lost much of their appeal not because they could not pay benefits but because the benefits they were ready to pay had lost so much of their purchasing power.

Sickness is an illusive phenomenon. Not only do individuals define it differently, which means that people do not all count the same objective symptoms as qualifying as sickness, but also all attempts to measure things deemed sickness are troubled by specifications. At one extreme, sickness might be acknowledged from the point at which people are prepared to complain to a friend about their health; at another, it might mean a condition requiring hospital care. For some observers the suitable specification is more extreme still; for authorities who believe that sickness rates track death rates, then death itself is the only sure evidence of sickness: it is the only proof that a sickness was grave. In all cases except the last, the count of sickness events and of sickness time will be influenced by many forces that affect whether something that people experience becomes a part of the record of things detected.

Toward the middle of these possible specifications stand two about which large bodies of historical evidence exist: the consultation of doctors and the amount of time taken off from work because of sickness. Each of

---

64. AOF, *Directory*, 1903, xlii–xliii. The AOF also made grants to courts in financial trouble.

65. Clearance was granted to members in good financial standing.

these narrows the specification considerably, without eliminating problems associated with it. Regarding a doctor's patients, are we to take the evidence of the patient's presenting as a sign of sickness, or only the doctor's judgment? How much are we to worry about the potential patient's access to a doctor? For work time lost, too, there are in practice factors that affect the specification. This chapter's purpose has been to survey those that influenced sickness as it was tallied by British friendly societies in the nineteenth and early twentieth centuries, more especially the Foresters in the period 1872–1910. The results of this survey show qualifications to the definition the friendly societies gave sickness. Identical qualifications are unlikely to obtain at another time or place. Hence, comparisons of sickness time between friendly society members in Britain in the nineteenth century and people at other times and places must, if they are to be made on the same terms, take these differing specifications into account.

On the whole, the specifications the sick clubs made reduced the number of episodes of ill health that would be counted as sickness, taking a narrow rather than an expansive view of when health problems were serious enough to warrant taking time off from work. The waiting period eliminated claims for most brief sicknesses, reducing in a consistent way the number of episodes that would be counted as sickness and, together with the requirement of certification by a doctor, eliminated instances in which absenteeism might have been concealed by an excuse of sickness. Earlier in the nineteenth century some societies declined to pay benefits for insanity. But the tendency in place by the 1870s was to explain emotional disorders by physical causes, which made them eligible for benefits. Still, some episodes of emotional disorder that disabled men and women for work probably were not allowed as claims. As time passed the physical demands of work diminished gradually, and the expectation that people should work into old age gave way to an expectation that they would retire around age sixty-five. Those changes, too, tended to reduce the number of claims made. But the AOF, like other friendly societies, refused to make a special case of the old in such a way that would curtail the health problems they could legitimately claim as sickness.

In the longer run the number of claims made was lowered also by inflationary inroads into the value of assets accumulated in the nineteenth century. The real value of benefits, however, was high enough to make claims worthwhile up to the 1920s. The friendly societies might also have reduced the number of claims their members could make by strictly enforcing their rules about behavior or by selecting new members with greater care. They might, for example, have refused to pay benefits for a longer initiation period, up to ten or fifteen years, or have ejected members who fell sick when they were young adults. But the fraternal sentiments of members overpowered the insurance instincts of officials: the societies neither monitored their member's behavior closely nor catered to the well.

Friendly societies defined sickness in a particular way. What matters here is whether the sickness claims of friendly society members provide a reasonable gauge of sickness, and whether those claims were recorded in a consistent way over time. Although time lost from work because of sickness is only one possible threshold for distinguishing sickness from wellness, it is an important and useful threshold that is captured by the claims that men made for benefits. Over time the AOF made some changes in its rules and procedures. But on major issues, which threatened to affect the sickness rate in a substantial way, AOF practice remained consistent over the period of this study. The changes that did occur were small in their effects. They threaten to make the interpretation of sickness and its trend difficult only if changes in sickness rates were also small.

CHAPTER 6

Health Patterns of the Foresters

THE HEALTH of the Foresters changed in the last decades of the nineteenth century and into the twentieth century, in two ways. They lived longer, and they were sick more of the time. Their higher sickness time joins their lower mortality as a measured outcome, one that can be assessed by statistical means to learn something about which factors played a part in changing patterns of health.

The health of a population can be assessed from both its mortality and its morbidity. Mortality rates gauge the likelihood of survival. Sickness incidence rates gauge the risk of falling sick. Sickness prevalence rates measure the overall amount of time spent in sickness, or the risk of being sick. Friendly society sources provide much evidence about trends in mortality and sickness time and some evidence about sickness incidence. Thus they allow conclusions to be reached about sickness trends. In turn, these conclusions influence judgments about the relationship between sickness time and mortality, the economic consequences of sickness trends, and the distribution of people within the population between frail and robust. Simple inferences have provocative implications about the well-being of workingmen.

The Ancient Order of Foresters published directories of its national, regional, and local units beginning in 1836. Those directories relate the vital statistics of the courts for fifty-one years, beginning in 1872: the number of members eligible for benefits, their average age, and the number of days sickness accumulated during the year, plus additional information.[1] Each directory refers to experience in the preceding year, so that this series

1. The directories also sum vital statistics by district and order but without providing the average age for those units. In *Foresters' Miscellany*, Jan. 1871, 276–84, Henry Tompkins argued that the only data required to show whether a friendly society was solvent consisted of an annual record of its number of members, their average age, receipts, expenditures, and assets. Presumably, the expansion of the directory to include these data was meant to address

of vital statistics covers the period from 1871 through 1921.[2] Two parts of this record are especially valuable. Many sources in the history of health, such as hospital and physician records, report how many people received treatment, but few report also the size of the population at risk. Lacking a denominator, a sickness rate cannot be calculated. Fewer sources still have anything to say about the age structure of the population at risk.

SICKNESS INCIDENCE, SICKNESS DURATION, AND SICKNESS PREVALENCE

Sickness can be measured in three basic ways. One way counts the number of new sickness events occurring within a certain period and divides that number by the population at risk. This mode of measurement produces an incidence rate, which is a statement about the risk of falling sick. It does not consider the temporal duration of sickness incidents. A second gauge focuses on how long each sickness lasts, calculating its duration or, across groups, its average duration.

A third gauge, the one most often used here, measures the amount of sickness time that people accumulate, that is, the period prevalence of sickness. Whereas duration measures the length of specific episodes, which may extend across several years, prevalence measures the amount of sickness time within a certain period, here usually a year. The actuary Francis G. P. Neison Jr.'s study of AOF experience during 1871–75 furnishes the information needed to calculate crude and age-specific rates of sickness incidence and prevalence for the entire order, following the rules Neison adopted for distinguishing new episodes of sickness from existing conditions. The AOF directories report the number of days of sickness and provide the information needed to calculate the amount of time during which members were exposed to risk. Those data make it possible to calculate rates of sickness time but not of incidence and to analyze sickness time rather than sickness events.

To see the difference between incidence and prevalence, consider the experience of two hypothetical courts, each with one hundred members of the same ages. In court A the hundred members file twenty-five separate claims during the year. Each claim refers to a distinct sickness episode, as specified by the rules of the AOF and the judgment of the doctors allowing

---

the point Tompkins had raised. However, Tompkins did not explain how to use those data to determine solvency.

2. To obtain all the information needed for analysis, years are paired, with the result that the experience described and analyzed here begins in 1872 rather than 1871.

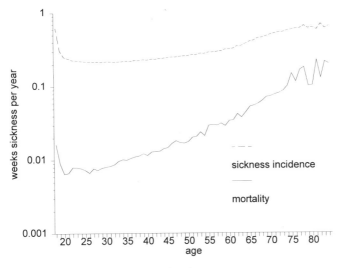

Fig. 6.1. Sickness Incidence and Mortality, by Age, 1871–1875
Source: Data from Neison, *Rates of Mortality and Sickness, 1871–1875*, 35–36, 55–56.

or disallowing claims. Each distinct sickness lasts an average of ten days, which is the average duration. From that information it is possible to calculate an incidence rate of sickness (25 members / 100 = 0.25) and a prevalence [(25 members × 10 days) / 100 = 2.5 days per member year].

In court B, however, the hundred members file only fifteen claims during the year, each of which lasts an average of 10 days except for one claim, which lasts the entire year, 365 days. In that court the incidence rate is lower, at 0.15, but sickness time is higher, at 5.05 days.[3] In the AOF, as figures 6.1 and 6.2 illustrate using Neison's data, the two forms describe very different risk curves. The risk of falling sick (sickness incidence) is portrayed in figure 6.1 as the proportion of claimants divided by all members at risk at each age.[4] It varies from a low of 21.4 percent at age twenty-nine to a high of more than 60 percent at age eighty. At age twenty-nine, an AOF member had slightly more than one chance in five of falling sick during the course of a year.[5]

3. That is,
$$[(14 \times 10) + (1 \times 365)] / 100 = 5.05.$$
The average duration of each episode is 33.7 days (14 episodes of 10 days each plus 1 of 365 days divided by 15 episodes).

4. It can also be calculated as the number of claimants divided by the number of well members at each age.

5. The same individual might enter more than one claim during a year, and Neison counted

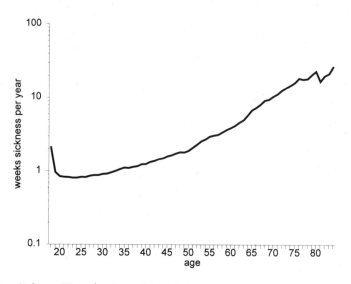

Fig. 6.2. Sickness Time, by Age, 1871–1875
Source: Data from Neison, *Rates of Mortality and Sickness, 1871–1875,* 35–36, 55–56.

Figure 6.2 shows a curve of the risk of being sick, which is measured as the number of weeks of sickness per member per year divided by the number of years at risk, and which has a more sharply defined association with age. Like the risk of death, which is measured by the proportion of deaths to years at risk, the risk of being sick rises sharply with age. The scale for sickness rates in the two figures is logarithmic, which signals that the risk of being sick rises in geometric progression while age rises in arithmetic progression. Between two ages, say thirty and sixty, the risk of being sick increases far more than suggested by the increase in years. The average duration of sickness episodes increases more with age than does the chance of contracting a new sickness. Hence, in assessing sickness time it is especially important to take age into account.

AGE AND AVERAGE AGE

The risk of being sick is associated with a number of characteristics that distinguish people from one another, including occupation, place of resi-

---

the number of claims rather than the number of individual claimants. He later reported similar data for the Rechabites, in Neison, *Rates of Mortality and Sickness, 1878–1887,* 30.

dence, sex, and age. Of these, age has the most profound influence. It has such a strong influence because more people contract more prolonged sicknesses as they age and because age captures some other effects that can rarely be observed directly. The most important of these unobserved effects is prior sickness patterns, which consist of sicknesses and injuries as well as other things that condition health. One purpose of this research is to investigate how characteristics other than age influenced patterns of sickness in Britain. Hence, it is essential that sickness rates be interpreted in a way that removes or diminishes the chance that variations attributable only to age will conceal variations that are due to other observable characteristics. That is, age as a factor must be controlled.

If age were not controlled, the meaning of sickness rates would be uncertain. For example, a rate of ten weeks' sickness a year per person would be extraordinarily high for a group of people aged twenty-five or for a group of adults with an average age of twenty-five. But it would be moderate for people in old age or for a group with an average age of about sixty-five.

The AOF directories report not the age of each member of a court or the range of ages among court members but the average age of all members of a court. Court officials calculated average age by summing the ages of members and dividing by the number of members.[6] Since age is so important and since the information available for relating the occurrence of sickness to age consists not of the specific ages of AOF members but the average age of all members in a court, it is necessary to consider how the average age of court members reflects the specific ages of individuals. The distribution of the overall AOF membership by age is known for some periods, because Foresters actuaries published that information, extracting it from manuscript reports.[7]

As figure 6.2 shows, age is a good predictor of sickness time. Is average age also a good predictor? Figure 6.3 compares Neison's schedule of age-specific rates during 1871–75 with average age rates for 1873–77, the first five years for which those rates are available from the AOF directories in complete form. Both curves rise with age in a manner that is regular for all the ages at which large numbers of people and courts are represented, and

6. E. g., AOF, Abthorpe Court papers, ZA1715.
7. Those records were not preserved, presumably because the AOF changed the location of its offices each year. Movable headquarters meant that many communities shared the reflected glory and economic advantage of hosting the annual meeting and housing the working staff of the order; but it also meant that the office had to be selective in the records it retained.

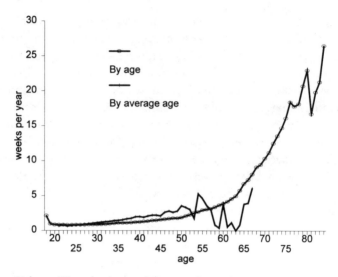

Fig. 6.3. Sickness Time, by Age and Average Age, 1871–1877
Source: Data from Neison, *Rates of Mortality and Sickness, 1871–1875,* 35–
36, 55–56; and AOF, *Directories,* 1875–79.

both break up at higher ages, where few individuals or courts are represented.[8] That visual image implies that a close statistical relation exists
between age and sickness time, a relationship that makes age a good
predictor of sickness time. By regressing sickness rates first on age and then
on average age, it is possible to assign values to the closeness of this
association. Considering only ages twenty-one to fifty-seven, at which
large numbers of individuals and courts are represented in each series, 85
percent of the variation around the mean of sickness rates in Neison's
schedule can be associated with age. Age predicts sickness time with considerable success, not because aging itself determines the likelihood of
being sick but because aging is associated with so many other factors that
influence this likelihood, and much of the force of those factors is captured
in the simple linear regression of sickness time on age. Both age-specific
and average age sickness rates show a substantial dispersion when measured by the variance of rates among individuals at each age or among
courts at each average age. That is, some individuals and groups experienced much more sickness than others. Figure 6.4 shows this for 1874 by
reporting the sickness time of all courts by average age.

8. On this issue, see appendix 2. Very few AOF courts had members with an average age
above fifty.

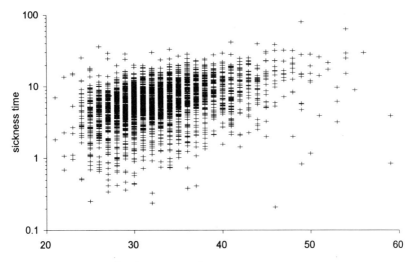

Fig. 6.4. Dispersion of Sickness Time, by Average Age, 1874
Source: Data from AOF, *Directory,* 1875.

The average age of court members should not be expected to be as accurate a predictor of sickness rates, if only because each court included people of many different ages. Nevertheless, an analogous regression of sick days on average age for the same ages, twenty-one to fifty-seven, shows that 80 percent of the variance can be associated with average age. Average age does not predict sickness time quite as successfully as age itself, but it is still a very good predictor.[9] Sickness risk is so closely related to the age of individuals (and to the average age of groups) that differences in age structure have to be taken into account in order to compare patterns of sickness in different groups on the same terms.

The average is a measure of central tendency, in this case the central tendency of ages among men aged from eighteen to extreme old age. It measures central tendency in circumstances that may differ from court to court. As study of the distribution of members by age in various courts reveals, there are two ways that average age could be misleading. First,

9. Both results, obtained by ordinary least squares regression, weaken when calculated for higher ages, where smaller numbers of members are included. The residuals increase sharply at higher ages, as the series break apart, and they show no trend. For low average ages, up to twenty-six or twenty-seven, the residuals steadily decrease. This reveals in another way the tendency for the dispersion of average ages among courts to increase with average age, as shown in figure 6.4. From other evidence it appears also that, in courts with a low average age, most members were concentrated at youthful ages, whereas as courts attained higher average ages the range of ages among their members increased.

members in different courts could be dispersed broadly or narrowly around the average age. Second, the average age could, if members' ages clustered at two or more different poles, represent an age at which there were few actual members. The key factor in the dispersion of members' ages around the average was found to be the age of the court, and the key factor influencing age clustering was found to be the rate at which new members joined. The AOF directories report both each court's founding date and the number of new members taken in each year, allowing these factors to be added to the equation. Appendix 2 provides a detailed explanation of reasons for controlling for age by these three factors: average age, the court's age, and the initiation rate.

ESTIMATING SICKNESS TIME

One aim of this research is to compare sickness time over the period 1872–1910 and in different regions of Britain while controlling for age. Hence, the point is to compare groups of courts in various regions. Were sickness rates higher in the 1880s than the 1870s, controlling for age? Were they higher in London than in Yorkshire for the same period? A two-step regression analysis has been employed to make that comparison. The first step produces estimates of sickness time and mortality for the AOF as a whole for each of four decades, from 1872 to 1910, drawing on the individual experience of all courts, controlling for average age, the court's age, and the initiation rate, and weighting the analysis by court size. The second step produces estimates of sickness time and mortality for all the AOF courts in individual counties in each decade.[10]

10. This describes the procedures employed to derive results reported in chapter 8, where geographical differences in patterns of health are examined. It is included here because the control variables and their implications are issues under review in this chapter.

The first stage produces coefficients for the three control variables, weighting for court size, and average values for the average age, years since court formation, and initiation rate. The second stage produces a separate set of coefficients that are specific to each county. An estimated sickness rate or mortality rate for each county is then derived by multiplying the coefficients for that county by the average value for each control variable (average age, years since court formation, and initiation rate) for that decade in the AOF as a whole. In that way it is possible to compare experience in all the courts in individual counties for specific periods, such as the 1870s, with experience in the AOF as a whole for the same period. From those differences I constructed, first, a table of percentage differences for each county in each decade, which is not shown, and, second, an overall average of the percentage differences for each county, which appears in chapter 8. It is necessary to weight for court size because the courts varied so much in size.

Results are construed as statistically significant if the null hypothesis that the regression

To illustrate: the sickness rate for the AOF as a whole in the period 1881–90, at the mean of each control variable,[11] is 10.6 days per year per member. Among counties in England, rates varied from a low of 7.2 days in Lincolnshire to a high of 13.5 days in Staffordshire. In other words, controlling for age and related characteristics, Staffordshire AOF members reported far more sickness than did Lincolnshire members. Given such a large variation—Lincolnshire's average was 32 percent below the overall average and Staffordshire's 27 percent above—it is apparent that sickness time was not evenly distributed across England. The same is true of Scotland and Wales. These figures do not provide any explanation for why sickness rates were higher in one region than in another. They merely provide a way to organize the data so as to discern regional variations.

This regression approach can be evaluated by examining whether it produces results that agree with other information and other approaches. The simplest test is to find whether courts with similar values for average age, age dispersion, and initiation rates show the same trends as those estimated via regression. That comparison gives the same results. Thus the trend of rising sickness time could be shown simply by grouping together courts with the same characteristics. But regression analysis has some big advantages. It allows regional comparisons among groups of courts that do not have similar characteristics in the three control variables, thus providing a much more flexible way to use data from the directories. Another way to check the regression analysis is to notice that the portrayal of rising sickness time it provides is proportional to the increase reported by actuaries of the Oddfellows, a friendly society similar to the Foresters. In sum, regression analysis can be relied on to extract year-by-year changes in sickness time and to capture regional differences.

---

coefficients taken in combination are equal to zero can be rejected. The groups of courts for which sickness rates have been estimated by the means explained here are not random samples of all courts. Hence, gauges of statistical significance cannot signify whether the distribution in one group fell close to the distribution within the entire population. Indeed, it is expected that the sickness rates (derived in the second stage) will vary from one group of courts to another.

George Alter suggested the use of weighted regression as a means of estimating values, discussed and explained the procedure, and referred me to Kmenta, *Elements of Econometrics*, 322–29.

11. For 1881–90 those means are:

Average age:	34.453 years
Years since court formation:	28.753 years
Initiation ratio:	0.077

THE SICKNESS TREND, 1840s–1910s

At first glance crude death rates seem to have remained stable in England and Wales from the 1820s to the 1870s. But progressively larger parts of the population lived in cities, where death rates were higher than in rural areas, and it is the changing proportion of people living in high- and low-risk areas that creates the appearance of stable mortality.[12] In the population at large and in the AOF, death rates declined among men living in rural areas and among men living in cities, but from different levels.[13] The risk of death was lower in rural areas than in cities. Not until the 1870s did the forces favoring mortality decline gain enough momentum to override the effects of continued increase in the proportion of people living in high-risk areas. Thus not until the 1870s does the national index of death rates show a decline, even though mortality was moving downward earlier.

If mortality declined, behind the cover of changing residential patterns, sickness time showed no clear trend between the 1840s, when the first reports from Foresters and Oddfellows actuaries appeared, and the 1870s. Sickness time increased in rural areas, controlling for age. But it decreased slightly in cities. Among the Oddfellows, according to the studies Henry Ratcliffe made of experience in three periods, 1846–48, 1856–60, and 1866–70, the average duration of sickness episodes at each age changed little.[14] The same thing was true among Foresters, as appears from a comparison of sickness times calculated by William Watkins for the period 1850–52 and those by Francis G. P. Neison Jr. for 1871–75. Standardizing for age, Foresters experienced 2 percent more sickness in 1871–75 than they had in 1850–52, an amount too small to suggest a trend.[15]

In the 1870s, however, death rates continued to decline and sickness time began to rise. Friendly society actuaries calculated these rates at individual ages and in age groups with narrow bands, drawing on reports

---

12. Woods, "Effects of Population Redistribution on the Level of Mortality."

13. Ratcliffe, *Observations on the Rate of Mortality & Sickness* (1850), 14; and [Ratcliffe], *Independent Order of Odd-Fellows*, 6, 29. The comparison is between 1848–50 and 1866–70.

14. Hardy, "Friendly Societies," 287–88, points out some shortcomings in Ratcliffe's tables.

15. Watkins, *Statistical Notes*, 6, 35; and Neison, *Rates of Mortality and Sickness, 1871–1875*, 43. The calculation refers only to men aged twenty to sixty-nine. Watkins worked with evidence concerning 22,572 members compared to Neison's 369,655.

Nineteenth-century actuarial reports often compared findings for different friendly societies or for groups of friendly societies without showing how different rules influenced the results for each.

from the officers of local units. At each age among men who belonged to the Oddfellows, sickness time increased and death rates decreased between 1866–70 and 1893–97.[16] The same trend was noticed by actuaries of the Loyal Order of Ancient Shepherds, although on the basis of a much less thorough investigation than the one done for the Oddfellows, and by actuaries working for other friendly societies.[17]

The actuaries closely monitored sickness and mortality statistics. They quickly noticed trends of both declining mortality and rising sickness time. They initially suspected that rising sickness time might be explained by changes in the composition of friendly society members, specifically by larger proportions of people living in high-risk areas or working in high-risk occupations. Thus their inquiries focused on issues of composition. The Oddfellows actuary Alfred Watson conducted a thorough investigation during the 1890s, exploring three factors: age, occupation, and residence. He concluded in 1903 that sickness time had increased at each age not because more members practiced more hazardous occupations or lived in risky areas but because sicknesses had become more protracted. AOF actuaries reached the same view earlier. Analyzing valuations received from individual courts in 1897, Samuel Hudson concluded that sickness time exceeded the expected amount by 16.5 percent because of heavy demands from members who were not dying. Even though he believed it "impossible to reconcile persistently heavy sickness with a low death rate," "this is just what has happened."[18]

Since the membership of the Oddfellows closely resembled that of the Foresters, and since the trend of the Oddfellows' experience was so similar to that in other friendly societies at points where direct comparisons can be made, persuasive reasons exist to infer that sickness time increased among friendly society members in general. But the Oddfellows records do not show how the course of sickness time and mortality developed from year to year, and they do not allow regional comparisons.

The AOF directories make it possible not only to reconstruct patterns of sickness between actuarial surveys but also to follow the course of these patterns after 1897, when the last great survey was completed. Figure 6.5 summarizes the AOF sickness trend by providing curves of sickness time

16. Findings from the investigations of Henry Ratcliffe and Alfred W. Watson are compared in Riley, "Ill Health during the English Mortality Decline."
17. [Abbott, Abbott, and Abbott], *Report*, xviii, xxii–xxiv; and Bowser, *Royal Berkshire Friendly Society*, 5.
18. Watson, *Sickness and Mortality Experience*, 17–80; for Hudson's views, AOF, *Statement of the Valuations of the Districts and Courts* (Norwich, 1897), v.

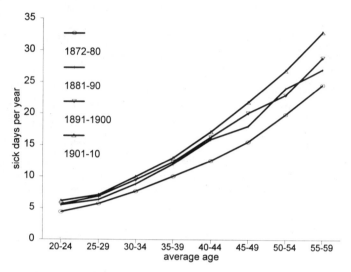

Fig. 6.5. Sickness Time by Age Group, Males, 1872–1910
Source: Data from AOF, *Directories,* 1873–1911.

for eight age groups across four decades.[19] The curves in these figures advance from each period to the next. With the sole exception of the fifty-to-fifty-four age group, in the 1890s, sickness time was always higher in succeeding periods. Among men belonging to the Foresters, as among male friendly society members in general, the passage of time brought more sickness.

In the same period, death rates decreased. Figure 6.6 displays curves of mortality for each five-year age group for the same four decades. It shows that the death rate dropped with almost the same uniformity that sickness time increased. By 1901–10, Foresters in courts where members had the same average age were much likelier to be sick but much less likely to die than had been the case in the 1870s.

These changes followed an uneven course. Annual values for sickness time among male members of the AOF in the period 1872–1911 appear in

19. This and the next figure report patterns of sickness and mortality in courts grouped by the average ages of their members. Thus, for example, the sickness rate for 1881–90, in figure 6.5 for the age group twenty to twenty four, which is 5.5 days per member per year, counting in six-day weeks, groups together all the experience in courts with an average age of twenty to twenty-four for its male members.

Groups with higher and lower ages are not pictured because the small number of courts with average ages of eighteen and nineteen or sixty and older make those rates unstable and unreliable.

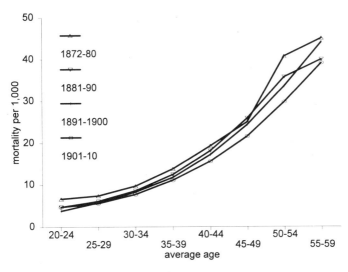

Fig. 6.6. Mortality by Age Group, Males, 1872–1910
Source: Data from AOF, *Directories,* 1873–1911.

figure 6.7, where they are expressed in terms of a standard population.[20] Sickness time increased in the long run, but not between the mid-1880s and around 1900, and it varied from year to year. By 1911 the standardized sickness time was 53 percent higher than it had been in 1872.

Standardized annual death rates appear in figure 6.8, where they are compared with standardized death rates for all males aged over twenty years in England and Wales.[21] Both curves follow the same downward path, and they follow it with a large degree of similarity in the short-run deviations they show. This strong similarity shows that, in mortality at least, the health patterns of AOF members closely tracked those of men in

20. This standard population is composed of courts distributed by the average age of their members during 1891–1900. In this case it is inappropriate to estimate annual sickness rates by the regression method outlined above, because the initiation rate and the number of years since court formation changed their relation to average age over time. Hence, estimating sickness rates for reference values for each of these factors would artificially suppress changes in patterns of health.

The 1873 AOF *Directory* reports numbers of new members and deaths but not the numbers of men who seceded in 1872. Thus, for 1872 alone the adjustment for secession occurs only as an effect of averaging the number of members at midyear. The net effect is to inflate the denominators and, thus, to deflate sickness and death rates. But the scale of these effects is too small to be of concern.

21. In this figure AOF death rates standardized on the average age of court members in 1891–1900 are compared to the death rates of adult males in England and Wales standardized on the age of that population in 1891. The display is given in index numbers in order to make the comparison on the same terms.

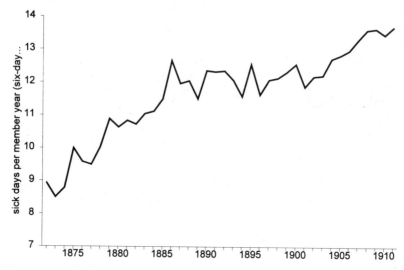

Fig. 6.7. Standardized Annual Sickness Time, AOF Males, 1872–1911
Source: Data from AOF, *Directories,* 1873–1911.

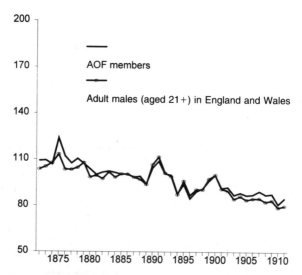

Fig. 6.8. Index of Death Rates, 1872–1911 (1900 = 100)
Source: Data from AOF, *Directories,* 1873–1911.

general. Sickness time cannot be observed in the overall male population. But the congruence of death rates in the two groups provides reason to suppose that sickness time in the AOF may accurately represent the trend and short-run variations of sickness time in the adult male population.

Among male Foresters and men in England and Wales in general, death rates decreased across the entire period. They fell with somewhat greater force between the 1870s and 1890s than later. Death rates varied more than sickness time, and certain years—1875, 1890–91, and 1900—were particularly hazardous. By 1911 the standardized death rate among AOF men was 22 percent lower than it had been in 1872, while among men in England and Wales in general it had dropped by 22.7 percent.

SICKNESS TIME, 1911–1930s

Female Sickness and Death Rates

From 1892 the AOF allowed the formation of courts for female members alone, and from 1902 existing all-male courts could admit women as members.[22] As a result of these rule changes, by 1902 the Foresters counted many courts that contained only male members, a few with male and female members, and a few with only female members. In 1911 the National Insurance Act designated a few friendly societies, including the AOF, to administer payments of insurance benefits from public revenues, a step that opened AOF courts to a new category called "state" members. State members might be males or females, so that from 1912 most AOF courts included female members.

Data from the friendly societies and modern investigations alike indicate that male and female patterns of health differ. Females are likelier to be sick, but males are likelier to die. What is problematic about the addition of female members to the AOF is that neither their number nor their average age was reported separately from the number and average age of male members. Thus courts that allowed females to join after 1902, and from 1912 many other formerly all-male courts, exhibited a mixture of characteristics, some having female characteristics (a propensity for higher sickness but lower death rates) and some male characteristics (a propensity for lower sickness but higher death rates). Yet the proportion of female

22. Independent female friendly societies were commonplace much earlier. See Jones, "Self-Help in Nineteenth-Century Wales." On women in the workforce, see Rose, *Limited Livelihoods*, esp. 76–101.

members in each court is unknown. Given the characteristics of female health patterns, the addition of women in large enough numbers would, by itself, push sickness time up and death rates down. In fact women did not join the AOF in large numbers until 1912 and thereafter. Nevertheless, the addition of female members may have affected the trend of morbidity and mortality in some courts in a substantial way, even though it probably had little effect in the overall AOF before 1912. In order to avoid the potential confusion of trend that follows from the admission of women as members, the sickness and death rates discussed above deal only with courts having an exclusively male membership.

From 1912 exclusively male courts admitted women as members, but the small number of exclusively female courts did not admit males. Thus from 1912 it is no longer possible to trace health patterns in a large group of exclusively male Foresters. The National Insurance Act also departed from friendly society practice in disallowing certain claims that friendly societies had covered and continued to cover, meaning that, everything else being equal, claims under the NIA tended to fall short of claims before 1912, when the act went into force.[23] What is more, World War I confused the size of the denominator in sickness and death rates. Many men joined the armed forces and served away from their homes and courts. While in service they were ineligible for benefits from the AOF, since the military assumed the burden of assisting these men when they were sick. But AOF courts regularly carried these men on their rolls, expecting them to resume membership and payments on their return. Thus during the war denominators were inflated by the inclusion of men who were neither present nor eligible for benefits. The result is that, even if the 1911 National Insurance Act had not by itself muddled the matter of interpreting patterns of health from the statistics reported by each court, World War I would have done so.[24]

If courts with mixed male and female memberships can no longer provide secure information about the trend of sickness and death rates, however, it is still possible to trace experience for a few years in courts with exclusively female members, disregarding the effects of new NIA claims

23. Claims made by people unable to perform their former work but able to perform another type of work were disallowed. Watson, "Analysis of a Sickness Experience," 15.

24. Thus, general friendly society sources do not provide the means necessary to test J. M. Winter's conclusion that civilian health did not deteriorate during the war. Winter, *Great War and the British People*, 105–6. However, that claim might be tested by individual-level data concerning the health of women and of men outside military-service ages.

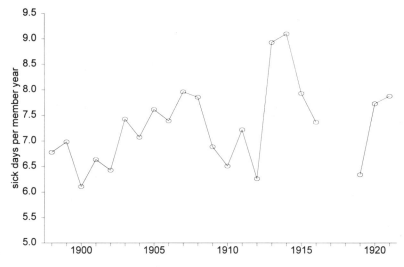

Fig. 6.9. Sickness Time, Females Aged 25–29, 1898–1921
Source: Data from AOF, *Directories,* 1898–1922.

rules. In theory it is possible to reconstruct female patterns of health from 1892, when female courts first appeared, to 1921, after which the AOF suspended publication of statistics for each court. But in practice the early coverage of female experience is unsatisfactory because so few female courts were formed.

Figure 6.9 shows annual sickness time from 1898 to 1921 for exclusively female courts having members who averaged twenty-five to twenty-nine years of age.[25] Sickness time continued to increase, and death rates to decrease, up to World War I, a finding consistent with what other sources suggest about friendly society claims experience. But it is not apparent whether it continued to increase during and after the war.

25. Years prior to 1898 have not been included because of the small number of female courts and members. Two years, 1917 and 1918, are not included because the 1918 *Directory,* reporting on 1917, was abridged due to the war. Since in the calculations for this figure, as in those for the experience of male courts, years have been paired in order to obtain a midyear estimate of the number of members at risk, the 1918 abridgment results in the loss of estimates for two years.

Sickness rates are presented for the average age group into which the largest number of courts fell across the period 1898–1921 rather than as standardized rates, because of rapid change in the age structure of female courts.

National Insurance Evidence

Claims under the 1911 National Insurance Act reached a temporary peak in 1912 and 1913 but diminished during World War I. After the war they increased and by the mid-1920s surpassed the levels of 1912–13. Claims continued to rise into the 1930s. Noel Whiteside, who investigated factors associated with this trend, concluded that it should be explained as an effect with several causes. Lower mortality did not leave the population in better health, and improved medical techniques resulted in the detection of diseases that would not have been diagnosed earlier. But according to Whiteside, the chief reason sickness claims continued to increase was the industrial recession. Higher rates of unemployment added to sickness lists men and women suffering from stress-related maladies, and it also drove the employees first laid off, who tended to be older and more infirm than employees kept on by their employers, to file for sickness as well as unemployment benefits.[26]

The different ways in which statistics were kept after 1911 plus the changed incentives of sickness claims under national insurance make it difficult to compare pre-1911 and post-1911 health patterns on the same terms. Whiteside's interpretation of the sickness trend from the 1920s and the 1930s is interesting chiefly because it lays so much stress on the possible effects of unemployment and on sickness claims as an expression of changes in the demand for labor. But it is at odds with the conclusion reached by the NIA and former Oddfellows actuary, Alfred Watson. Watson detected a decline in the incidence of new sickness claims at each age but a continued rise in the average duration of claims episodes and stressed the effects of better medical care rather than the business cycle.[27] In sum, Watson found that, adjusting for age, death rates declined within the insured population, sickness incidence also declined, and sickness time increased.

After showing no distinctive trend between the 1840s and the 1870s, sickness time among Foresters and among members of other friendly societies increased between the 1870s and 1911. It continued to increase thereafter. The health patterns of friendly society members and men in general undoubtedly improved between the 1840s and the 1930s, in terms

26. Whiteside, "Counting the Cost." On a related issue, see also Winter, "Unemployment, Nutrition, and Infant Mortality."
27. Watson, "National Health Insurance: A Statistical Review," 449–50.

of survival prospects. But that improvement coincided with a substantial increase in the proportion of an adult life spent in sickness.

THE INVERSE ASSOCIATION OF SICKNESS TIME AND MORTALITY

In 1837 William Farr expressed a commonsense assessment of medicine and sickness. He expected that "medical art" would shorten the course of sickness or increase the likelihood of recovery. Hence, evidence about the duration of diseases would show something about the efficacy of different medical regimes.[28] Farr's expectations are often encountered in the history of health, but the data presented in figures 6.5–6.9 suggest that they are misleading. The "medical art" and some other forces, too, increased the likelihood of recovery in sickness, just as Farr expected. But sickness time increased rather than diminished. As all five figures show, sickness time and death rates changed over time in inverse rather than parallel directions. As the likelihood that a Forester would die at any particular age diminished, the likelihood that he or she would be sick increased.

Two views existed about the association of sickness and mortality in the nineteenth century. In 1832 T. R. Edmonds, who had made a superficial study of the matter, proclaimed: "that death and sickness simultaneously increase and decrease . . . is a proposition which few people will be inclined to dispute."[29] Some years later, after the first reports on sickness and death rates among friendly society members had been published and analyzed, F. G. P. Neison Sr. and Henry Rumsey took a contrary view. Neison found that sickness time and death rates did not move in a parallel manner, as Edmonds had claimed.[30] And Rumsey observed that sickness would increase as the prevalence of chronic sickness rose.[31]

Edmonds's view remains a common one, but Rumsey's characterization more accurately describes experience in Britain in the second half of the nineteenth century and into the twentieth. Higher survival rates were accompanied not by less sickness time but by more. Although Farr expected good doctors to be able to shorten the length of sickness episodes,

28. Farr, "Danger and Duration of Diseases," 72.
29. Edmonds, *Life Tables*, xxxix.
30. Neison, *Contributions to Vital Statistics*, 17–27, 410.
31. Rumsey, *Essays and Papers*, 5 (reprinting an essay written earlier).

friendly society evidence suggests that the forces influencing sickness combined not to abbreviate it but to prolong it. Good doctoring and the other forces at work deferred death as well as curing sickness. The people who did not die in the emerging lower-mortality regime were sick for longer periods. And the people who did die took a longer time to reach the crisis of their illnesses. Indeed, Farr discovered exactly this effect investigating the experience of people admitted to the London Small-pox Hospital. He found that the odds of death in any episode diminished as the duration of the episode increased.[32] The effect of hospital treatment was not to curtail the duration of smallpox cases but to improve the chances of recovery. Treatment at the hospital transferred more and more patients into the group of those who survived the disease and therefore whose sicknesses lasted longer. Declining smallpox mortality promoted more sickness time.

The Foresters counted as sickness any ailment that, in the opinion of the members themselves and of their doctors, rendered a member unable to work. Under that definition sickness time might rise because either the number of episodes or the average duration of episodes increased. Since the AOF directories report the total number of sickness days but not the number of episodes, they fail to show whether sickness time increased because more claims were filed or because on average the claims that were filed lasted longer. This is a key issue and a key distinction.

Death rates record the proportion of sickness episodes that end in death. That proportion might decline either because the number of sickness episodes diminished or because the average duration of sickness episodes increased. If the number of sickness episodes diminished, then it follows that declining death rates signal that the population has become healthier. Fewer people fell sick in the later period than in earlier periods, taking age and gender into account. Has health improved, however, if the rate of new sickness episodes decreased but the average duration of those episodes increased? In those circumstances it can be said that people fell sick less often, but when they did fall sick they were sick for longer periods.

Oddfellows actuaries attempted to measure both the incidence and the duration of sickness. To measure incidence they had to adopt conventions about how to distinguish episodes. When is a second sickness claim to be counted as a new episode and when as a relapse? Is sickness continuing into a new year a new episode? A consistent body of conventions was worked out by the first Oddfellows statistician, Henry Ratcliffe, who

32. Ibid., 74–77.

compiled data for three periods, 1846–48, 1856–60, and 1866–70. But Ratcliffe's successor, Watson, who studied patterns during 1893–97, altered the conventions, with the result that his inferences regarding sickness incidence cannot be compared with Ratcliffe's inferences on the same terms. Comparing the dissimilar measures, it appears that the incidence of sickness among the Oddfellows changed very little between 1866–70 and 1893–97.

Ratcliffe's and Watson's tables fail to show clearly how the incidence rate of sickness changed. But they do show very clearly that, among Oddfellows, the average duration of sickness episodes increased. Hence it is apparent that sickness time increased chiefly because the average episode lasted longer; its resolution, in recovery or death, was deferred. It is still not clear whether the incidence rate of sickness contributed to that effect or took away from it. Perhaps incidence also increased, albeit at a more modest rate. Perhaps incidence diminished. The trend of sickness incidence is an important issue because it weighs so heavily in interpreting the meaning of sickness. Sickness rates could rise because people had more sicknesses, holding everything else equal; because people and their doctors interpreted more experiences as sickness; or because sicknesses lasted longer.

To learn more about the form and force of changes in sickness rates, it is necessary to turn to the more detailed records of a single court where secretaries kept sickness ledgers, recording both the number of days for which benefits were paid and the timing of sickness episodes for each member. The records of one club, the AOF court situated in Abthorpe, a farming and shoe-making village near Northampton, have been reconstructed for each individual member. Across the period 1863–1922, Abthorpe Foresters accumulated 10,654.7 years at risk to sickness, a figure showing an average annual membership of 178 men. In those sixty years the members claimed 273,317 sickness days in 3,736 episodes. Hence the average episode lasted seventy-three days, about 10.5 weeks. But the average is pushed well above the mode—seven to fourteen working days—by a few very long sicknesses. For the typical member, comparatively brief sicknesses recurred intermittently through life. Only 160 of the 3,736 episodes ended in death. Hence the chances of dying while sick were less than one in twenty.[33]

33. One hundred sixty men died while sick, and an additional thirty-four died suddenly; their deaths are not counted as episodes.

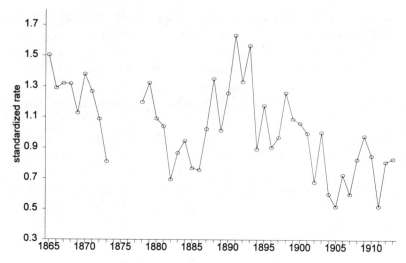

Fig. 6.10. Sickness Incidence among Abthorpe Foresters, 1865–1913
Source: Data from AOF, Abthorpe Court papers, ZA1586–1604, ZA1611.

Sickness incidence among the Abthorpe Foresters decreased sharply, as figure 6.10 shows for the period 1865–1912.[34] Watson failed to notice this trend because he counted each year within a protracted episode as a new sickness, artificially inflating the number of events as sickness duration rose. In sum, the Oddfellows actuarial studies indicate that sickness time increased only because episodes became more prolonged. Evidence from the Abthorpe Foresters, which measures incidents more accurately and for that reason is more convincing, shows that sickness time increased enough to offset a decline in new episodes. These men experienced longer sicknesses, even as they also experienced fewer sicknesses. Therefore, sickness time did not increase either because people fell sick more often or counted more episodes as sickness. It increased because the fewer sicknesses they reported each lasted longer.

LIFE EXPECTANCY AND HEALTH EXPECTANCY

Life expectancy measures the number of years people can be expected to live, while health expectancy assesses the number of years that will be spent in good health. Most people live many more years of wellness than of

34. The ledgers are incomplete for 1863–64, and the period after 1912 is omitted because national insurance changed the incentives.

sickness, so that health expectancy at birth is not many years less than life expectancy.

For friendly society members it is possible to calculate both values and, more to the point, to examine how they changed over time. Oddfellows actuaries provide the information necessary to make this calculation between two periods, 1866–70 and 1893–97. In that space of just less than three decades Oddfellows aged twenty-one added 2.3 years to their working life expectancy, an abridged measure that looks only at a working life from ages twenty-one to seventy-one.[35] Of that, they added 1.7 years of wellness and 0.6 years of sickness, so that nearly one-third of the gain was accounted for by sickness time. What is important to notice is that their sickness expectation was rising faster than their wellness expectation. The same calculations cannot be made for the Foresters, but it is apparent from the evidence discussed in this chapter that their experience closely paralleled that of the Oddfellows. For friendly society members in general, a small but rising share of time gained in life expectation was spent in sickness.

THE SICKEST SICK

Sorting and resorting the evidence at his disposal, Francis G. P. Neison Jr. found that he could divide the Foresters of 1871–75 into three groups: men who were not sick, men who were sick, and men who died. The patterns of sickness of each were distinctive. Figure 6.11 illustrates Neison's findings by showing four sickness curves and implying a fifth. The implied curve consists of the sickness record of men who were not sick during the survey period and whose sickness rates were zero at each age. The sicknesses of the sick raised those rates to the levels depicted in curve 1, which shows the average sickness time of all members. The average sickness time of members who were sick appears in curve 2, and that of the members who died in curve 3. As Neison could see, health problems were concentrated in a fraction of the AOF membership, and severe problems in a smaller fraction still. A total of 52.4 percent of the members had been sick at some point during the five years of the survey, and of course they accounted for all of the sickness. But the Foresters who died, who made up only 3.5 percent of the members, accounted for 19.7 percent of all sickness.[36]

35. Riley, "Working Health Time."
36. Neison, *Rates of Mortality and Sickness, 1871–1875*, 81–85. The proportions given here are based on years at risk.

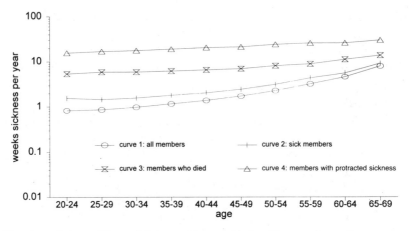

Fig. 6.11. Sickness Time of Sickness Groups, by Age Group, 1871–1875
Source: Data from Neison, *Rates of Mortality and Sickness, 1871–1875*, 35–36, 81–85.

Still more concentrated were the sicknesses of men who experienced protracted episodes. A total of 7,719 men had suffered protracted episodes, which Neison defined as sicknesses lasting at least a half year (twenty-six weeks). Their sickness time appears in figure 6.11 as curve 4. Neison could further identify 1,262 members who had been sick for the entire survey period, or up to their death during the survey period. Secretaries of individual courts answered his questions about the causes of these men's sicknesses, and the most common reasons were "limbs lost or broken through accident, blindness, lunacy, paralysis, rheumatism" and associated disorders.[37] But, as Neison further noted, the strongest determinant of protracted sickness that he could isolate was age. In young adulthood, at ages twenty to twenty-four, 93 percent of all sickness claims would take up twenty-six weeks or less. That proportion dropped steadily to 24.5 percent at ages seventy-five to seventy-nine, while the part of sickness lasting longer than a half year rose to 75.5 percent. Although Neison did not explore the point, his investigations do show the distribution of risk within the pool of members. A few Foresters would draw large sums from the sick fund. For them the fund would be a crucial means of support in their last sicknesses or for the prolonged convalescence and the disability

37. Ibid., 90–99, quote from 96. Neison counted all members sick for at least twenty-six weeks within a year as sick for twenty-six continuous weeks, though in fact that group would include some members who had suffered two or more independent spells.

associated with accidents, muscular disorders, and some other diseases.

Neison's investigations show the form of an important change in the pattern of health that occurs as a cohort ages. At birth most of the cohort is healthy, in that it is able to carry out activities associated with early infancy and lacks manifest signs of poor health. Only a small fraction—perhaps 1 percent—of a cohort displays anomalies that compromise health, even though many members may show temporary signs of sickness. As the cohort ages the fraction of people with congenital anomalies that compromise health shrinks, because so many members of that group die. But the share of the cohort showing signs of persistent ill health rises. The sickest sick, who among the Foresters accounted for such a large share of sickness time, emerge within the cohort. In this way the members of a cohort of Foresters divided into groups of the well and the sick, and the latter group grew as the men aged.

THE ECONOMIC TOLL OF SICKNESS

Building on work done earlier by William Farr, James Niven tried in 1911 to assess the costs of sickness to the British economy.[38] He had in mind a measurement based on the costs of sickness to the worker and the cost to the employer of work done poorly by a sick worker. James Burn Russell used friendly society sickness rates in a broader manner to estimate the daily prevalence of ill health among British adults and the costs of sickness to the British economy. Taking the aggregate Oddfellows average of nine working days lost per year to stand for the working population (males and females aged fifteen to sixty-five), Russell estimated that 572 thousand adults were absent from work because of sickness on any given day. Estimating wages at 10s. a week, he calculated the annual loss in wages at £14,886,000.[39] Russell believed that most of this sickness was preventable and sought to describe the conditions of life in Glasgow that caused excess sickness. For him the most important contributors to high morbidity and mortality were overcrowding, more than one adult per three hundred cubic feet of interior space; poor lighting and ventilation; inadequate privies; an unsatisfactory water supply; and lack of access to bathing and washing facilities.[40]

38. Niven, "Cost of Disease."
39. Russell, *Public Health Administration*, 291. On Russell, see Pennington, "Mortality, Public Health, and Medical Improvements."
40. Russell, *Public Health Administration*, 37–42.

Both Niven and Russell wanted to equate lost time with lost production or income and disregarded sickness as a source of employment: to perform the same work employers with higher sickness rates in their workforce will hire more workers than will employers with lower rates, even though their wage bill may be the same. Where employers pay no benefits to men out of work because of injuries or illnesses, which was the case for most workers in nineteenth-century Britain, costs of sickness are borne by the worker. The man or woman who did not belong to a friendly society carried the entire burden, aside from charity or poor law relief, while the worker who did belong to such a society shared this burden with fellow members. For most of them, even membership in a society that reliably paid benefits was not enough to cover the costs of sickness, because benefits totaled only a fraction of the wages lost. Since AOF members seldom received more than 40 percent of their wages in sickness benefits and got less than that if they were sick for long periods or if they earned high wages,[41] they carried the largest share of the financial burden of sickness. Assuming a rather low average wage of 3s. a day for adult males and compensation during sickness at 40 percent of that rate, or 1.2s. out of the 3s., then the cost to workers of their sicknesses was quite substantial. At an annual average of 636,688.4 days of sickness benefit among AOF members in 1871–75, the lost wages they had to absorb amounted to more than £57,000 for AOF members and a much larger figure for the working population as a whole.[42]

A rising trend of sickness time had several economic implications. At least among larger employers, it promoted higher rates of employment than would otherwise have obtained, because bosses had to hire more people to maintain the same level of staffing, and, for employers, it involved higher costs for training than would have obtained in a world of stable sickness. For workers, the rising trend of sickness time, especially when coupled with a shrinking real value of benefits,[43] meant a greater burden in making ends meet. They had to absorb larger and larger losses, compared to earlier counterparts. For the economy as a whole, rising sickness time threatened to cut into the discretionary buying power of working-class consumers. Both substitute workers, who filled in for the sick, and the sick themselves experienced rising sickness time and therefore had less to spend.

41. See chapter 5.
42. Neison, *Rates of Mortality and Sickness, 1871–1875,* 12, supplies the number of weeks lost for the five-year period 1871–75.
43. See chapter 3.

That development was countered to some degree by rising proportions of workers belonging to friendly societies. As that proportion grew so did the share of the labor force that received some compensation for lost wages.

Nevertheless, rising sickness time counteracted some part of the trend of rising real wages and left working people with less discretionary spending power than they would have had if the lower sickness time of the 1870s had continued to prevail. The British economy suffered not so much because employers and firms lost the productivity of workers, as Niven and Russell argued, but because workers had to absorb so much of the cost of sickness absence.

SICKNESS, MORTALITY, AND ECONOMIC TRENDS

Current explanations of mortality decline in England and Wales in the decades following the 1870s emphasize three contributing forces and assign little importance to a fourth. In the mainstream interpretation, higher life expectancy is explained by a rising standard of living and by improvements in public health amenities. Some scholars have argued that what mattered most within the rising standard of living was the quantity of food, insofar as better nutrition improved resistance to disease.[44] Few scholars any longer assign importance to medical therapy, which for a long time had been accepted as a major contributor to lower mortality.

These conclusions rest heavily on the association observed between mortality and certain economic indicators, especially real wages and per capita income, and on knowledge about the timing of public health reforms, especially improvements in urban sewerage collection and water purification made in the 1870s and thereafter. In England and Wales the decline of mortality coincided with rises in wages and income. The coincidence was so close, and the theoretical grounds for expecting higher income to provide people with ways to reduce hazards to survival so strong, that the conclusion that a better standard of living promoted lower mortality seems unavoidable.

Figure 6.12 plots changes over time in the three measures of health

44. See especially McKeown, *Modern Rise of Population*, where the case for food quantity is put and reasons given for rejecting the idea that medical therapies helped lessen mortality; and Fogel, "Conquest of High Mortality and Hunger." Guha, "Importance of Social Intervention," finds grounds for the case for a nutrition link in the declining lethality of diseases.

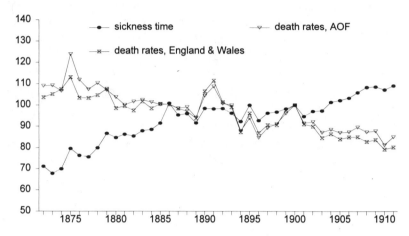

Fig. 6.12. Index of Sickness Time and Mortality, 1872–1911 (1900 = 100)
Source: Data from AOF, *Directories,* 1873–1911.

status discussed above—sickness time and mortality in the AOF and mortality among adult males in England and Wales. Figures 6.13–6.15 plot some economic indicators. Figure 6.13 shows trends in the cost of living and three leading items within it: food, clothing, and alcohol and tobacco. Food and clothing prices, and the cost of living as a whole, dropped sharply from the 1870s into the 1890s, then rose. The falling prices of the period up to 1895 suggest that consumers were spending smaller and smaller portions of their income for the same quantity and quality of food and clothing. These relative gains created an opportunity to spend more on items that enhanced survival prospects or on other things. But consumers had to spend more on rents and taxes, as figure 6.14 shows. Nevertheless, prices in general rose at a slower pace than did wages. Expressed in constant values, wages increased up to the latter 1890s. Until nearly 1900, workingmen in England and Wales shared the economy's gains. Gross domestic product per capita and wages alike increased. Throughout, unemployment remained highly variable, as figure 6.15 shows by converting unemployment rates into index numbers.

These figures suggest, in sum, that workingmen and their families gained, at least into the 1890s, by getting control over a larger share of their income to spend as they elected. How they spent this share may have influenced their survival. Higher taxes paid for water and sewerage improvements. Working people may also have bought more spacious housing, more or better food, soap, and detergents, additional changes of clothing, and other items that improved their survival prospects. But it is

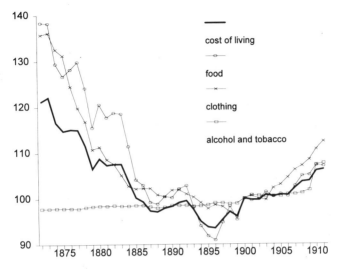

Fig. 6.13. Index of Prices of Consumption Items, 1872–1911 (1900 = 100)
Source: Data from Feinstein, "New Look at the Cost of Living," 170–71.

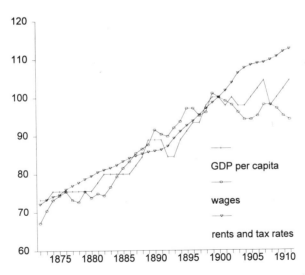

Fig. 6.14. Index of GDP, Wages, and Rents, 1872–1911 (1900 = 100)
Source: Data from Feinstein, *Statistical Tables,* T42–43, T140; Feinstein, "New Look at the Cost of Living," 170–71.

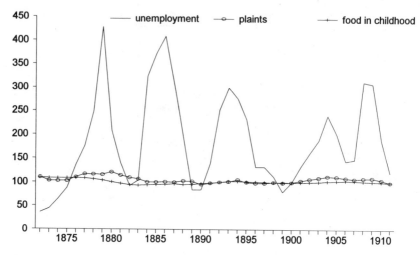

Fig. 6.15. Index of Unemployment, Plaints, and Food Prices in Childhood, 1872–1911 (1900 = 100)
Source: Data from Feinstein, *Statistical Tables*, T125–26; Johnson, "Small Debts and Economic Distress in England and Wales," 65–87 (with a series of plaints supplied by Johnson's collaborator, Humphrey Southall); Mitchell, *British Historical Statistics*, 722–23.

important to notice that the trend toward lower mortality continued after the late 1890s, when real wages began to shrink. It is also important to notice that mortality fluctuated without describing a trend in the period 1885–1900, whereas real wages and thus discretionary spending power rose during most of those years. At first glance, economic gains— improvements in the living standard—look like a powerful force behind gains in survivorship across the whole period. Upon closer inspection, they seem to have had much less power after 1885 than before. From visual inspection of these trends, economic explanations for the mortality decline lose power.

In figure 6.12 the trend of sickness time is nearly a mirror image of mortality. It rose in the first phase, when mortality declined; it fluctuated without describing a trend in the second phase, when mortality did the same; and in the third phase it rose again as mortality declined. This inverse association suggests that mortality change may have been responsible for some portion of the changes in sickness time. An inverse association did not obtain, except perhaps in rural England and Wales, from the 1840s to the 1870s, and in the years 1885–1900 sickness time changes from year to year generally tracked mortality changes rather than running inverse to them. More was going on than the more prolonged survival of men with fatal sicknesses, even though, as the actuaries concluded, that was itself an important development in patterns of health.

The strong trends apparent in figures 6.12–6.14 complicate the task of using statistical means to determine which economic forces were associated with sickness time and mortality by giving an artificial addition of power to explanatory variables that, like sickness time and mortality, exhibit strong trends. The standard way out of this dilemma is to extract the trend and search for associations that remain.[45] These factors are under consideration: unemployment, the level of real wages, an index of small-debt plaints developed recently by Paul Johnson and Humphrey Southall as a gauge of economic distress, and food prices in the early life of AOF members, a variable included to look for a deferred effect of nutritional deprivation.[46] The detailed results appear in appendix 3.

For sickness time the most important implication from this statistical analysis is that economic forces played a small role in year-to-year varia-

45. In the initial forms of the model the dependent variables—sickness time and mortality in the AOF and mortality among adult males in England and Wales—are suspected of being associated with unemployment, real wages, the rate of plaints for small debts, and prices thirty-five years earlier. Three more complex forms of the autoregressive model are discussed here:

1. $ST = f(STlag1 + STlag2 + DR + Unem + Unemlag1 + Unemlag2 + Wage + Failindx + Prcmvav)$
2. $DR = f(DRlag1 + DRlag2 + Unem + Unemlag1 + Unemlag2 + Wage + Failindx + Prcmvav)$ and
3. $EWDR = f(EWDRlag1 + EWDRlag2 + Unem + Unemlag1 + Unemlag2 + Wage + Failindx + Prcmvav)$

where:
ST = sickness time
DR = mortality in the AOF
$EWDR$ = mortality of adult males in England and Wales
$UNEM$ = the unemployment rate in those trades reporting such information
$Wage$ = the real wage
$Failindx$ = the rate of plaints for recovery of small debts
$Prcmvav$ = an eleven-year moving average of food prices centered on thirty-five years earlier and
$lag1 \ldots lag2$ = lagged forms of individual variables.
In each case, lagged versions of the dependent variable are included as a means of detrending.

46. Feinstein, *Statistical Tables*, T18–19, T42–43, T125–26, and T140; Feinstein, "New Look at the Cost of Living," 170–71; Johnson, "Small Debts and Economic Distress in England and Wales" (with the series of plaints supplied by Johnson's collaborator, Humphrey Southall); Mitchell, *British Historical Statistics*, 12–13 and 722–23; and AOF, *Directories, 1872–1911*. In addition, on unemployment consult Burnett, *Idle Hands*, esp. 149–53. The average of the average ages of AOF members rose from 32.6 years in 1872 to 36 years in 1896. Here, the food price variable consists of a moving average of prices thirty-five years earlier. Humphrey Southall supplied me with an annual series of small-debt plaints in England and Wales, which I turned into a rate by dividing it by the population.

tions. Higher unemployment can be associated with higher sickness time, perhaps because some AOF members pleaded sickness when in fact they were out of work but not sick and certainly because the stress of losing a job and being unemployed added to sickness. But the contribution of unemployment was small. Higher mortality appears to add to higher sickness time, although in terms of statistical significance the association is marginal. What is implied is that years of high mortality often coincided with years of heavy sickness, but the two did not coincide systematically. Other associations are weak.

For mortality it is possible to analyze the same variables for two outcomes: mortality in the AOF and mortality among adult males in England and Wales. Both forms suggest quite similar things. Higher wages promoted lower mortality: over time, men earning more were able to improve their safeguards to death. Similarly, a higher rate of plaints to recover small debts—mostly shopkeepers entering claims against working-class customers who had run up bills—can be associated with lower mortality. As Southall and Gilbert suggest, the plaints appear to have been filed when times were improving and when, therefore, shopkeepers thought their chances of recovering debts were higher.[47] In that case, the plaint index serves less as a measure of economic distress, as was initially intended, than as a gauge of recovery. The association suggests that, in periods of recovery in working-class household finance, men could find ways to further limit the mortality risks they faced. Too much cannot be made of this association, but it does suggest an interesting hypothesis: the capacity of workingmen to control mortality risk waxed and waned with their own business cycle, in ways independent of unemployment. Higher unemployment—both in the same year and in previous years—is associated with lower mortality. The association is not statistically significant, but it is consistent in scale and sign, which tends to undermine the idea that unemployment in the few trades for which data have yet been recovered signaled higher risks to survival among workingmen in general.

This statistical analysis also gives implied support to the idea that AOF experience is a representative microcosm of the experience of adult males in general. In the visual analysis, shown in figure 6.12, it can be seen that AOF mortality closely tracked adult male mortality in England and Wales. That impression is affirmed in appendix 3, where the same variables are seen to have closely similar associations with the two mortality outcomes.

47. Southall and Gilbert, "A Good Time to Wed."

In sum, the detrended time series analysis suggests that higher wages and the phase at which a working-class household stood in its business cycle played an important role in mortality in the period 1872–1911. Except for unemployment, however, economic forces had a smaller part to play in sickness time. There, the effect noticed may be chiefly a sign of the health consequences of losing a job or being out of work.

POPULATION FRAILTY

Several commentators have suggested that sickness rates may change over time as mortality alters the composition of the population with respect to its susceptibility to health risks, a characteristic called frailty. Such effects have been posited at advanced ages when, it is sometimes held, the frailest members of a population have died and those who remain are markedly more vigorous. In that form, the hypothesis attempts to explain why survival rates do not continue to decrease in old age at the stable pace usually observed at ages forty-five to sixty-five or so but instead decrease at a lower rate. However, it is also possible that what changes at advanced ages is not the composition of the population with respect to frailty but the reliability of statements about age. If, as many researchers suspect, people increasingly overstate their ages as they grow old, then survivorship may only appear to decrease at a lower rate.

Another case where population composition unambiguously changes in ways that alter the level of frailty is provided by some epidemics. People who are particularly susceptible to falling sick die in unusually large numbers in certain epidemics, carrying off a disproportionate share of the frail. In those circumstances the population's level of frailty drops during the epidemic but gradually recovers in subsequent months. For a time, mortality, and presumably also sickness, are distorted by deviations in population frailty.[48]

If death rates can be distorted by changes in the composition of a population in certain circumstances, then sickness rates, too, may sometimes deviate because of changes in population frailty rather than because of actual changes in health experience. In the present case there is little question of age misrepresentation, because the ages of friendly society members were recorded in young adulthood, when there is no tendency to exaggerate age.

48. Foster, "Are Cohort Mortality Rates Autocorrelated?"

In nineteenth-century Britain declining mortality added "new survivors" to the population, people who would have died in the earlier mortality regime but who lived longer in the new regime. New survivors cannot be identified individually, but they appear on average to have experienced more sickness time than their counterparts, the "old survivors." Hence, population frailty did change because of mortality, if not also for other reasons. It rose.

Early analyses of frailty viewed it as a characteristic fixed at birth and interpreted later changes in population frailty as an effect of shocks or other circumstances that promoted higher mortality among frailer individuals. If frailty quotients are present at birth, it is also likely that life experiences add or take away from each individual's risk of death or sickness.[49] Insults, which add to the frailty quotient, may accumulate. Life experiences such as vaccinations and some types of surgery augment an individual's ability to resist sickness or defer death. The degree to which levels of frailty actually changed in Britain in the period under study here is, of course, outside observation.

The principal way that frailty enters this study lies in the inference that decreasing mortality contributed to rising sickness time. Sickness time increased at each age not because the physical environment deteriorated, making people sick more often, but at least in substantial part because people's susceptibility to being sick rose. Frailty rose in two chief forms. First, there was some substitution of maladies, chronic diseases taking the place of acute diseases. Sickness time rose as the disease profile shifted more toward protracted maladies, an issue that is explored in more depth in the following chapter. In that case, added frailty took the form of fewer sickness events—that is, sickness incidence retreated—but more sickness time. Second, friendly society members survived longer when sick. In that case, added frailty took the form of additional survival time for people in the midst of fatal episodes.

The finding in this chapter that sickness incidence declined is crucial. It shows that the disease and injury environment was improving, a finding consistent with what is known about mortality, economic gains, public health improvements, changes in behavior, and other factors that should have enhanced people's health. A leading form that better health took was the enhanced survival of the sick, as well as an enhanced capacity to avoid

49. Manton and Stallard, *Recent Trends in Mortality Analysis;* and Alter and Riley, "Frailty, Sickness, and Death."

becoming sick in the first place. AOF records document the growing capacity of workingmen to be sick rather than dead.

Sicknesses became more protracted among friendly society members in the period 1872–1911 and probably also among men in Britain in general. The decline of mortality among adults, which augmented life expectancy, added both years of wellness and years of sickness. For friendly society members, as for adults in general, the years already lived had been overwhelmingly years of wellness. But the years added were more evenly divided between wellness and sickness. Among them, sickness time accumulated faster than wellness time.

The mortality decline added to the population men who fell sick less often yet stayed sick for longer periods, men whose deaths were deferred but more often in sickness than in wellness. As sickness time increased, workers had to absorb a growing burden of lost wages. For friendly society members the burden was shared between the sick and the well, but sickness benefits covered less than half of the wages lost. Individually, the sick had much less to spend than did the well and much less economic power to avoid the hazards to survival usually grouped under the heading of standard of living. As a group their numbers increased, so that for the society as a whole increased sickness time meant a depletion of discretionary spending. Over time, higher wages provided some means to protect against threats to survival, an effect that shows up in more protracted sickness. Sickness meant a loss of economic power, because benefits amounted to only a fraction of wages. Even a fraction, however, was better than what men who did not belong to friendly societies received. Unless relieved by charity or the poor law, they had to work when sick; if forced to give up work, they earned nothing.

The patterns of health experienced by the Foresters can be measured over time and can be assessed in three ways. The decline of mortality among them, and the fall in sickness incidence in the Abthorpe court, a telling case study, suggest that health improved. Men lived longer, and they fell sick less often. The evidence about sickness time seems at first glance to contradict this portrayal. Men lived longer and spent more time sick. More sickness time meant that the gains in life expectancy were counterbalanced in some degree by survival time spent in sickness rather than wellness. But the larger point is that men in the AOF and other friendly societies survived to be sick, rather than dying earlier.

CHAPTER 7

Sickness Profiles,
Sickness Thresholds,
Sickness Hazards

SICKNESS DESCRIBED its own trends in nineteenth- and early-twentieth-century Britain, separate from the trend of mortality. Sickness also possessed its own profile of causes, one that overlapped the causes of death that have figured importantly in reconstructing patterns of sickness in that period but was also distinct from the mortality profile. Did the sickness and mortality profiles differ because of the sickness threshold? That is, did the workingmen whose ailments can be recovered plead sickness and enter claims only for maladies bearing a high risk of death or associated with serious discomfort? Or was the sickness profile different because of epidemiologic factors?

Friendly society advisors, especially the actuaries, worried about accepting as members men who practiced trades that exposed them to unusual health risks. The investigation of occupational health showed both the existence of grades of risk and, over the later nineteenth century, a closure of differences among them. The results of these investigations can be used to divide commonplace occupations into categories of occupations more or less likely to bear a heavy burden of sickness and to explore which trades brought stable or even improving and which deteriorating health conditions as their practitioners aged.

PROFILES OF SICKNESS AND DEATH

Sickness profiles, unlike profiles of causes of death, are shaped by the threshold employed to distinguish wellness from sickness. Each point of entry into sickness—self-medication or treatment, consulting a doctor, seeking the club doctor's certification to declare on friendly society benefits, or entering a hospital, among others—captures a different perspective. Friendly society testimony already discussed suggests that workingmen who were not friendly society members did not call a doctor in the earliest stages of illness but waited until their malady was serious.[1] If this is true, then records of doctors' consultations with such people would contain an unobserved waiting period, during which some recovered and some remained sick to the point where they consulted a doctor.

A waiting period is suggested also in some hospital records. At the Gloucester County Hospital, where summary statistics were compiled for the period 1834–44, most in-patients had suffered from their ailments for months, sometimes even years, before entering the hospital. Among 148 men and women admitted for treatment of skin diseases, for example, the illness had lasted an average of two years and three months. In-patient treatment took an average of four and a half months.[2] If this information is more or less accurate, and that depends on the probably defective memory of patients admitted, then it follows that for some maladies most of the sickness episode goes unobserved in hospital records even when they carefully remark dates of admission and discharge. At Gloucester, the proportions were summed in three categories. For accidents the average treatment lasted one month three weeks and followed immediately on the injury. But for surgical cases treatment made up only 16 percent of the average duration of a reported episode, and for medical cases only 21 percent.

Friendly society records, too, portray sicknesses after a brief waiting period of three to six days, three days in the AOF. Members could not claim benefits until their sickness had lasted through the waiting period, whereupon they were compensated for all the sickness time. In such circumstances it is difficult to compare patterns of sickness representing different thresholds—from the hospital to the friendly society—on terms similar enough to lead to meaningful conclusions. Hospitals served much smaller numbers of individuals in sickness than did friendly societies, and they served them under a sharply different definition of sickness. Here the coverage focuses on records of work time lost because of sickness and on the profile of sicknesses suggested by the friendly society threshold.

Many of the same diseases and injuries caused sickness as caused death

1. See chapter 2.
2. Gloucester County Hospital, in-patient records, 17563.

in nineteenth- and early-twentieth-century Britain. The two profiles differ not so much in the identity of the ailments as in their relative importance. Some diseases loomed much larger as causes of death than as causes of sickness, and the reverse is also true. To explore these differences, data have been collected to construct three profiles. The first is the most familiar. It derives from the causes of death reported to the registrar general in 1908, a not atypical year in the midst of a period in which far more precious data have been gathered from manuscript sources about causes of sickness. The second relates the causes of sickness identified in three friendly society sources dating from 1906–14 and 1919, intentionally excluding years of war. The third shows causes of sickness among men working for the Great North of Scotland Railway in the period 1902–13. Not much is known about the social lives of these railway employees, but it is likely that some belonged to friendly societies and some did not.

The three profiles may capture three different views of the health problems workingmen faced. The registrar general's report, which provides separate statistics for deaths at ages fifteen and above for each of 188 causes, shows the diseases and injuries likeliest to cause the deaths of adult males from all social classes. Some of the diseases and injuries listed there have been combined for this comparison, and the most far-reaching combination allocates all accidental deaths to a single category. Table 7.1 lists eleven leading causes among the 169,334 deaths that occurred in 1908 to males aged fifteen and up.[3] Together, these eleven causes accounted for 75.8 percent of deaths, which is an initial signal that deaths among adults were attributed to a narrower range of causes than deaths among children, a range that excluded most infectious diseases.

Although heart disease and tuberculosis lead this list, closer inspection of the data shows how important respiratory diseases other than tuberculosis were. Together, pneumonia and bronchitis accounted for 14.2 percent of all deaths, nearly the same proportion as the leading cause of death, heart disease. Four respiratory diseases together—tuberculosis, bronchitis, pneumonia, and influenza—account for nearly the same proportion of all deaths as do the organ diseases taken together—heart disease, can-

3. The next leading cause accounted for less than 2 percent of all deaths. Valvular disease, angina pectoris, dilation of the heart, fatty degeneration of the heart, syncope, and unspecified heart diseases are combined in the category *heart disease,* and pulmonary tuberculosis, phthisis, and other forms of tuberculosis are combined in the category *tuberculosis.*

During 1910–12, the closest available dates, men aged fifteen and up in occupational categories III–VIII, skilled workmen to agricultural laborers, showed virtually identical distributions. Great Britain, *Mortality of Men in Certain Occupations,* 4–6.

Table 7.1
LEADING CAUSES OF DEATH IN ENGLAND
AND WALES IN 1908

Cause	Percent of total
Heart disease	14.26
Tuberculosis	13.88
Old age	8.30
Cancer	8.13
Bronchitis	7.20
Pneumonia	6.97
Cerebral hemorrhage	4.64
Accidents	4.58
Chronic Bright's disease, albuminuria	3.12
Influenza	2.56
Apoplexy	2.18

Source: Data from Great Britain, Registrar General of Births, Deaths, and Marriages, *Seventy-First Annual Report* (1909), 291–310, using the data for males only.

cer, cerebral hemorrhage, chronic Bright's disease, and apoplexy. This list testifies to the general importance of respiratory disease, but it is also probably the case, as Arthur Newsholme argued, that doctors often did not recognize tuberculosis until it reached an advanced stage, diagnosing it earlier as bronchitis.[4]

In recording the sicknesses of their members, many friendly societies used preprinted books containing a column for cause of sickness. Few secretaries consistently entered information in this column. Some entered causes occasionally, most probably in ways that bias any attempt to use those entries to compile an inventory of causes of sickness. They mentioned most often a few diseases, such as influenza. The likelihood of finding diseases identified in friendly society records increases with time, presumably because the societies became more accustomed to asking the club doctor not merely to certify sickness but also to identify it, and the secretary copied that identification from the doctor's certification slip into the society's sickness ledger. In the mid-nineteenth century doctors typically signed a certification without giving a diagnosis, but by the end of the century they often added diagnostic information.

Other secretaries seem to have asked the sick member about the cause of his sickness. That would explain why the Oddfellows found it necessary to

4. Newsholme, *Fifty Years in Public Health,* 264.

Table 7.2
LEADING CAUSES OF SICKNESS IN THREE FRIENDLY SOCIETIES, 1896–1919

Cause	Proportion of cases (percent) (1)	Average duration (in days) (2)	Prevalence (1) × (2) (3)
Accidents	15.78	33.4	527.1
Poorly identified	13.48	38.7	521.7
Influenza and catarrh	13.30	20.6	274.0
Bronchitis	8.69	58.3	506.6
Rheumatism	3.72	54.4	202.4
Lumbago	3.55	35.0	124.3
Gastritis	2.48	33.1	82.1
Carbuncle	1.59	12.0	19.1
Tonsillitis	1.42	20.7	29.4
Skin ulcers	1.42	68.7	97.6

Source: Data from Bristol City Sick Benefit and Dividing Friendly Society papers, 40126/f/1/b, ledger of contributions and sick pay, 1919; AOF, Abthorpe Court papers, ZA1600, benefits, 1896–1910; and IOOF, Loyal Vale of Clun Lodge papers, 1927/1, resolution book, 1908–14.

publish Carruthers Corfield's *A Handbook of Medical Terms* and why the *Foresters' Miscellany* mentioned *The Family Physician* as a source of information about health.[5] In the expanded edition of 1892, *The Family Physician* provides a dictionary of diseases and treatments. It would have been helpful in clarifying a garbled disease identification, but club secretaries could not easily have constructed an accurate diagnosis from nothing more than a list of symptoms. Uncertainty about the diagnosis may explain why even sickness ledgers compiled after 1900 contain a significant number of cases where the diagnosis column has been left blank or where the ailment is described by symptoms.

Table 7.2 combines information from three sources that report causes for most sickness episodes, giving the leading causes of sickness among 564 members of friendly societies in Bristol, Abthorpe (Northamptonshire), and Clun (Shropshire).[6] The age profile of members of two of the three societies is unknown, but the evidence clearly indicates that they were, on average, older than the adult male population in general.[7] Thus

5. Respectively, Corfield, *Handbook of Medical Terms;* and *Foresters' Miscellany,* Sept. 1887, 272. The reference is to *Family Physician* (1866) or perhaps a later edition (London, [1873]).

6. Since the longest sickness episode in this sample lasted a year, it is likely that some cases reported in these sources are truncated.

7. Abthorpe Foresters averaged 56.13 years of age in the period when their ailments were recorded.

Table 7.3
LEADING CAUSES OF SICKNESS ABSENCE AMONG GREAT NORTH OF SCOTLAND
RAILWAY EMPLOYEES, 1902–1913

Cause	Proportion (percent) (1)	Average duration (in days) (2)	Prevalence (1) × (2) (3)
Poorly identified	23.9	11.9	284.4
Accidents	21.3	20.6	438.8
Influenza and catarrh	15.6	9.5	148.2
Colds	7.3	7.8	56.9
Lumbago	2.1	12.0	25.2
Rheumatism	2.0	20.9	41.8
Bronchitis	1.7	27.8	47.3
Tonsillitis	1.0	10.7	10.7
Sore throat	1.0	9.6	9.6
Appendicitis	0.9	32.3	29.1
Measles	0.9	9.7	8.7

Source: Data from Great North of Scotland Railway Passenger Department papers, register of staff off duty, vol. 2, 1902–13.

their sicknesses should be expected to have lasted longer than would be the case in a stratified sample, and the profile of ailments must also accentuate the maladies of older men, especially in its inclusion of rheumatism, lumbago, and skin ulcers. In this profile ten causes account for 65.4 percent of the total, signaling that for sicknesses, too, the range of recognized maladies among adults was restricted. Here the data can be arranged in two ways. The primary ranking in table 7.2 groups ailments according to incidence, which implies that the diseases and injuries that occur in the largest numbers of people are the most important. A secondary ranking, constructed by weighting the diseases by their duration, appears in column 2 of table 7.2. That ranking, which more successfully captures the effects of sickness time on an economy, elevates the importance of bronchitis and skin ulcers. Sicknesses in those categories were unusually protracted; they contributed significantly more to the average duration of sicknesses, and thus to sickness prevalence, than they did to incidence.

Officials of the Great North of Scotland Railway kept registers of staff who went off duty for health reasons in the period 1897 to 1926, and the second volume in the series, dealing with 2,655 cases in 1902–13, is summarized in table 7.3.[8] Although ages of some individuals can be recov-

8. The register reveals the name of the employee who went off duty, his post, the date he

ered from other sources within the collection, most of the approximately six hundred separate men who appear in the register cannot be assigned an age. It is nevertheless clear that they were younger than men in the sample of three friendly societies, and their sicknesses were shorter. Furthermore, sicknesses of short duration figure more prominently in the railway employees sample, in which ailments were recorded even when they did not lead to work absence and in which many employees lost work for fewer days than were required to qualify for friendly society benefits.

All these profiles exhibit uncertainty surrounding identification of some causes of death and sickness, cause-of-death statistics in the form of entries for "old age," and cause-of-sickness data in the category "poorly identified," which combines cases left blank, those assigned to ailments that were described by their signs and symptoms, and other ill-defined conditions. For the rest, and despite differences in age and the circumstances of work loss, the sickness profiles are remarkable both for their similarity to one another and for their distinctiveness from the profile of causes of death in 1908.

Adult males in England and Wales in 1908 died chiefly as a result of organ disease. Table 7.1 probably understates that by assigning such a large proportion of deaths to old age, a category likely to include additional cases of heart and circulatory diseases and neoplasms.[9] In contrast, both sickness profiles accentuate respiratory diseases, musculature disorders, and accidents.[10] Together, those categories accounted for 45 percent of all sicknesses in the friendly society sample, and 50 percent in the railway sample, but only 35 percent among 1,908 causes of death. Tuberculosis in one form or another was often listed as a cause of death, but it does not often appear in either sickness profile. Given the stigma associated with it, this diagnosis may have been withheld from the sufferer and therefore also from his employer or friendly society.

But it is also possible that, except in its final stage, tuberculosis did not always disable men for work. In Southall's mapping of the trajectories of sickness among a few engineering workers in the 1830s and 1840s, what is

went off duty, the date he returned, and the disease or injury that occasioned work loss. Individuals who went off duty for reasons other than sickness are not considered. For example, A. Will ran away. Where two or more ailments were identified, the case was classified by the first. Cases of catarrh are joined with influenza and German measles with measles; three varieties of colds—ordinary, severe, and bad—are combined.

Leneman, "Lives and Limbs," analyzes injuries.

9. Gage, "Decline of Mortality in England and Wales."

10. Among schoolteachers in the same period, too, respiratory diseases led as causes of sickness. See Hart, "Investigation of Sickness Data," 351.

striking is, first, the prolonged course of sickness among men who died of tuberculosis and, second, the merely intermittent occurrence of work loss in the months and years before death.[11] Tuberculosis was a chronic but not necessarily a disabling disease, and it was a disease that began with vague symptoms: listlessness and chest pains. Arthur Newsholme maintained that successful diagnosis needed "a skilled overhauling of each patient with persistent and repeated cough" but did not explain further what should be looked for.[12] Only gradually, after months or longer, did tuberculosis advance to the distinctive final symptoms: coughing, purulent sputum, fever, and light sweating.[13]

Tables 7.1–7.3 suggest further that accidents resulting in cuts, broken bones, and other damage played the leading role in well-identified causes of sickness but a much smaller role as causes of death. They also show how large muscular disorders loomed in the everyday working life of adult males in the early twentieth century. Men were often sick with rheumatism or lumbago, but they did not often die from those disorders. All three tables show profiles in which infectious diseases played only a modest part.

Adding duration to the ranking of important sicknesses changes the rank order. It does not, however, change the composition of the leading causes of sickness in either the friendly society or the railway profile. Although in full form each profile contains other maladies, none was sufficiently protracted to promote it to these lists. The inference to be drawn is not only that the duration profile of causes of sickness differed from the profile of causes of death but also that the incidence of diseases causing sickness differed substantially from that of diseases causing death.

Finally, these tables suggest two forms of *epidemiologic transition,* a

11. Southall, "Morbidity and Mortality among Early-Nineteenth-Century Engineering Workers." Tuberculosis patients were often advised to exercise, and during the second and third decades of the twentieth century one leading therapy put patients to work. See Bryder, *Below the Magic Mountain,* 157–73.

12. Newsholme, *Fifty Years in Public Health,* 264.

13. Smith, *The People's Health,* 287–88. Smith (291–92) cites three case studies in which the patient continued to work after a diagnosis of tuberculosis but argues (291) that "breadwinner victims [of tuberculosis] had to cease working long before they died."

The interpretation that it did not always disable is suggested also by the patterns of sickness and mortality of London customs agents in the period 1857–74 in reports filed by their medical officer, Walter Dickson, who presumably identified tuberculosis (phthisis) even when he did not reveal that diagnosis to his patient. Among customs agents, phthisis accounted for 31 percent of all deaths but only 1.4 percent of the number of sicknesses and 8 percent of sickness time. Rheumatism and associated diseases, in contrast, caused only 0.4 percent of deaths but 14 percent of time lost from work. Dickson, *On the Numerical Ratio of Disease,* 8. Ballard, "Report," 10, provides some additional information about the disease profile in Islington in the years 1857–68.

term coined to describe the passage from a regime of causes of death led by infectious diseases to a regime led by degenerative diseases.[14] In the mortality transition, infectious diseases had already lost place as a leading cause of death among adult males well before 1900; respiratory diseases, which had become dominant in the nineteenth century, were waning in force; and organ diseases were taking over. Tuberculosis dropped sharply as a cause of death in the first decades of the twentieth century.[15] In the sickness transition, however, infectious diseases played little part by the early twentieth century in the sicknesses that men suffered, while respiratory diseases still loomed large. Taking the respiratory diseases together, they did not account for as large a proportion of all causes of sickness as did respiratory diseases among causes of death. But they did account for the largest category, surpassing accidents, the poorly identified group comprising organ diseases, musculature diseases, and infections. As well, they continued to account for a large share of sickness for several decades into the new century.[16]

One medical diarist who commented on the profile of his patients' ailments, Harry Pearson Taylor, who practiced in the Shetlands, reported that they suffered from much the same maladies in the 1940s as in the 1890s.[17] At each step of the mortality transition, from infectious to respiratory and from respiratory to chronic organ diseases, a new profile emerged chiefly because the hazards associated with leading causes of death in the old profile diminished, allowing another part of the underlying structure of mortality to come into prominence.

Two important conclusions, one familiar and one not, follow. The shift from short to long illnesses and from infectious to chronic diseases, which is what the epidemiologic transition in its conventional meaning describes, proposes that sicknesses must have become more prolonged. In this sense the epidemiologic transition predicts that sickness time increased while mortality decreased, insofar at least as the greater length of sickness episodes outran their smaller number. This prediction is upheld by the sickness profiles examined here. The maladies that friendly society members and railway workers contracted in the early years of the twentieth century, especially bronchitis and rheumatism, often required prolonged convales-

14. Omran, "Epidemiologic Transition"; and Riley and Alter, "Epidemiologic Transition and Morbidity." Smith, "Health," describes specific features of change in Britain.
15. Bryder, *Below the Magic Mountain*, 1–2, 7.
16. Fry, *Profiles of Disease*, 10–11.
17. Taylor, *Shetland Parish Doctor*, 72.

cence. These chronic episodes weighed more heavily in the overall profile of sickness.

Second, the new profile dominated by organ diseases emerged more slowly in relation to sickness than in relation to death. Taken together, organ diseases waxed in prominence as causes of death into the twentieth century, while respiratory diseases waned. As causes of death these prevailing diseases were controlled not by means that reduced susceptibility but by means that promoted recovery. In other words, the evidence gathered here implies not only that the sick gained access to some means of controlling the resolution of respiratory diseases but also that the way the sick and perhaps also their doctors dealt with sicknesses mattered more than did modes of controlling exposure. Anne Hardy has pointed out that the leading adult infectious diseases of the second half of the nineteenth century were amenable to preventive intervention, whereas the leading childhood infections were not.[18] The evidence introduced here suggests that explanations for the reduction in adult mortality should attend to both prevention and treatment but also that they should be focused on disease management. With the help of their doctors, working people learned how to manage many of the respiratory and organ diseases they contracted.[19] For adult diseases, and perhaps also for injuries, the most significant change in the latter decades of the nineteenth century was neither the prevention nor the cure of sickness. It was, instead, the management of sickness in such a way that episodes that formerly ended in death carried forward through a longer duration.

THE SERIOUSNESS OF SICKNESS: THRESHOLDS THEN AND NOW

Between the nineteenth century and the present, it is sometimes argued (or more often assumed), people came to take their sicknesses more seriously, specifically, to act as though they were sick in circumstances that would not have induced their counterparts in the earlier period to act sick. Dividing patients into categories of traditional and modern, Edward Shorter claims that "traditional patients sought treatment or took time off for relatively few of their symptoms: only the most alarming ones, such as

18. Hardy, *Epidemic Streets*, 290.
19. Bynum, *Science and the Practice of Medicine*, 226, discusses doctors' success at managing tuberculosis, which certainly played a role in the rising average duration of sickness time and the length of sickness episodes. But tuberculosis was not the only disease being managed.

coughing up blood or abdominal edema, or only the most disabling ones, such as broken bones or immobile joints." He believes that, in a transitional stage, which began early in the nineteenth century, patients developed greater sensitivity to bodily symptoms and gained more confidence in the doctor's ability to cure. Only after 1960 did patients define symptoms as illness and regularly seek help for their illnesses.[20] For Shorter, the nineteenth century was an important period of transition, in which patients lowered the threshold at which they considered themselves sick. But the blatant changes in threshold did not occur until after 1960, when there was an enormous increase in the variety of symptoms for which patients sought relief. In sum, Shorter fashions a metahistory in which dramatic contrasts should exist between the complaints people made when they missed work or consulted doctors in the nineteenth century and the complaints they made after 1960.

Sheila Johansson makes this argument in another form. Her view is that sickness rates rise because of "the cultural inflation of morbidity": people report more diseases, but the diseases are less severe.[21] According to Shorter, sickness rates rise because people count more trivial experiences as sickness. Johansson refers explicitly to the lethality of disease, implying that sickness rates are inflated by the addition of both more trivial diseases and diseases with waning case fatality rates. The lethality of familiar diseases diminished in the period 1872–1910 among AOF members and in the British population in general. But it did so for reasons having little to do with beliefs about what constituted sickness and much to do with changing economic, public health, and medical circumstances. Given this decline in lethality, the key issue that the sickness profiles address is whether, in the friendly society definition, sickness time increased because more trivial complaints were added. The previous chapter has shown that the incidence of new episodes diminished, an important finding that requires rejection of part of the claims that Shorter and Johansson make. What remains to be considered is the profile of complaints.

Shorter and Johansson stress the effect of cultural forces on the sickness threshold. People decide at what point they will take action about bodily symptoms, and their decisions are influenced, even determined, by an

20. Shorter, *Bedside Manners,* 24, 57, and 75–110, quote from 57. For sickness profiles from the late eighteenth century, see Loudon, *Medical Care and the General Practitioner,* 54–62.

21. Johansson, "Health Transition." Also Riley, "From a High Mortality Regime to a High Morbidity Regime"; and Johansson's response, "Measuring the Cultural Inflation of Morbidity."

unspoken agreement that is part of the culture. Here most of the evidence that can be considered sets the threshold between sickness and wellness at the point where people decide, subject to a doctor's approval, whether to go to work or not, in circumstances in which everyone whose decisions can be observed faced a similar set of financial costs and benefits. The question is, what manner of sicknesses seemed, to late-nineteenth-century friendly society members, who included the central ranks of the British working classes, sufficient to justify taking time off from work?

The threshold is difficult to specify in a precise way, since descriptions of the warrant that allows us to consider ourselves sick today, like descriptions from the nineteenth century, appear so often in relative terms. As J. W. Northey explained in an 1873 article in the *Foresters' Miscellany,* "every degree of bodily condition causing only occasional or slight discomfort is conventionally termed [a matter of] health."[22] The editors of *The Family Physician,* the dictionary of diseases and treatments mentioned in the *Foresters' Miscellany,* open with a definition similar in its breadth to that given in article 1 of the 1948 Constitution of the World Health Organization: "Health is a state of complete physical, mental, and social well-being and not merely the absence of disease or infirmity."[23] According to *The Family Physician,* "disease may be defined as being any condition of the organism which limits life in either its powers, enjoyments, or duration." Health "implies freedom from pain and sickness, and freedom from all those changes in the natural fabric of the body that endanger life or impede the easy, regular, and effectual exercise of the vital functions." "A corn is a disease, and so is a cancer."[24] According to this testimony, late-nineteenth-century doctors and laypeople alike counted minor as well as grave ailments as sickness.

Nineteenth-century commentators, like many of their late-twentieth-century counterparts, also believed that people were extraordinarily sensitive about their health. An anonymous writer in the *Foresters' Miscellany,* probably the editor, John Hinchcliffe, suggested in 1876 that "one of the most distinctive traits of this generation is its almost fidgety care about its health."[25] People worried about how much they should eat; they fretted about what they should drink and in what quantity. They worried, too,

22. *Foresters' Miscellany,* Apr. 1873, 437.
23. WHO, *First Ten Years,* 459, quoting the constitution adopted in 1948. The chief difference between the two definitions is that the WHO definition promotes a more positive conception.
24. *Family Physician,* xi–xii.
25. "Stimulants."

about identifying and following rules for a long life. Was the secret moderation in all things, as the Greeks had held? Was it, according to the testimony of an American attorney named Kent, the avoidance of study in youth? (Kent claimed he had not studied until he was twenty-four but then studied hard during the rest of a long and successful life.)

Was the secret a faithful following of the rules of life urged by late-nineteenth-century doctors, such as explained by one named Combe in the *Foresters' Miscellany* in January 1872: ventilate living quarters; exercise; avoid heated rooms, late hours, and foods that disagree; wear sufficient clothing; wash or air clothing; wash the body; avoid excitement; and sleep soundly.[26] Combe wished especially to warn his readers about the insidious and cumulative effect of violating rules of health. No penalty will follow in the short run, but in the long run the abuses will build up to a long sickness. The testimony of old people seemed contradictory, except perhaps about the efficacy of exercise and moderation in drink or the great value of being born to long-lived and vigorous parents.[27]

Nineteenth-century observers also believed they were living in an age of tension and anxiety sufficiently intense and at a pace of life harried enough to affect health. J. S. Swan included in his "Hints upon Some of the Advantages of Friendly Societies" their capacity to lessen anxiety about financial emergencies.[28]

Individual doctors kept ledgers where they entered the charges they made and where, sometimes, they specified each item charged for, including individual medications. But their ledgers do not often reveal what sicknesses the medications and procedures were meant to treat. The case study records of some physicians and surgeons, and more often of hospital doctors, survive, but those are often collections of atypical cases, either those the physician or surgeon found unusual and therefore interesting or those admitted to hospital and therefore skewed toward injuries and surgery cases. Loose within a ledger from his practice at Thorne, West Riding, John Stephen Taylor preserved a list of dates and diagnoses that refer to one of his patients. In eighteen episodes he treated this patient for urethritis twice, bronchitis three times, tonsillitis twice, indigestion twice, and injuries three times. He also treated him for toothache, hoarseness, a swollen knee, and hair loss; twice Taylor recorded the medication but not the

26. Combe, "The Preservation of Health."
27. "Happy and Healthy Old Men."
28. Swan, "Hints upon Some of the Advantages."

diagnosis.[29] The profile is not modern, in the sense that few late-twentieth-century adults would expect to call on their doctor for these disorders. But the mildness of many of the symptoms is striking. Taylor had treated this patient for several ailments that posed no threat to life and for some that posed no prospect of pain.

Dr. Phillipson of the Newcastle Infirmary recorded in 1868 that he had treated Jane Johnson, a married women aged thirty-eight, on thirteen occasions as an outpatient over a five-month period for hoarseness, a dry mouth, and costive bowels (i.e., constipation).[30] Eventually she recovered. In the same period he treated James Riley, a married laborer from Gateshead, for a persistent cough, weight loss, and night sweating. Riley does not seem to have recovered, but the record stops on September 2 with an entry for a medication. Phillipson often concerned himself with the status of his patients' tongues and bowels.

These few cases have limited meaning. But they show that some patients called doctors or visited infirmaries for a broad spectrum of maladies and conditions, major and minor. Whereas Britain's cause of death profile suggests the gravity of the people's health condition, Taylor's cause-of-sickness profile for this single patient suggests that people called doctors for many ailments that were not life threatening. If mortality is the yardstick, the sickness profile by its very nature deals chiefly with "minor" ailments. In the Abthorpe court, for example, only 160 of 3,736 episodes—fewer than 5 percent—in the period 1863–1922 ended in death.

Tables 7.2 and 7.3 affirm the "minor" quality, in this sense, of the leading causes of sickness among members of three friendly societies and employees of a single railway. Many of the men took time off from work and sought treatment for abrasions; colds, differentiated as ordinary, severe, and bad; and other minor ailments. Among 72,272 claims filed under the National Insurance Act in 1924, respiratory diseases, muscular disorders, and injuries accounted for 59.6 percent.[31] The profile of causes of sickness in that year closely resembles the evidence presented above for the beginning of the century and, like the profiles of members of three friendly societies and railway employees, it features such disorders as headaches

29. John Stephen Taylor Collection, D/597, loose between pages 100 and 101. The list was compiled in connection with the patient's application for life insurance (see D/582).

30. Dr. Phillipson's casebook, 1868–69.

31. Hill, "Investigation of Sickness in Various Industrial Occupations," 184. That is, the sum of the categories influenza, bronchitis and related diseases, pneumonia and other respiratory diseases, injuries and accidents, and lumbago.

and colds. So, too, do other sources, most of which describe causes less systematically. Sick stewards of the Amalgamated Society of Wood-workers in 1892–1900 often accepted claims from men with colds and with ill-defined inflammations.[32] In the Eversholt Friendly Society the secretary recorded diagnoses irregularly in the period 1864–83, but the most common ailment he noted was a cold.

In sum, for doctors and laypeople alike high mortality and the lethality of some commonplace diseases did not dominate the conception of sick-ness, as they have dominated it for historical demographers and for some social historians. For people who were sick and for the doctors who treated them, it mattered also that a person felt ill, suffered a corn or a cold or indigestion, or in some other way felt indisposed. As *The Family Physi-cian* acknowledged, diseases could be graded in importance not only ac-cording to the threat they posed to life but also according to how much they limited the utility or enjoyment of life.[33] Sicknesses that compromised the quality of life warranted relief by medical treatment and sickness benefits.

What is remarkable about the nineteenth-century profile is not its dis-similarity but its similarity to the late-twentieth-century profile in terms of the banal nature of many complaints. Shorter imagined that sharp differ-ences would exist between the ailments that prompted nineteenth-century and early-twentieth-century patients to visit doctors or take time off from work and the conditions that made people miss work in the late twentieth century. But the differences are mild rather than sharp. Nineteenth-century observers already believed that people were finicky about their health, and they were correct. Friendly society members did not wait until death threatened to declare themselves sick.

The past cannot be imagined accurately. It is an error to claim that rising sickness time within the period 1872–1910 can be explained by either the trivialization or the cultural inflation of sickness.

THE HAZARDS OF OCCUPATIONS

Early investigators of friendly society sickness patterns surmised that some occupations exposed the person employed in them to greater-than-ordinary hazards in the workplace. Friendly society statisticians also came

---

32. Amalgamated Society of Woodworkers, acc. 4685/112.
33. *Family Physician,* xii.

to appreciate that the issue of occupational hazards was not entirely straightforward. It introduced a secondary threshold, consisting of what a job demands in the way of activity. People with the same degree of incapacity may be unable to work in one trade but able to work in another. Over a lifetime the tasks people do in one trade may change to accommodate some deterioration in health, allowing people to continue to work even though their health no longer allows them to perform the same tasks they could when younger. People with health limitations may change jobs in search of tasks they can still perform. Furthermore, the hazards associated with a given occupation change over time with the technology and circumstances of work and with its pay, both absolute and relative. Moreover, people sort themselves out to some degree in taking jobs. In one study, Henry Ratcliffe's analysis of Oddfellows data for 1846–48,[34] clerks had abridged life expectancies already in their twenties, even though their jobs per se carried no marked risks. Presumably they brought the characteristics that abbreviated their lives to their jobs rather than acquiring those characteristics from their jobs.

Friendly society statisticians approached this issue chiefly as a problem of distinguishing unhealthy from ordinary occupations and rarely introduced the additional evidence necessary to control for confounding factors.[35] Nevertheless, their investigations of occupational hazards illustrate relationships between mortality and morbidity and the differential effects of occupation upon health. They also show that the men who collected evidence about patterns of sickness and mortality kept a close watch on occupational composition, knowing that any shift toward or away from hazardous occupations would affect patterns of health.[36]

Ratcliffe explored this issue in some detail in 1850, using the patterns of sickness and mortality of the Oddfellows in 1846–48.[37] Together, he and

34. See below, this chapter.

35. Another problem lies in the imprecision of occupational terms, which makes it difficult to compare sickness and death rates provided by different authorities unless they also provide a detailed explanation of the terms they use to describe occupations.

36. Watson, *Sickness and Mortality Experience*, 17. Problems in collecting and using occupational data are discussed further at 28 ff; and Haines, "Conditions of Work."

In the early decades of the nineteenth century, friendly societies were sometimes formed either to exclude men in hazardous trades or to provide benefits specifically for such workers. Affiliated societies, such as the Foresters and Oddfellows, generally admitted men regardless of trade.

37. Ratcliffe, *Observations on the Rate of Mortality & Sickness* (1850), 38–120. See also Richard Wall's comments in the introduction to *Mortality in Mid-Nineteenth-Century Britain*, where Ratcliffe's book is reprinted. Ratcliffe assumed that there was no selection among men entering occupations, either for age or health. Also helpful on occupational health are

Francis G. P. Neison Sr., who took up the issue in 1857,[38] created a counterpoint to analyses by physicians, in which assessments of relative health status were sometimes made for individual occupations by focusing on diseases associated with them. In 1831 Charles Turner Thackrah, a young surgeon strongly impressed by the sick men he had seen rather than by the sick and the well, fashioned a nosology of occupational diseases, intending to warn doctors about the need to ask patients the occupation they followed to better anticipate the man's ailments. Thackrah believed that all working-class occupations bore some hazard to life or health, but he lacked the data necessary to quantify these.[39]

Ratcliffe used Oddfellows statistics to estimate both mean sickness and death rates by age and trade and the degree of deviation from the mean. He found distinctive hierarchies of mortality and sickness time. At every age, from men of twenty who had practiced their occupations only for a few years to men of sixty who had (at least in many cases) practiced their occupations for several decades, Ratcliffe found substantial variations for the twenty-six occupations for which he had enough evidence to make comparisons. At one extreme stood carpenters, whose survival exceeded the Oddfellows norm by an average of 23 percent and whose sickness time fell short of the average by 19 percent. At the other extreme stood miners, who experienced more mortality and more sickness time than the average.[40] The lives of miners were short and marred by rheumatism, ruptures,

---

Hunter, *Diseases of Occupations*, esp. 119–39; and the essays in Weindling, *Social History of Occupational Health*. Ratcliffe presumably used information about occupations provided by club secretaries, who must have differed one from another in the care they took to update employment records. Hence, some men associated with each occupation may have practiced it when they joined the society but not throughout their working lives. Nevertheless, most of the records presumably refer to current occupations.

38. Neison, *Contributions to Vital Statistics*, substantially expanding the content of work first published in 1845. Watkins, *Statistical Notes*, 45–54, also derived occupation-specific rates, but on far smaller numbers. Francis G. P. Neison Jr. wanted to investigate occupational experience among Foresters in the period 1871–75, but AOF officers balked. AOF, *Second Quarterly Report of the Fifty-First Executive Council*, 9.

39. Thackrah, *Effects of Arts, Trades, and Professions*. His conclusions are sometimes sharply at odds with Ratcliffe's findings and sometimes in close agreement. For example, Thackrah believed that butchers lived short lives because they overate (64), whereas Ratcliffe found them long-lived. Thackrah's conclusions appear to have been based partly on his own clinical practice and partly on his reading, but most are offered without references to sources. Rule, *Experience of Labor in Eighteenth-Century Industry*, 74–94, reviews evidence on the ill effects of factory work and the diseases associated with certain occupations.

40. The mortality averages are based on average deviations from normative sickness rates at each of five ages for which Ratcliffe summarized his findings. The morbidity comparisons are based on cumulative sickness time from ages twenty to sixty. Ratcliffe, *Observations on the Rate of Mortality & Sickness*, (1850), 38 and 41.

Table 7.4
RELATIVE HAZARDS OF OCCUPATIONS, 1846–1848

	Life Expectancy (% +/− norm)	Sickness Time (% +/− norm)
Group 1: Long lives, low sickness time		
Bakers	2.8	−4.2
Butchers	3.5	−33.1
Carpenters and joiners	23.2	−19.0
Rural laborers	13.9	−2.6
Millwrights	1.1	−25.5
Servants	5.3	−19.5
Wheelwrights	1.8	−39.2
Group 2: Long lives, high sickness time		
Hatters	0.4	7.9
Weavers	9.4	11.2
Group 3: Short lives, high sickness time		
Bricklayers	−19.2	2.6
Coopers	−5.6	23.9
Dyers	−3.5	5.0
Urban laborers	−0.4	6.4
Miners	−7.3	67.7
Plumbers	−6.1	18.4
Potters	−6.0	56.5
Printers and compositors	−16.2	8.0
Spinners	−7.8	23.0
Stonemasons	−4.0	32.3
Woolcombers	−3.4	20.5
Group 4: Short lives, low sickness time		
Blacksmiths	−7.4	−4.1
Clerks and schoolmasters	−18.0	−37.5
Mill operatives	−14.2	−6.6
Sawyers	−2.8	−20.1
Shoemakers	−0.7	−11.8
Tailors	−8.0	−15.0

Source: Data from Ratcliffe, *Observations on the Rate of Mortality & Sickness,* (1850), 37–120.

and lung disease,[41] whereas the lives of carpenters, according to Ratcliffe's study, were long and comparatively sickness free. The sicknesses that miners suffered lasted no longer, on average, than did those of men in other trades. But, as later investigations showed, miners suffered more episodes, chiefly because of a higher rate of accidents.[42]

Table 7.4 divides Ratcliffe's twenty-six occupational groups into four categories comprising each possible combination of sickness time and life

41. Benson, *British Coalminers in the Nineteenth Century,* 44–47.
42. Watson, *Sickness and Mortality Experience,* 65.

expectancy. Only one occupational group in the table represents unambiguously favorable circumstances: group 1 (bakers et al.) lived longer lives with less sickness time. The other three groups represent mixed circumstances or unambiguous disadvantages. Hatters and weavers (group 2) lived long lives but were often sick. Group 3 (bricklayers et al.) experienced short lives marred by frequent sickness. Group 4 (blacksmiths et al.) lived short lives with comparatively infrequent sickness. Ratcliffe's work highlights the existence of favored and unfavored occupations. It also points up differential patterns of sickness among men with short lives. Some men were seldom sick, and others accumulated high quotients of sickness time. The men whose lives were short did not follow the same health paths through life.

Examining Ratcliffe's tables, scholars have sometimes been struck by the incongruence between patterns of sickness and of mortality and have taken that incongruence as a reason to have misgivings about Ratcliffe's data or methods. But factors affecting mortality and morbidity operated in different ways among these occupations, creating a complex rather than a simple picture of occupational health. Certainly, the work a man did mattered to his health. Men who worked amidst mineral dust—miners, potters, and stonemasons—all suffered for it, living short lives with frequent sickness.[43] So, too, did urban laborers, bricklayers, and men in some other trades. Nor was occupation the only factor influencing the distribution in table 7.4. Ratcliffe recognized that the city played a role, for he divided laborers into two groups, rural and urban, depending on the size of the place where they lived. But he did not acknowledge the fourfold complexity of the problem before him, and he also did not directly attack the issue of identifying other factors exercising influence. At the end of the century J. T. Arlidge refocused the issue away from the statistics of sickness and mortality toward the pathology of occupational diseases, so that Ratcliffe's approach languished.[44]

Ratcliffe's own willingness to pursue the issue of occupational health must have been tested by his findings in a subsequent investigation based

---

43. The risk obtained also for men in occupations about which Ratcliffe had too few cases to include. See, e.g., Inkster, "Marginal Men," 143–44, regarding grinders; Matsumura, *Labour Aristocracy Revisited*, 39–43; and Haines, "Conditions of Work." See further Arlidge, *Hygiene, Diseases, and Mortality*, 245–353; Dupree, *Family Structure in the Staffordshire Potteries*, 82 and 84–86; and Lewchuck, "Industrialization and Occupational Mortality," 344–66, for an alternative approach that stresses the effect of fatigue, a factor that Ratcliffe could not assess.

44. Arlidge, *Hygiene, Diseases, and Mortality*, 1.

on Oddfellows statistics for the period 1856–60. Those findings reaffirmed some of the conclusions suggested by the 1846–48 data, especially those showing sharp differences in mortality or morbidity. But for occupations with milder differences, his earlier findings did not always hold up.[45] Occupation was a forceful enough factor to distinguish miners from workingmen in general, and Ratcliffe took the occasion to prepare detailed premium tables for miners. But he was too cautious to suggest the same thing for other trades. Neither did he propose the creation of separate premium tables for men practicing distinctively healthy occupations.

Ratcliffe and Neison set the terms of investigation into the statistics of occupational health. For them what mattered most was the division of friendly society members into occupations associated with long or short lives. By implication, their question was this: should some members pay higher premiums because they engage in occupations that carry a higher risk of death? That question remained important in friendly society debates for several decades. In often heated debates, risk-minded officials, members, and observers warned that accepting men working in hazardous occupations raised the cost of friendly society benefits to all other members, in proportion to their part of the total. Fraternal-minded members responded with a plea of working-class solidarity. A man's occupation does not, they held, fall into the same category of characteristics as those that allow clubs to deny admission to men already in poor health or to refuse benefits to members who fell sick because they were drunk or started fights. It is morally neutral. Men practicing hazardous trades deserve to be included.

In sum, Foresters and Oddfellows rejected the advice of risk-minded observers by arguing the insurance principle: risks should be shared. In return, their advisers pointed out the need to charge higher premiums in clubs where men working in hazardous occupations were numerous, and they constructed separate premium tables for hazardous trades.[46] By the 1880s mortality statistics showed that the risks associated with mining

45. Ratcliffe, *Observations on the Rate of Mortality and Sickness* (1862), 39–83. In his next investigation, concerning experience in 1866–70, Ratcliffe repeated the separate calculations for miners but omitted those for other trades. [Ratcliffe], *Independent Order of Odd-Fellows.* Watson, *Sickness and Mortality Experience*, 30–75, returned to the issue but elected to group occupations into three classes that showed differences in risk more forcefully.

46. For discussions of these and other points at issue, see "The Proposed Advance of Twenty-five Per Cent," Nov. 1888, plus letters on the topic, 360–64; "The Proposed Advance of Twenty-five Per Cent," Dec. 1888; "Inadequate Contributions" and the letters on this topic, 395–400; and *Foresters' Miscellany*, in the 1873, 1878, 1880, and 1889 issues.

had dropped sharply from what they had been in Ratcliffe's day.[47] In such circumstances higher premiums no longer seemed an important issue.

The friendly societies approached differing occupational experiences as a problem of risk and effects rather than as a problem of health and causes. Their members accepted the differentials they discovered fatalistically rather than seeing them as grounds for identifying the causes behind health differentials or for making the differentials an issue in debates on public health. On one hand, therefore, Ratcliffe's data highlight the existence of complex determinants of health and the need to know more than Ratcliffe did about the characteristics of men practicing different occupations.

On the other hand, Ratcliffe's data also point to the existence of health factors that accumulated. In some of the twenty-six occupations he studied for 1846–48, no pattern of change is apparent from young adulthood to old age.[48] Other occupations fall into the distinctive categories of gainers and losers, as depicted in table 7.5.

Compared to all Oddfellows, the group including weavers and servants gained an advantage in life expectancy as they aged, so that in their sixties the members of this group had a greater advantage than they had had at earlier ages. Tailors, mill operatives, and bricklayers, in contrast, lost position. Tailors aged twenty had a life expectancy 4 percent below the norm. But tailors aged sixty had an expectation 23 percent below the norm. Shoemakers and wheelwrights gained an advantage in sickness time as they aged, relative to their peers, whereas the group including bricklayers and dyers suffered progressively more sickness time.

Certain jobs appear to have exposed the men who practiced them to accumulating insults that led to a progressive deterioration of health. Potters, stonemasons, printers, and others lost standing in either mortality or morbidity as they aged, but bricklayers and mill operatives lost standing in both. In terms solely of changing health status, those were the worst jobs a man could hold. Other jobs apparently protected the men who followed them from insult accumulation, in one form or another rather than in both. Weavers, servants, potters, rural laborers, carpenters, and butchers gained in life expectancy as they aged, compared to other Oddfellows. A different group—shoemakers and wheelwrights—gained in terms of sick-

47. *Foresters' Miscellany,* Nov. 1888, 329.
48. This analysis assumes that most of the men about whom Ratcliffe had information had practiced the occupation they were following in 1846–48 throughout their working lives. Spree, *Health and Social Class in Imperial Germany,* 53–54, finds that the ill effects of working in industrial jobs accumulated.

Table 7.5
COSTS AND BENEFITS OF STAYING IN A TRADE, 1846–1848

	Life Expectancy	Sickness Time
Gainers	Weavers	Shoemakers
	Servants	Wheelwrights
	Potters	
	Rural laborers	
	Carpenters and joiners	
	Butchers	
Losers	Tailors	Bricklayers
	Mill operatives	Dyers
	Bricklayers	Mill operatives
		Potters
		Printers and compositors
		Stonemasons

Source: Data from Ratcliffe, *Observations on the Rate of Mortality & Sickness* (1850), 37–120.

ness time. Bricklayers and mill operatives had no counterparts; that is, no occupational group gained in both mortality and morbidity. Ratcliffe noticed these changes in relative position and pointed them out to his readers. But the cumulative effect of an occupation did not become a central element in his discussion of occupational hazard. Nor did Ratcliffe pursue this point in analyzing Oddfellows data for 1856–60, even though most of the trends toward advantage or disadvantage found in his 1846–48 data held up in the 1856–60 data.

Nevertheless, Ratcliffe's mode of analysis offers a way to distinguish jobs that carried hazards at any time from jobs in which hazards accumulated over time. Groups 3 and 4 in table 7.4 include the jobs with higher hazards. They make up most of the jobs men in his sample held. Table 7.5 identifies the jobs in which health deteriorated as their holders aged. From the point of view of table 7.4, one of the worst jobs to hold was in mining. But miners suffered higher mortality and sickness time in a consistent way as they aged. In contrast, bricklayers, potters, stonemasons, mill operatives, printers, and dyers suffered progressively deteriorating health. Mining was a more dangerous job to take, but those others were more dangerous jobs to hold.[49]

49. The Shropshire Provident Society charged miners higher premiums but allowed former miners to pay the lower premiums for nonhazardous trades. That is, by implication if not intent, the directors of this friendly society did not expect mining to have deferred effects. Shropshire Provident Society, 436/6728, minutes, Jan. 1, 1870.

The diseases and injuries that workingmen suffered in the late nineteenth and early twentieth centuries did not cause death in the same proportions that they caused sickness. In the cause-of-death profile, organ diseases already dominated by 1900, but in the profile of causes of sickness, accidents and respiratory diseases led, followed by muscular disorders. In the epidemiologic transition death had already made a shift away from infectious diseases through respiratory diseases to chronic organ diseases. A lagged transition was under way in sickness. Judging from data about time lost from work, men continued to suffer often from respiratory diseases for some time after those diseases had lost their leading roles as causes of death. This lag suggests the form of a health transition as experienced by adult males. Men stopped dying as often as they had in the past from respiratory diseases well before they stopped getting sick from the same diseases. The circumstances of health changed not so much in ways that affected men's exposure as in ways that affected their ability to manage their diseases. Something of a revolution was under way in the years around 1908. The lethality of disease declined more than did the prevalence, and the likeliest candidate to explain that is better disease management.

In the nineteenth century men pleaded sickness and missed work for minor colds and cut fingers as well as for bronchitis, influenza, and broken limbs. Comparisons are difficult to make on the same terms, so that it is not possible to say that "minor" ailments were either more or less common in the profile of complaints then than in the middle to late twentieth century. What can be said for the moment is that what appear to have been minor ailments loomed large in the things that people worried about and took time off from work for, in the nineteenth and early twentieth centuries. Whereas friendly society members sometimes described themselves as people who worked through their sicknesses and took time off from work only when forced to do so, their opinions about how serious their health problems needed to be to warrant being called "sickness" seem strikingly modern.

If they were sensitive to health, good and bad, however, they seem to have been insensitive to the implications of their experience. Already in 1850 Henry Ratcliffe, the Oddfellows statistician, could measure the added risks accompanying some occupations. His research was used to press the case for premium schedules adjusted for risk but not to fashion arguments in favor of compensation for those risks or to devise public policies that reduced the risks. Nor did men in the friendly societies, trade unions, or other working-class organizations make much of the evidence Ratcliffe assembled about how, in certain trades, risks accumulated at a notably faster pace the longer a man practiced them. Toward century's end protective programs were introduced, especially in the form of legislation intended to safeguard men in hazardous trades or to oblige employers to pay benefits to men injured on the job. But the friendly societies took little part in arguing for those benefits or making a case about the cumulative ill health effects of some occupations.

Friendly society members managed to do some things that prolonged their survival when sick. Covertly, perhaps in negotiations with their doctors, they found ways to live longer despite sickness. Ironically, they did not seize the opportunity Ratcliffe made apparent. They did not also demand compensation from employers or from the public for the hazardous trades many of them followed, either those with an outright penalty or those with a cumulative penalty. Ratcliffe's statistics made the case for workers' compensation a half century before compensation was gained.

CHAPTER 8

The Geography of the Foresters' Health

GOOD HEALTH and the ability to work, like their inverse, bad health and the inability to work, were not spread evenly over Britain. In some regions men belonging to the AOF were sick much less of the time than their counterparts in other regions. This chapter explores these regional differences in patterns of sickness, controlling for age and differences in the distribution of members by age.[1] It complements the chapter that follows, which investigates why some regions were unhealthier than others.

AOF GEOGRAPHY

Map 8.1 gives the locations of more than four thousand AOF courts situated in 2,876 different villages, towns, cities, and other sites across mainland Britain active between 1872 and 1910.[2] In 1872 the AOF had

1. Appendix 4 discusses how problems associated with county boundaries have been dealt with. In sum, the AOF system, which located courts in the ancient county system, has been adapted to the system of administrative counties for purposes of drawing maps and to the system of registration counties for purposes of analysis. Near county boundaries, some court members must have lived in counties other than where the court was located. Their numbers are assumed to have been too small to influence results.

2. Drawing heavily on advice from Naomi Williams, Randy Johnson constructed this map, using Bickmore et al., *Atlas of Britain and Northern Ireland,* to draw the boundaries established in 1888. See Freeman-Grenville, *Atlas of British History,* 122, 140, for a comparison of the boundaries of administrative counties as drawn in 1888 with those redrawn in 1972–73.

AOF courts are located by the longitude and latitude of the site where they were situated, as indicated by Great Britain, *Ordnance Survey Gazetteer.* Altogether, eighty-nine courts, 1.8 percent of the total, could not be located, chiefly because two or three sites in the same county shared the same name and insufficient information was available to decide in which of them the court was located. Many problems in situating courts were resolved by using the *Gazetteer of the British Isles,* which describes situations and reports distances from neighboring

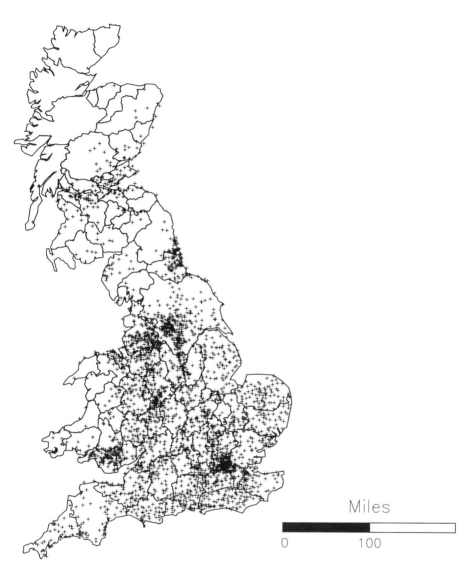

Map 8.1. AOF Court Locations, 1872–1910
Source: AOF, *Directories*, 1873–1911.

---

villages, towns, and cities; and England and Wales, Office of Population Censuses and
Surveys, *Census 1971: Index of Place Names.*

   Locations off the mainland are not considered. The Soke of Peterborough and the Isle of
Ely have been joined with, respectively, Northamptonshire and Cambridgeshire. Sussex,
Suffolk, Lincolnshire, and Yorkshire are treated as single counties rather than by the subdivi-
sions introduced in the administrative county system.

   Southall, "Unionization," maps locations of some trade friendly societies; and Purvis,
"Popular Institutions," discusses regional strengths of the AOF and the Oddfellows.

397,973 members in 3,701 active courts distributed across England, Scotland, and Wales. By 1911 its British membership totaled 601,435 in 3,729 active courts.[3] Membership was broadly distributed across the land. Except for Scotland in the 1870s, most counties not only had AOF courts but also had enough courts and members, and stable enough patterns of health, to provide statistically acceptable estimates of sickness and death rates.[4] In England, AOF courts were distributed more or less in proportion to population; they were thick on the ground in all areas but the north. But that was not true in Scotland or Wales. As would be expected, in Scotland courts were most numerous in the populous region stretching from Glasgow to Edinburgh. Some highland counties lacked courts altogether, other counties contained only one or two, and still others had so few courts that the results of examining morbidity and mortality in them are unreliable in statistical terms for the earliest decade, the 1870s. In Wales there were comparatively few courts in the west, and there, too, it is sometimes necessary to combine experience from courts located in adjacent counties in order to obtain satisfactory statistical results.[5] Two counties in England, Rutland and Westmorland, contained so few courts that they have been joined with Leicestershire and Cumberland, respectively.

Each year, each court supplied a reading about the health of its members in reporting to the compilers of the directory. Thus, the locations of AOF courts illustrate the data set that has been constructed to show regional differences in patterns of sickness in this chapter and, in the next, to support an analysis of reasons for those differences. Historians often grumble about having too little information from the past, but it is possible also to have too much information. The AOF directories bring this problem to life by furnishing data for each court in each year from 1871 through 1921. It is therefore possible to discuss regional differences in patterns of health each year. Indeed, it is possible to discuss annual differences in the morbidity and mortality experience of each court. Such a detailed discussion would be useful if the health statistics of individual courts jumped around or if differences in experience within regions varied

3. AOF, *Directory*, 1913, 665.
4. Thus, comparisons of differences in patterns of health at the county level for the most part satisfy high standards of statistical reliability. Unless otherwise indicated, the comparisons reported below for sickness rates are significant at the 0.01 level; often the level of significance is more precise still. Those for death rates are significant at the 0.05 level.
5. In each case these groupings combine adjacent counties on a basis of composing groups of the smallest number of counties that need to be joined in order to produce acceptable statistical results. Many other scholars, for example, Lee, "Regional Inequalities in Infant Mortality," have preferred official groupings of Scottish and Welsh counties.

much from year to year. They do not. Thus it is possible, when considering differences in experience at the level of counties, to collect experience within administrative units, summarizing what happened to men belonging to different courts situated in the same county, and to combine experience across groups of years, 1872–80, 1881–90, 1891–00, and 1901–10. Because many relationships remained stable over that entire period, it is possible in some cases to compress the analysis still further by considering regional differences for the period 1872–1910 as a whole.

REGIONAL PATTERNS IN THE ADMINISTRATIVE COUNTIES

Sickness and death rates among men who belonged to the AOF often differed substantially from one county to another. Considered in terms of sickness rates, some counties can be deemed healthy and some unhealthy. The same is true of death rates, except that the grouping of healthy and unhealthy counties is only partly the same. Some counties were unhealthy in terms of sickness rates but healthy in terms of death rates. The inverse is also true. Sickness cannot otherwise be observed, but death rates from the AOF directories correspond closely in their differences from county to county with the death rates reported by the registrar general. At least for mortality, basic patterns that obtained for Foresters in trend and regional differences also obtained for the adult population at large.[6]

Comparisons of patterns of sickness and death within decades rely on techniques explained in chapter 6. The important point is to control for age in order to bring into focus the differences that should be explained by factors other than age. Neither a court's average age nor its indicators of the distribution of members by age—the initiation rate and the number of years since a court was formed—changed much within a decade. Hence it is possible to compare patterns within decades, using decennial averages. But the point is to make comparisons across space and time. To obtain reliable values across decades, decennial averages for counties have been compared with overall AOF experience in each decade by calculating a percentage difference. For example, in the 1880s the death rate in County

6. The registrar general did not publish mortality data for males of the age groups of men belonging to the AOF, so this comparison is for both sexes. AOF, *Directories, 1889, 1890*; Great Britain, Registrar General of Births, Deaths, and Marriages, *Fifty-First Annual Report* (1888) and *Fifty-Second Annual Report* (1889).

Durham was 0.5 percent below the death rate estimated for the whole AOF at the mean for the average age, initiation rate, and years since court formation in the Foresters as a whole. In contrast, the death rate in Cornwall was 29.4 percent lower, and that in Lancashire 33.3 percent higher, than the AOF average. Calculating percentage differences makes it possible to transform the comparison from differences within each decade to differences among decades. In this way counties can be distributed according to whether their sickness and death rates were high or low for the period 1872–1910 as a whole, as well as for each decade within those years. For example, the average percentage difference in County Durham's death rates across the four decades was +1.6 percent, Cornwall's −22.2 percent, and Lancashire's +36.6 percent. Across the entire period, County Durham's death rates slightly exceeded the AOF average, Cornwall's fell substantially below the average, and Lancashire's substantially exceeded the average.[7]

AOF members in England enjoyed favored health. Their sickness and death rates were lower than the average for British members as a whole. Wales was a decidedly unhealthy area, with persistently higher sickness and death rates. Scotland was healthier than the average in sickness, but its mortality was higher than the British average. And unlike England and Wales, Scotland changed relative position between the 1870s and the second decade of the twentieth century. Through the 1890s its health patterns were more favorable than the British average or than England's average. But Scotland lost that favored status in the decade 1901–10 and lost it in such a demonstrative manner that, for the four decades as a whole, Scotland's experience was worse than England's. Table 8.1 shows the extent to which each area deviated from the British average in each decade and for the period 1872–1910 as a whole. Because so many AOF members lived there, England dominates the British average. But a noteworthy feature of table 8.1 is the degree to which sickness and death rates in Scotland and especially in Wales deviated from the overall average and from the English average. Considering merely these three areas, it is apparent that differences in patterns of health within Britain were large.

Table 8.1 also suggests that, for Welsh and Scots AOF members, health deteriorated over time, at least in relative terms. Wales moved further away from the British average in each decade; there, sickness time increased more sharply than it did in England. Scots members shifted from

7. Within each decade the averages, weighted by the number of members in each county, sum to zero, except for rounding errors. The same thing is true across decades. But no attempt is made here to weight county averages by the number of members.

Table 8.1
SICKNESS AND DEATH RATES IN ENGLAND, WALES, AND SCOTLAND, 1872–1910
(PERCENT DIFFERENCE FROM AOF AVERAGE)

	1872–80	1881–90	1891–1900	1901–10	average
			Sickness Time		
England	−1.4	−1.2	−0.2	−1.0	−1.0
Wales	23.8	24.3	26.8	29.1	26.0
Scotland	−1.5	−9.9	−6.4	9.5	−2.1
			Mortality		
England	−1.8	−2.5	−1.4	−1.8	−1.9
Wales	15.3	14.1	20.2	25.4	18.8
Scotland	−2.1	0.0	2.8	10.6	2.8

Source: Data from AOF, *Directories,* 1873–1911.

positions more favorable than those of their English counterparts to positions less favorable; there too, sickness time increased more than it did in England. Death rates for Scots members of the AOF rose above English rates in the 1880s, and sickness rates did so in the decade 1901–10.

In most cases individual counties show consistent deviations from overall AOF experience from decade to decade. Thus it is possible to summarize their experience across the four decades and to discuss in more detail only those cases where a county's position shifted.

England

Maps 8.2 and 8.3 can be examined in association with maps I.1 and I.2, which identify counties. Maps 8.2 and 8.3 show the distribution of all counties and groups of counties by their differences in sickness time and death rates across the period 1872–1910.[8] The scale used to construct these maps clusters counties with similar experience within groups, moving from proportions substantially above the mean, represented by darkly shaded areas, to proportions below the mean, represented by lightly shaded areas.[9]

8. A few counties lack stable values for the 1870s, and those have been left out of these calculations.
9. The scaling technique maximizes goodness of variance fit, using a Fisher-Jenks iterative method that is incorporated in the software used to produce these maps. Overall goodness of

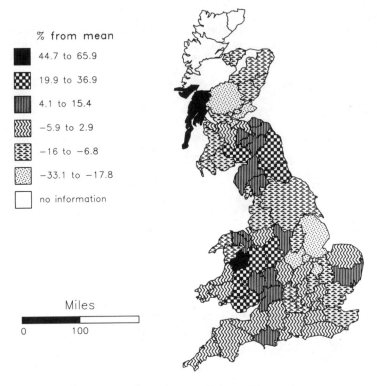

% from mean
- ■ 44.7 to 65.9
- ▨ 19.9 to 36.9
- ▥ 4.1 to 15.4
- ▨ −5.9 to 2.9
- ▨ −16 to −6.8
- ▨ −33.1 to −17.8
- ☐ no information

Miles

0   100

Map 8.2. Overall Variations from Average Sickness Time, 1872–1910
Source: AOF, *Directories,* 1873–1911.

From map 8.2, which deals with sickness patterns, it is apparent that neighboring counties usually shared similar health patterns. Counties with unfavorable experience are grouped together in two regions, one comprising the border area of Wales and England and the other the border area of England and Scotland. Counties with favorable experience are likewise clustered, with the most favored areas centering on Lincolnshire in England and Perthshire in Scotland.

In map 8.3, which deals with mortality, all counties in Scotland and Wales are taken together. English counties with higher death rates are clustered in the north, creating a north-south divide, which is a familiar part of discussion about patterns of mortality in Britain and indeed of some other factors in the nineteenth century and, according to the Black

---

fit is measured from 0 to 1, with values close to 1 having the desirable property of being tightly clustered. For sickness rates the overall fit is 0.958, and for death rates it is 0.982.

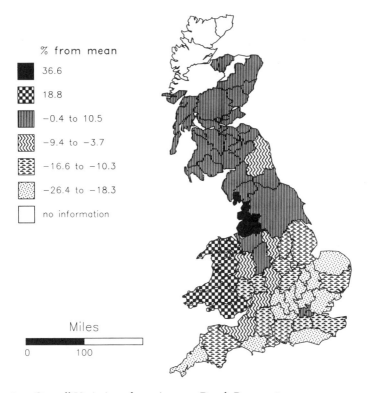

% from mean

36.6

18.8

−0.4 to 10.5

−9.4 to −3.7

−16.6 to −10.3

−26.4 to −18.3

no information

Miles

0   100

Map 8.3. Overall Variations from Average Death Rates, 1872–1910
Source: AOF, *Directories,* 1873–1911.

Report, still a fixture.[10] But sickness rates differed within England alone, and in Britain, too, along an east-west divide, counties with heavier morbidity being grouped in the west.

Counties with particularly low or high relative sickness and death rates are identified in tables 8.2 and 8.3.[11] Some counties enjoyed consistently low morbidity and mortality: Cambridgeshire, Huntingdonshire, Kent, Leicestershire and Rutland, Lincolnshire, Nottinghamshire, and Oxfordshire. Others changed position in a noteworthy way across the period

10. Southall, "Origins of the Depressed Areas," discloses a north-south divide in unemployment that was evident from the 1880s, which he discusses further in his "Poor Law Statistics." For the more recent period, see Great Britain, "Black Report," and "Health Divide," esp. 49–50. Mortality patterns within England are also discussed in Woods and Hinde, "Mortality in Victorian England," 39–41, 47.

11. Sickness rates for Nottinghamshire are unstable in the 1880s and 1890s; death rates are unstable for Cornwall in the 1870s and 1880s and Herefordshire in the 1870s.

Table 8.2
ENGLISH COUNTIES WITH MARKEDLY LOWER OR HIGHER
SICKNESS RATES, 1872–1910

	Low	High
+/− 30 percent	Lincolnshire	Northumberland
+/− 20–29.9 percent	Huntingdonshire	Durham
		Staffordshire
+/− 15–19.9 percent	Leicestershire and Rutland	Derbyshire
	Nottinghamshire	Shropshire
+/− 10–14.9 percent	Cambridgeshire	Gloucestershire
	Lancashire	Herefordshire
	Kent	Worcestershire
	Oxfordshire	
	Yorkshire	

Source: Data from AOF *Directories,* 1873–1911.

1872–1910, gaining or losing ground in comparison to the overall averages. The following list identifies counties where the change in sickness-time position was sharpest and shows the degree of change (in number of steps) between the 1870s and the first decade of the twentieth century.[12]

Gainers	Losers
Bedfordshire (3)	Buckinghamshire (2)
Cumberland and Westmorland (2)	Cheshire (5)
Hampshire (2)	Derbyshire (4)
Hertfordshire (2)	Dorsetshire (3)
Huntingdonshire (2)	Herefordshire (3)
Middlesex (3)	Leicestershire and Rutland (2)
Suffolk (2)	Worcestershire (4)
Sussex (3)	

Cheshire lost ground in the most pronounced way, moving from sickness time well below the AOF average through five steps to rates above the average, and Bedfordshire gained notably, moving from sickness time already below the average through three steps to rates nearly as low as any found in Britain. For both sickness and death rates, English counties tend-

12. Data from AOF, *Directories,* 1875–1911. Steps mean that boundaries have been crossed among categories of sickness time, decreasing or increasing from +/−0 to 4.9 percent from the average, 5 to 9.9 percent, 10 to 14.9 percent, 15 to 19.9 percent, 20 to 29.9 percent, and 30 or more percent difference. In short, the point is to distinguish counties that changed relative position rather than to report the quantity of change.

Table 8.3
ENGLISH COUNTIES WITH MARKEDLY LOWER
OR HIGHER DEATH RATES, 1872–1910

	Low	High
+/− 30 percent		Lancashire
+/− 20–29.9 percent	Bedfordshire	
	Berkshire	
	Buckinghamshire	
	Cambridgeshire	
	Cornwall	
	Essex	
	Huntingdonshire	
	Norfolk	
	Oxfordshire	
+/− 15–19.9 percent	Dorsetshire	
	Herefordshire	
	Hertfordshire	
	Kent	
	Nottinghamshire	
	Sussex	
	Wiltshire	
+/− 10–14.9 percent	Devon	Yorkshire
	Hampshire	
	Leicestershire and Rutland	
	Lincolnshire	
	Northumberland	
	Suffolk	
	Surrey	
	Worcestershire	

Source: Data from AOF, *Directories,* 1873–1911.

ed to move closer to overall averages over time, signaling that the degree of regional variation was shrinking among AOF members, as it was also in the death rates of the population at large.

Wales and Scotland

Maps 8.4 and 8.5 show that five Welsh counties—Brecknock, Montgomery, and Radnor plus the two most populous counties, Monmouth and Glamorgan—had sickness rates well above the British average for the period 1872–1910, as did Wales as a whole. Montgomery was the least-favored county in Wales; its sickness rates exceeded the AOF average in the 1870s by 49.7 percent and in the 1880s by 75.9 percent before falling toward the average in the first decade of the new century (at only 15.5

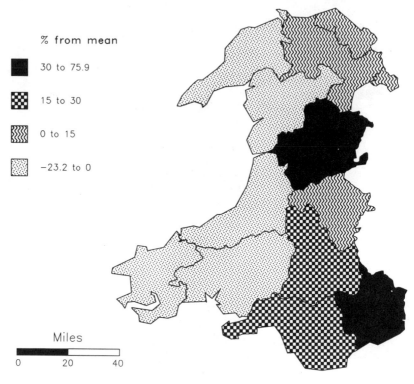

% from mean

30 to 75.9

15 to 30

0 to 15

−23.2 to 0

Miles

0   20   40

Map 8.4. Sickness in Wales, 1881–1890
Source: AOF, *Directories*, 1873–1911.

percent above). In Wales only the counties of Caernarvon and Merioneth, combined here in order to produce stable estimates, experienced sickness rates below the British average for the period as a whole, although some counties and groups had below-average rates for some decades.[13]

Wales's relative position deteriorated over time, which can be seen by comparing map 8.4 with map 8.5. The first, showing each county's position in the 1880s, reveals that sickness time in Wales was higher than the overall British average in seven counties and lower in five. By 1901–10, however, morbidity was higher than the overall average in ten out of twelve counties. The pair Caernarvon and Merioneth had gained. Montgomery moved from a position of immoderately high to one of only mod-

13. These were Flint in the 1870s and the group comprising Cardigan, Carmarthen, and Pembroke in the 1870s, 1880s, and 1890s but not for the entire period. Caernarvon and Merioneth sickness rates for the 1870s are unstable and have not been considered.

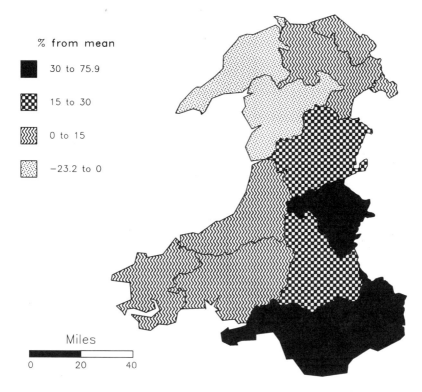

% from mean

■ 30 to 75.9

▦ 15 to 30

▨ 0 to 15

▦ −23.2 to 0

Miles

0   20   40

Map 8.5. Sickness in Wales, 1901–1910
Source: AOF, *Directories,* 1873–1911.

erately high sickness. But Glamorgan, Radnor, and the group Cardigan, Pembroke, and Carmarthen all lost position. At the beginning of the twentieth century Wales was, in terms of what is measured here, a decidedly unhealthy region and a region whose relative position in health was deteriorating.

The least-favored county in all Britain was Argyll, where sickness rates far exceeded the AOF average in every decade: in the 1880s by 57.6 percent, in the 1890s by 73.5 percent, and during 1901–10 by 66.6 percent.[14] Like Wales, Scotland was an area of marked contrasts in relative morbidity. During the period when Scotland as a whole fell below the overall British average in sickness time, some counties (Berwick and East

14. The excess for the 1870s, when the AOF counted few Scots members, was more pronounced still, at 251.4 percent.

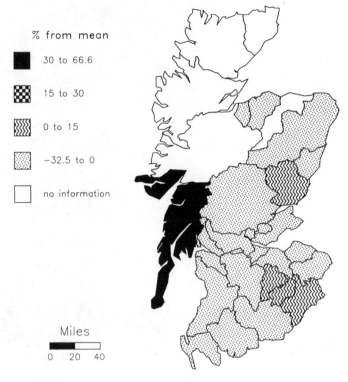

% from mean

30 to 66.6

15 to 30

0 to 15

−32.5 to 0

no information

Miles

0   20   40

Map 8.6. Sickness in Scotland, 1881–1890
Source: AOF, *Directories,* 1873–1911.

Lothian, Argyll, Dumfries, and Forfar) notably exceeded the average.[15]
Maps 8.6 and 8.7 show the counties where sickness rates improved or
deteriorated between the 1880s and 1901–10 relative to overall averages.
Although Forfar and the group Peeble, Roxburgh, and Selkirk gained
substantially, most counties lost position. Some, especially Berwick and
East Lothian, Dumfries, and Midlothian, took huge steps toward higher
relative sickness time. And, as has already been remarked, Scotland as a
whole lost position. In 1901–10 Scotland approached Wales as a region of
pronounced high sickness time, although it had previously been a region of
low relative morbidity.

Given the inverse trends of mortality and the duration of sicknesses,
Scotland's greater gain in sickness time might be considered an advantage.

15. Sickness rates for Angus and the group Aberdeenshire, Kincardineshire, Morayshire,
and Nairnshire are unstable for the 1870s.

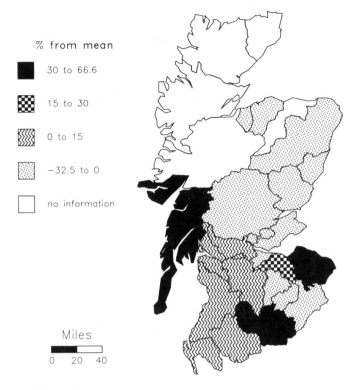

Map 8.7. Sickness in Scotland, 1901–10
Source: AOF, *Directories,* 1873–1911.

But that would be so only in absolute terms and only if mortality declined simultaneously. Death rates among Scotland's AOF members did decline, and sickness time increased, as they did also in England and Wales. But the contrast drawn here is a relative one. Compared with England and Wales, Scotland's position deteriorated. To some extent Scotland's loss of position was an artifact of different structures of AOF membership. In the parts of Scotland where friendly society membership was most widespread, employment in heavy industry and coal mining was more commonplace than in Britain as a whole.[16] Furthermore, in Scotland as in Wales, population shifted toward industrial areas and occupations toward industrial jobs in the period 1872–1910, while in England the pace of industrial growth slowed.[17]

16. Watson, *Sickness and Mortality Experience,* 27.
17. Eilidh Garrett and Alice Reed called this point to my attention.

But much of the explanation lies in the gradual deterioration of Scotland's position in leading indicators of the quality of life and, in particular, in a sharpened rate of deterioration around 1900. Compared to England, Scottish wages decreased yet prices increased.[18] Crowding in housing, on which Scottish statistics show improvement into the 1880s, afterwards stabilized, losing relative ground. The focus of high unemployment within Britain shifted to add Scotland to the list of regions that suffered most in depression periods. And in several regions of Scotland infant mortality increased.[19] In these various and important ways the quality of life in Scotland deteriorated sharply at the beginning of the twentieth century.

Great Britain

Sickness time and mortality constitute discrete hazards. In combination, the two hazards pose four possible outcomes, compared to the overall average of AOF experience: sickness time and mortality both below average, sickness time below average and mortality above average, sickness time above average and mortality below average, and sickness time and morality both above average. One region may hold a favored position on both gauges, it may be favored on one but not the other, or it may be unfavored on both. Clearly, one outcome—low sickness time and low mortality—is distinctly preferred, and its opposite—high on both indexes—is unwelcome. For reasons explained further in chapter 9, high mortality with low sickness time signals that maladies end earlier in death, whereas low mortality together with high sickness time signals more protracted maladies and more frequent recoveries, as opposed to deaths. The other two combinations can also be ranked in order of desirability, with this overall order:

1. low sickness time   low mortality
2. high sickness time   low mortality
3. low sickness time   high mortality
4. high sickness time   high mortality

Using combined experience across the period 1872–1910, map 8.8. distributes the counties of Britain into these four ranks, showing distinctly favored, favored, unfavored, and distinctly unfavored counties. With the

18. Rodger, "Invisible Hand," esp. 197.
19. Lee, "Regional Inequalities in Infant Mortality," 64; Smout, *Century of the Scottish People*, 113; Chalmers, *Health of Glasgow,* 47; and Southall, "Origins of the Depressed Areas," 257.

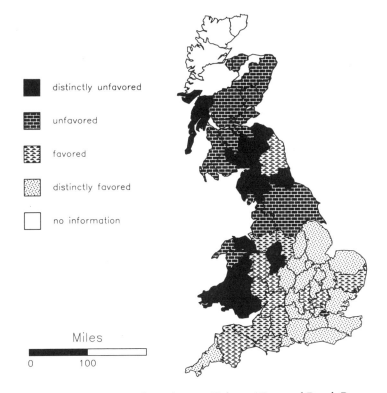

distinctly unfavored

unfavored

favored

distinctly favored

no information

Miles

0   100

Map 8.8. Overall Variations from Average Sickness Time and Death Rates Combined, 1872–1910
Source: AOF, *Directories,* 1873–1911.

notable exceptions of London and Northumberland,[20] this map highlights sharp regional differences in health. Distinctly favored counties are concentrated in the southeast, and favored counties in southwestern England. Unfavored counties appear in Wales, northern England, and Scotland, plus Staffordshire. Great Britain was a land of marked regional disparities in health.

HEALTH DIFFERENTIALS AT THE LOCAL LEVEL

Descriptive information about the regional distribution of high and low sickness and death rates, and about changes in relative position over time,

20. Considered in terms of the sum of percentage differences in sickness time and mortality, Northumberland falls into the category of unfavored counties.

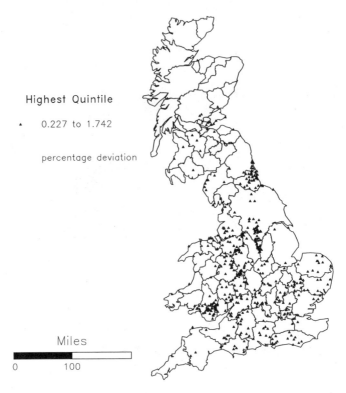

Highest Quintile

▲   0.227 to 1.742

percentage deviation

Miles

0   100

Map 8.9. Sickness: Highest Quintile, 1872–1910
Source: AOF, *Directories,* 1873–1911.

highlights the importance of searching for determinants of county-level differences, which is the objective of chapter 9. But it is also worthwhile to investigate the degree to which these differences are matters of location within counties. To what degree did individual counties encapsulate both high and low sickness and death rates?

Maps 8.9 and 8.10 give the locations of AOF courts in the highest and lowest quintiles of sickness time in the period 1887–95. The quintiles consist in each case of one-fifth of the 2,345 locales in which active courts existed in this period. Sickness and death rates have been aggregated for all locales and compared to overall AOF experience, following the same procedures as those employed to differentiate counties, except that the discussion is limited to experience in a period of nine years centered on 1891.[21]

21. The maps in this section exclude courts that accumulated fewer than fifty member-years at risk to sickness and death. Where locales had more than one court, the experience of those courts has been combined, weighting for size. Reasons for choosing this period are explained in chapter 9.

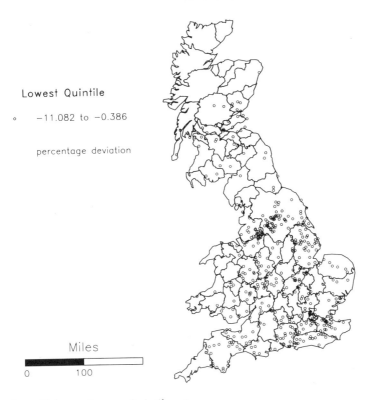

Lowest Quintile

o   −11.082 to −0.386

percentage deviation

Miles

0   100

Map 8.10. Sickness: Lowest Quintile, 1872–1910
Source: AOF, *Directories,* 1873–1911.

Except for Scotland, where the health of AOF members deteriorated relative to England and Wales, the broad stability of position of different regions and counties suggests that this particular test period will produce results that can be cast backward and forward in time.[22]

These maps show how rarely areas within counties with low sickness time overlapped areas with high sickness time. Although in London—the city and the county—locales with both low and high rates appear, in most of the remainder of Britain the two maps depict separate zones. For example, Durham, Northumberland, and South Wales contained only a few locales with low sickness time but many with high. Except for a seam of high sickness time extending south from the West Riding of Yorkshire

22. A shorter period would produce results more heavily influenced by regional differences in influenza morbidity and mortality rather than differences in overall sickness and death. A longer period would cause the control variables employed to compare courts and locales on the same terms—average age of members, years since court formation, and initiation rate—to lose meaning.

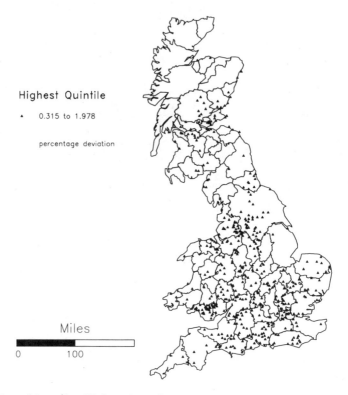

Map 8.11. Mortality: Highest Quintile, 1872–1910
Source: AOF, *Directories,* 1873–1911.

along the border of Derbyshire and Nottinghamshire, Yorkshire and Lincolnshire constituted an area of unusually low sickness time. Map 8.9,
which shows the highest quintile of morbidity, reveals distinctive regional
clusters, some of which can be associated with mineral deposits and mining, especially coal mining. Even before undertaking a statistical analysis,
it seems likely that occupations in mining must have played a large part in
determining which AOF courts and which locales had high morbidity. But
the same map shows clusters of high morbidity that do not coincide with
mineral deposits. And, more precisely to the point, a comparison of maps
8.9 and 8.10 shows that most British counties had locales with both high
and low sickness rates. Although in the aggregate, Britain was a country of
marked regional disparities in health, few counties were so unfavored that
they lacked pockets of good health, nor so favored that they lacked pockets of bad health.

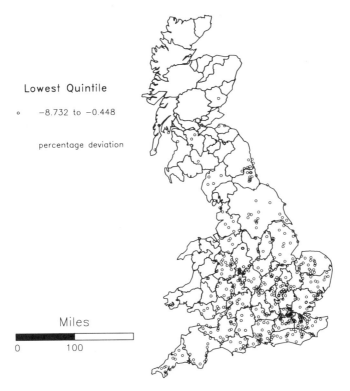

Map 8.12. Mortality: Lowest Quintile, 1872–1910
Source: AOF, *Directories,* 1873–1911.

Maps 8.11 and 8.12 provide information in the same form for mortality. Once more, London shows a cluster of locales and neighborhoods with both high and low mortality. But in the remainder of Britain, low-mortality locales cluster separately from high-mortality locales, and the clusterings often fail to follow county boundaries. Moreover, Scotland and Wales both exhibit only a few locales with low mortality.

Across the period 1872–1910, England gained relative position in health standing; its mortality fell more and its sickness time rose less. Scotland and Wales, especially Scotland, lost standing. A north-south divide distinguished healthy from unhealthy regions in mortality, but the divide in sickness time ran on an east-west line. When sickness time and mortality are considered together, both divides appear. Southeastern England was the most-favored region, with low sickness time and mortality, while in Wales and the border counties high mortality and high sickness time combined to give a least-favored health profile. Northwestern England, with its concentration of cotton textile manufacturing, appears in these descriptions as a region of heavy mortality but low sickness time. Whether it was a region favored or unfavored in health awaits further analysis in the chapter that follows.

This descriptive information about the regional distribution of high and low sickness and death rates and of changes in relative position over time points up a leading question: why did sickness time and mortality vary so sharply among the regions of Britain? In the next chapter attention shifts from description to analysis and from the administrative counties to three other units: registration counties, registration districts, and municipalities. Now that more is known about which areas and locales were favored and unfavored in their patterns of health, the objective is to discover why, concentrating on England and Wales.

CHAPTER 9

Determinants of Sickness Time and Mortality

S ICKNESS AND DEATH rates varied sharply among AOF members depending on where they lived in Britain. Some of the variations seem predictable. Regions where coal was mined stand out in the maps given in the previous chapter for their higher rates.[1] Similarly, some sparsely populated rural regions where agriculture was the leading occupation are conspicuous for their low sickness and death rates. Other regional differences are unexpected. Sickness time in Lancashire, for example, was lower than would be predicted on the strength of that county's concentration of manufacturing, its rapid urban growth, and its high death rates, plus the oft-made assumption that sickness parallels mortality. This chapter describes the results of a statistical search for explanations for regional differences in sickness and death rates and explains why the assumption that sickness parallels mortality should not be made.

The aim in the analysis of factors thought to influence an outcome, in this case sickness time or mortality, can be conceptualized as an attempt to isolate a few factors that exhibit a strong statistical association, one that makes them prospective predictors of the effects under study. All factors considered in any approach that relies first on identifying plausible candidates are likely to show some association. In such circumstances the point is to distinguish the variables having the strongest effect, in either theoretical or historical circumstances. In theoretical circumstances the most important factors are those that determine sickness time or mortality to a substantial degree—those which appear to push sickness time or mortality up or down with particular force and consistency—regardless of the circumstances of the moment. Age is the strongest of these. It looms so large

---

1. Coal-mining areas are identified in Pope, *Atlas of British Social and Economic History,* 71.

because age captures both physiological changes across the lifetime and a big share of the health history of the individual and the group, factors that otherwise stand in the background here, where attention focuses on current and recent socioeconomic and environmental influences. The aim is to identify other factors besides age that show a strong statistical association with sickness time or mortality. Statistical analysis in this form can also provide a way to focus attention on factors that played a large role in changes in sickness time and mortality in specific historical circumstances. Which factors actually drove changes in sickness time and mortality in Britain in the late nineteenth century?

Each explanatory factor considered in an equation may be positively or negatively associated with mortality or sickness time. The associations may match, so that factors promoting lower sickness time also promote lower mortality. But the associations may also be at odds, so that, for example, factors that promote lower rates for sickness time may promote higher rates for mortality.[2] This possibility is the most interesting, both in theory and practice. If important variables are associated in opposing directions, then this finding promotes two leading conclusions. First, opposing associations suggest the essential separateness of sickness time and mortality. Such a finding would show that it is fundamentally unsatisfactory to substitute data about mortality in analyses of sickness prevalence, as scholars have often done, or to try to modify sickness prevalence by manipulating variables selected because of their known associations with mortality. Second, opposing associations would highlight the difficulties involved in selecting policies that promote both lower mortality and less sickness time.

Lower mortality and less sickness time are both desirable effects. One way to understand the objective of this chapter is to imagine that it could be possible to use hindsight in the service of the past, rather than merely of the present. If this were so, it would be possible, investigating circumstances in the AOF and in Britain around 1891 and in the period 1872–1910, to study how potential explanatory factors were associated with sickness and mortality with the aim of designing a reactive strategy. That strategy would enable public authorities in the 1890s to adopt a superior plan for promoting both higher life expectancy and less sickness time among the men who belonged to friendly societies, and perhaps among

---

2. Ways in which lower death rates may promote more sickness time are explored in Alter and Riley, "Frailty, Sickness, and Death"; and Riley, "Morbidity Trends in Four Countries."

people in general. Of course, this notion is the stuff of fiction. We cannot intervene in the past. But it is not entirely outrageous. The information and some of the statistical procedures used here were available at the end of the nineteenth century and might have been brought to bear on the problem of selecting an optimal health policy. British public health administrators and other observers aimed to reduce the incidence and lethality of disease.[3] In an 1884 address the influential surgeon James Paget explained the need to devise a national strategy for health maintenance and used friendly society records in his own analysis of ways in which sickness undermined national income.[4]

HOW ACTUARIES EXPLAINED REGIONAL DIFFERENCES IN SICKNESS AND MORTALITY

The statisticians and actuaries who studied mortality and patterns of sickness in the friendly societies in the nineteenth century noticed variations among different courts and sought to explain them. They noticed that age was a powerful force distinguishing sickness and death rates and organized their search for other explanatory factors by controlling for age. Two other factors—town size and occupation—seemed most important. Influenced by studies such as E. H. Greenhow's investigation of reasons for the urban penalty in mortality and by William Farr's claim to have uncovered a law of mortality and population density,[5] friendly society actuaries and statisticians equated town size with mortality risk, dividing settlements into three categories: rural areas with fewer than five thousand inhabitants, towns of between five thousand and thirty thousand, and cities of thirty thousand and more. They expected an urban hazard to obtain also in morbidity, an assumption some historians have since adopted.[6] The actuaries observed that occupations could be divided into two types, hazardous and not, the former being associated with much higher death rates. As a result of the tedious work they did constructing mortality and sick-

3. Hardy, *Epidemic Streets,* 1.
4. Paget, "National Health and National Work," 381, 392–95.
5. Greenhow, *Papers Relating to the Sanitary State of the People of England;* and Russell, *Public Health Administration,* 138–39, which discusses Farr's law ("the mortality in two places is as the sixth root of their densities") in order to modify it.
6. Floud, "Medicine and the Decline of Mortality." On different patterns of mortality within the city, see Kearns, "Biology, Class, and the Urban Penalty." In 1903, Alfred Watson (*Sickness and Mortality Experience,* 23–24) pointed out that urban sickness time did not systematically exceed rural except at higher ages.

ness time averages for town size and occupation, each controlling for age, the actuaries were able to reliably advise friendly societies on how to set premiums that would earn enough revenue to pay sickness and burial benefits.

Those sensible steps of analysis take us a substantial distance toward understanding why patterns of health varied so much from region to region. The mix of levels of urbanization and the proportion of jobs that can be deemed hazardous varied across Britain. But these explanations are also inadequate. Sickness and death rates may have varied for reasons other than town size and occupation, even if it can be shown, as the friendly society actuaries repeatedly demonstrated, that town size and occupation each, by itself, did matter. In terms of the statistical techniques now available, but only beginning to be developed when the friendly society actuaries did their work, the largest reservation about accepting the actuaries' results arises from their dependence on explanations in each of which only two factors were considered: age and town size or age and occupation.

Here, the aim is to press the search further along two particular avenues. First, it is useful to consider more factors, drawing on modern theories about health risks to identify forces that may have influenced sickness and death rates in the AOF and searching for information that allows those forces to be included in a statistical analysis. Second, the search may be conducted by different means, adopting regression analysis as a way of assessing the statistical associations between potential explanatory factors and sickness and death rates while considering a large number of factors at once.[7] The same groups of factors are considered in separate analyses, making it possible to discover how each factor interacts with sickness time and mortality while controlling for all other factors included in the analy-

7. There are no entirely satisfactory statistical techniques for analyzing either sickness time or mortality. For sickness time the best method available is ordinary least squares. Sickness time cannot satisfactorily be analyzed by logistic regression because it cannot be assumed that the likelihood of one day of a member's sickness was independent from the likelihood of another day.

For examination of factors affecting mortality, there are good reasons to choose logistic regression, but there are also good reasons to prefer ordinary least squares. Logistic regression is better suited to a bounded dependent variable, which, like the death rate, can be expected to exhibit a curvilinear, rather than a linear, path. But ordinary least squares is a candidate because deaths are observed within groups rather than at the individual level. Mortality results will be reported below in some detail for logistic regression, together with a comparison of what ordinary least squares shows.

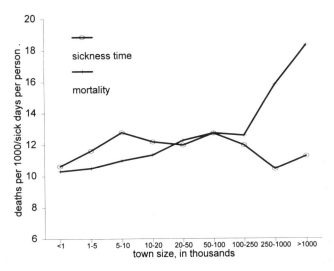

Fig. 9.1. Sickness Time and Mortality, by Town Size
Source: Data from AOF, *Directories,* 1872–1911; Great Britain, *Parliamentary Papers,* 1893–94, CIV, 31, 51–530; 1893–94, CV, v, xxxv–xxxvii, 3–1165; 1893–94, CVI, 9–545.

sis. For purposes of this analysis AOF experience is deemed a sample of all male friendly society experience.

A closer examination of town size and health in the years around 1891 shows that this relationship was more complex than the actuaries thought. Figure 9.1 tracks how sickness time and mortality among AOF members varied according to town size.[8] Mortality increased as towns grew in size and jumped to much higher levels in large cities. But the curve for sickness time does not follow the same path. It resembles an inverted U. Rising sickness time coincided with rising mortality, which is the least desirable association, in the early part of the spectrum, moving from villages to small towns. For cities of a hundred thousand to a million, in contrast, the two trends moved in opposite directions: sickness time diminished, while mortality increased. The average number of days that AOF members lost to sickness each year was highest in towns and small cities and lowest in cities of 250 thousand to a million, a category including Sheffield, Leeds,

8. These findings are based on regression analysis in which sickness time and mortality have been predicted by town size after controlling for age and age dispersion.

Birmingham, Manchester, and Liverpool.[9] By considering only three categories, most friendly society actuaries failed to notice that sickness time did not continue to increase as towns grew in size and, moreover, that mortality and sickness time followed divergent paths in Britain's largest cities.

An increase in town size tended to promote higher sickness rates in a definitive way only in the lower part of the spectrum, up to towns with somewhere between twenty thousand and one hundred thousand inhabitants. For cities with between one hundred thousand and one million inhabitants, sickness time tended to decline as town size rose. To interpret this relationship, it is useful to consider the curve for mortality as an assessment of both the relation between town size and the risk of death and that between town size and sickness incidence. When considered as an indication of sickness risk, the mortality curve in figure 9.1 indicates that the risk of falling sick increased with population size, especially between large towns and cities. This sharp upward trend in mortality and incidence, together with the decline in sickness time, means that the average duration of sickness episodes must have been shorter in cities than in villages. Perhaps because their episodes came more often in close succession, and because living in a city also meant having a poorer health history, the sicknesses of city dwellers were more often cut short by death.

That poorer health history of urban residents also emerges from friendly society records, which show that the sickness insults to which urban dwellers were exposed accumulated. Figures 9.2 and 9.3 depict urban and rural sickness and death rates among Foresters in the years 1871–75.[10] Sickness and mortality risks increased with age at a faster pace in cities than in rural areas, as shown by the widening gap between the urban and rural curves as age advances. Living in a city exposed workingmen to accumulating risks and damaged their health in a progressively more aggravated manner.[11]

9. For town size and other variables whose relationship with sickness time or mortality is nonlinear, quadratic terms have been employed in the linear regression equations.

10. Oddfellows statistics, also reported by Neison, *Rates of Mortality and Sickness, 1871–1875,* 42–43, 346–47, show the same effect.

11. This inference assumes that most friendly society members were long-term residents of rural or urban areas, which is true according to my study of entries and exits in individual courts. Some friendly society members migrated, obtaining clearances from their home court, and others seceded at one place and joined another sick club elsewhere. Many of the migrants took with them health histories gained in another type of locale, usually taking rural experience to urban districts. For adults, however, the AOF statistics are dominated by health histories gained in the locale of record, because long-term members were so numerous.

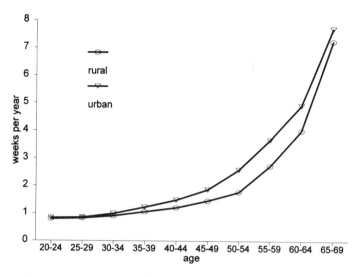

Fig. 9.2. Insult Accumulation, Sickness, by Age
Source: Data from Neison, *Rates of Mortality and Sickness, 1871–1875*, 42–43.

These two figures promote an important inference about the relationship between sickness time and mortality. What appears at first glance to be a paradox—that sickness time should decrease in cities the size of Manchester and Liverpool as mortality increased—turns out to reveal an intricacy in the use of sickness time as a measure of health status. On the one hand, lower sickness time is a desirable outcome, but only if it is associated with lower mortality. If sickness time is reduced by the earlier death of individuals, the effect is instead undesirable. On the other hand, higher sickness time will, if associated with lower mortality, signal that the resolution of sickness episodes ending in death has more often been deferred. In this sense, higher sickness time is a desirable outcome, to the degree that survival in sickness is more desirable than earlier death in sickness. To interpret the sickness time outcome for any one variable it is necessary to look also at the mortality outcome for that variable. This more complex association explains why some regions depicted in chapter

---

However, it must be the case that many members brought different childhood patterns of health and residence to the site where they lived as adults, with the result that court records exhibit a mixture of experience. The practical effect of this is to homogenize patterns of health, producing smaller differences in the contrasts noted here than would obtain if members could be studied at the individual level and divided by place of birth and childhood residence.

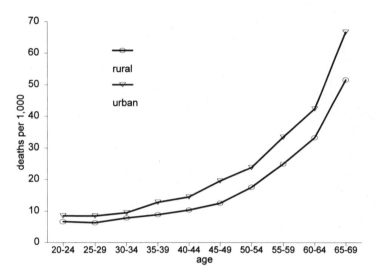

Fig. 9.3. Insult Accumulation, Mortality, by Age
Source: Data from Neison, *Rates of Mortality and Sickness, 1871–1875,*
42–43.

8 as areas of high mortality and low sickness, such as Lancashire and
Yorkshire, should be seen as regions of disadvantage. Those counties suffered high mortality, and the sicknesses among friendly society members
living there were unusually short. They were distinctly unfavored areas.

Figure 9.1 suggests further that town size produced desirable patterns of
health only at the lowest end of the spectrum. Reading the curves right to
left, from large town size to small, mortality and sickness time both diminished in the shift from London, the outlier with a population of more than
four million, to the next category of city size; perhaps in a weakly simultaneous decline from cities of fifty to one hundred thousand to those of
twenty thousand to fifty thousand; and more certainly in a simultaneous
decline in both measures in the shift from towns to villages. In 1891
Britain, health authorities might have promoted less sickness time, and
perhaps also lower mortality, by inducing people to migrate to towns and
villages, by preventing further growth of the metropolis, and by fostering
the formation of new villages.

Reorganizing their data, friendly society actuaries noticed that certain
occupations—especially mining—consistently posed more health risks.
But they did not take the further step of determining whether health risks
varied when age, town size, and occupation were all considered at once.

And, having found some answers to their question about why health risks varied from region to region, they did not press the search further.

A NEW EXPLANATION FOR REGIONAL DIFFERENCES

Sources and Approaches

Census authorities periodically surveyed certain vital statistics of England and Wales, and separately of Scotland, reporting their findings for each region as a whole and for several subdivisions. Four censuses were conducted within the period for which AOF experience is known, in 1881, 1891, 1901, and 1911. Each is most generous in the information it reports about the nation as a whole or its major areas. But those divisions provide an inadequate means of differentiating among courts. For England and Wales the censuses give a narrower range of information about the vital statistics of people living in counties and registration districts, the smallest units for which data are reported for most factors. The same is true of other sources, the annual reports of the Registrar General of Births, Deaths, and Marriages and historical studies or reconstructions that provide evidence about such specific factors as wages. As a result, most AOF courts must be associated not with the characteristics of people belonging to them or of people living in their immediate vicinity but with the characteristics of people living in the county or registration district in which the court was located.

The expansion of the search to include more explanatory factors than friendly society actuaries considered necessarily means a loss of intimacy in the association of characteristics to AOF members. Men belonging to courts in London certainly helped compose the statistical characteristics of the county of London or the particular registration district in which they lived. But their part in those characteristics is diluted by the inclusion of so many other people who did not belong to those London courts.

Determinants of sickness time and mortality can be explored at three levels for the 3,954 AOF courts. At the first level, the relationship between town size and health risks is examined. Individual courts are associated with the 1,690 municipal boroughs and civil parishes in which they were located[12] and with information about the population of each locale and

---

12. Census authorities reported town population only for the 303 towns designated as municipal boroughs in the 1891 census. For other communities, the census reported for

the number of inhabited houses, from which data the average number of residents per house has been calculated. This first level should be the most revealing, because it provides the closest link between court and community. But only a few explanatory factors can be considered at this level.

About registration districts, of which 582 out of 633 had AOF courts, census authorities reported information on marital status and the spatial density of the population. At this level more explanatory factors can be considered, but the distance between the court and its community grows as courts are associated with larger areas.[13]

At the third level, each court is associated with a further group of characteristics of each of the fifty-five counties in England and Wales in which courts were located, leaving out the island of Anglesey off the northwest coast of Wales.[14] Here, the range of information is broader, for the census reports the number of people practicing each of a large number of occupations for each county.[15] But the association of each factor with AOF courts is more remote. The most important limitation of this analysis arises from the need to associate courts with communities as large as the counties.

In earlier chapters patterns of health of AOF members were approached in a chronological manner, constructing annual rates to show the trends of sickness time and mortality and comparing regional differences for each decade between the 1870s and the decade 1901–10. To press the search further along this path would limit it to whatever information can be gathered on an annual basis for part or all of the period 1872–1910, of

administrative subdivisions, of which the most important are sanitary districts (for which a distinction between urban and rural was made but in a way the authorities admitted was often misleading) and civil parishes, 14,684 districts in which poor law taxes were levied. Neither is necessarily contiguous with the boundaries of a village, town, or city. Moreover, some AOF courts were situated in towns that did not have separate status as sanitary districts or civil parishes. Of the 3,954 courts whose health risks are considered here, 3,151 can be associated with municipal boroughs or civil parishes and, therefore, with a population size and housing density. Health risks for the courts that could not be assigned to a municipal borough or a civil parish are distributed in a manner similar to those in courts that could be assigned, indicating that the missing values do not introduce any bias.

13. Here, too, some courts cannot be considered because they cannot be placed in a given registration district. A total of 287 courts cannot be assigned to registration districts because of inadequate information. These courts do not appear in analyses that include information available only for registration districts, but in each case the sickness time and mortality values are randomly distributed, indicating that their exclusion does not bias results.

14. In a few cases the number is smaller still, for some data are available only for three groups of counties: Yorkshire rather than the three Ridings; and North and South Wales rather than their constituent counties.

15. See Great Britain, *Parliamentary Papers*, 1893–94, CIV, 325–50, for a discussion of limitations of the occupational data.

which the largest part concerns causes of death. Because data are more extensively available for single years, the search is instead reoriented to a single period.

In the former orientation what begged for explanation were differences from year to year, and sometimes also from region to region, in sickness and death rates. In the new orientation what beg for explanation are differences in the health risks of the groups of men belonging to each court. Therefore, in place of the national or regional AOF sickness and death rates that have been studied to this point, attention shifts now to differences among individual courts. The period chosen stands at the middle of the years for which AOF health statistics are known and is centered on 1891. Sickness and death rates and information about the ages of members in each court have been averaged for the nine years 1887–95, a step that transforms the potentially unstable sickness and death rates of individual years into stable values. This period is nine years long in order to submerge the effects of the influenza epidemic of 1890–91 and other short-term factors. In sum, sickness and death rates in 3,954 courts in the period 1887–95 are examined in terms of population size and other census statistics reported for April 1891, when the census was carried out, and other data that relate to 1891 or nearby years.[16]

Because the health data under study cover experience during nine years, more than five million years of experience are included, apportioned among the 3,954 courts by weight. Thus each court, and the characteristics associated with it, has an impact in proportion to the number of years of exposure to risk. This process of weighting is desirable because of substantial differences in the sizes of courts, of which during the period 1887–95 the smallest accumulated only eight years of exposure, and the largest 13,257 years.

This analysis assumes that Foresters shared the circumstances of the communities in which they lived strongly enough to allow those community characteristics, which can be reconstructed, to stand for characteristics of the Foresters, which cannot be recaptured. Two bases exist for that assumption. First, earlier parts of this book show that AOF members as a whole closely resembled the central ranks of the working population in Britain, which implies that they did so also in most local communities. Second, the likelihood that the experience of men drawn from the central

---

16. However, some values are missing for given courts, which means that they will not appear in the analysis. Most of these losses occur because courts cannot be assigned to municipal boroughs or civil parishes.

ranks of the working population would resemble the experience of the community in general rises with the number of people and groups under observation.

The AOF enrolled several hundred thousand members. In many villages the AOF court was the only friendly society and enrolled a large part of the male working population. In most towns and cities and in all registration districts and counties, the AOF was represented by two or more courts, the number rising to 494 courts in London. In 1891 the Foresters made up 7.3 percent of the adult male population of Great Britain. The lowest proportions in counties, as low as 0.7 percent in Buteshire and 0.5 percent in Morayshire, occurred in Scotland, which has been excluded from this analysis. Within England and Wales higher proportions prevailed, ranging up to nearly 20 percent in Surrey. Only two counties—Cardiganshire (1.8 percent) and Merionethshire (1.5 percent)—counted fewer than 2 percent of their adult male populations as Foresters. Yet it remains true that the degree of association between court members and the characteristics of a locale may differ from one variable to another in ways that cannot be detected. In sum, it is worthwhile to explore relationships between patterns of health in the AOF and characteristics of the communities in which members of the AOF lived. But, like other forms of historical investigation, the results should be regarded as suggestive rather than conclusive.

Theories about Why Health Risks Vary

Long study of the decline of mortality in Britain and other countries since the eighteenth century has armed historians, demographers, epidemiologists, and others with well-developed ideas about why mortality rates diminished. Certain factors played a leading role. The prose version of the explanation for mortality decline, which is the version that can be used in statistical analysis, identifies the factors to which most weight is assigned and sometimes also attempts to rank those factors. The algebraic version of this explanation converts each factor into something that can be measured. Almost always the algebraic version of the explanation sacrifices some precision for the sake of quantification. If, for example, the supply of medical services is believed to have played a role in the mortality decline, scholars wanting a quantitative version of that hypothesis may invoke the ratio of physicians to the population. This step sacrifices precision, in that medical services may be provided by people other than physicians and may also be provided with differing levels of skill by physicians.

But it gains something, too. In the quantitative form, it is possible to use statistical procedures to test whether communities with more physicians in fact enjoyed lower mortality, controlling for other possible explanations that can be included in the model, or whether, over time, additions to the stock of physicians can be associated statistically with lower mortality. In this way statistical analysis provides a means to test ideas held to be plausible for reasons independent of the statistical procedures. In the real world, which exists apart from either the prose or the algebraic version of explanations for events, it is not so much the singularity of causes that matters as the complexity and interrelatedness of causation. In sum, what often matters is the distinctive contribution of a specific cause to an effect having many causes, and that is the question statistical analysis attempts to answer by including all identified causal factors in the analysis.

Much less is known about the determinants of sickness. This is true, in the first place, because for so long most scholars assumed that sickness risks are reliably approximated by mortality risks. For that reason and because of the difficulty of finding sources that report about health in a similar way over time, sickness incidence and prevalence were rarely considered as outcome variables. The AOF records make it possible to test the assumption that mortality is a good proxy for sickness and to search out the particular factors related to sickness time. Research on causes of mortality change is an important source about factors that should be considered. Further guidance in identifying potentially important factors comes from the analysis of modern sickness surveys. Those show, for example, that sickness prevalence diminishes as socioeconomic status rises and that married people experience less sickness than unmarried people and thereby imply that socioeconomic and marital status are important determinants at other times and places.[17]

The search for determinants of regional differences in patterns of health in 1891 begins, therefore, with theory informed by historical and modern experience. In some ways the discussion that follows is, like Preston and Haines's investigation of infant and maternal mortality in Britain and the United States in the late nineteenth century,[18] a study about whether the determinants found to be closely associated with health risks in recent years were also closely associated with those risks in the late nineteenth century, insofar at least as those factors can be depicted from late-nineteenth-century sources.

17. On socioeconomic differences in health in recent times, see Great Britain, "Black Report," 53–55; and North, "Explaining Socioeconomic Differences in Sickness Absence."
18. Preston and Haines, *Fatal Years.*

Determinants

Three types of factors have been considered as possible determinants. The first group is composed of the now familiar variables dealing with age and the dispersion of members across the possible range of ages: average age of court members, years since court formation, and the rate at which new members were added. By including these variables, the experience of each court can be compared while controlling for age. A second group of factors represents the eleven census divisions in England and Wales. Dichotomous variables for these regions are included in an effort to capture effects that are regional in scope but are not associated with factors that are specified. A strong association between any single region and either sickness time or mortality indicates that some still unidentified feature or features of that region influenced the outcomes.

A third group of factors consists of variables expected, on the basis of theoretical considerations, to have either positive or negative effects on health. These factors identify characteristics of regional populations that may promote poorer or better health. They occur in three subgroups: (a) socioeconomic and other characteristics of the locale, registration district, or county; (b) occupations suspected, on grounds of prior findings by friendly society actuaries or because of the known characteristics of the job, to be related to higher- or lower-than-ordinary health risks; and (c) causes of death, based on death rates in each county from specific diseases. These factors, except for that of the last subgroup, causes of death, are identified and the considerations underlying the inclusion of each are explained in appendix 5.[19] Disease-specific death rates for each county turned out to be unrevealing, and their associations are not reported here.[20] Class differences do not emerge in this analysis, since all AOF members belonged to the working class and because it is not clear that

19. In preliminary analyses, other occupational groups and categories were included in an effort to identify unanticipated associations. At that stage, for example, it became apparent that the number of people engaged in making and selling tobacco products had no association with sickness time or mortality. Hence, in what follows dealers in tobacco products are included in a broader category of retailers rather than separately as a proxy for hazards associated with tobacco use.

20. The associations lack statistical significance, even between sickness time and mortality from diseases with a prolonged course. Diagnostic practices differed widely across Britain, and many causes of death were assigned to the category of unknown or inadequately described diseases. The absence from the list of causes of death of many ailments that have been identified subsequently as specific to occupations, such as silicosis to coal mining, must also contribute to these weak results.

interregional differences in wages, which will be considered, capture anything about social class.

Occupational risks preoccupied friendly society actuaries, who were able to confirm and assign weights to hazards associated with particular trades.[21] In explaining the decline of mortality in Britain, historians have been more interested in the standard of living, public health, epidemiologic trends, and medicine. Overturning earlier explanations that stressed the role of medicine in reducing the risk of death, Thomas McKeown has argued that most of the gain in life expectancy occurred because the standard of living improved and, within that, most particularly because, from the eighteenth century into the twentieth, people were progressively better fed.[22] McKeown reached that conclusion more by casting doubt on other possible explanations than by identifying specific improvements in nutrition that lowered mortality. He cast his argument chiefly in terms of nutritional bulk, calories consumed per capita, and in that way related it to the cost of food and to wages. More recent work has employed another gauge of nutritional status, height near the completion of growth.[23] Data are as yet unavailable for average height by county or registration district.[24] McKeown's earlier work stressed the importance of sanitary improvements, an interpretation recently given new force by Simon Szreter, who argues that public health improvements played a leading role in mortality decline.[25] Some scholars have also emphasized such epidemiologic factors as a putative change in the virulence of disease organisms.

Each of those interpretations stresses changes over time, which can be captured in the present analysis only to the degree that some counties consistently led or lagged in the indicators available for analysis, such as the proportion of sanitary workers or the wage level. Regional differences in Britain abounded, but they are ill suited for testing explanations for the mortality decline in the forms suggested by McKeown and Szreter. Instead,

21. See chapter 8.
22. McKeown, *Modern Rise of Population.* Guha, "Importance of Social Intervention," reasserts McKeown's case, interpreting evidence from the friendly societies.
23. Floud, Wachter, and Gregory, *Height, Health, and History;* and Fogel, "Nutrition and the Decline of Mortality since 1700."
24. John Beddoe gathered such information in 1866, but his findings are too distant in time and relate to too few counties to give reliable results here. Riley, "Height, Nutrition, and Mortality Risk Reconsidered." Heights and weights of school children are reported for some areas in 1908–11 by Greenwood, *Health and Physique of School Children,* but the coverage is uneven. Some counties are omitted, and most results derive from rural county council areas.
25. Szreter, "Importance of Social Intervention."

the analysis reported here focuses on features of experience that can be measured for each county, registration district, or town.[26]

RESULTS

Detailed results from the statistical analyses appear in appendix 6.[27] Table A6.1 shows the mean value of all variables. Tables A6.2 and A6.3 show the coefficients estimated for each variable and identify which individual factors contributed most forcefully to higher or lower sickness time or mortality by giving a column of elasticities. The elasticities can be compared to one another within each separate analysis but not between the two analyses. They show how much a given movement in a factor affects sickness time or mortality. In this way, for example, age and the dispersion of court members by age are seen to have exerted a large effect. Indeed, age by itself accounts for most of the power of this attempt to identify determinants of sickness time and mortality. The effect of the three age variables is also statistically significant, a characteristic shown in tables A6.2 and A6.3 by level of significance.

All other factors made smaller contributions than the variables controlling for age, and some have associations that are neither statistically significant nor sizable. Hence, tables A6.2 and A6.3 identify some factors that seem to matter and others that do not. Most factors that have a large effect also have a statistically significant effect, making it possible to focus attention on a few that played a major role as determinants of sickness time and mortality among AOF members.[28] Other factors appear to exert a large

26. Lee, "Regional Inequalities in Infant Mortality in Britain," takes an approach similar to that followed here.

27. Tables A6.2 and A6.3 identify the factors considered, show the coefficients calculated for each, give elasticities for each factor to gauge the scale of effect, and report statistical significance. For sickness time the products sum to an estimate of 10.535 days of sickness per member per year, close to the weighted mean of sickness time for all courts (11.67 days). For death rates, the products sum to a log odds value of -4.535, which indicates a probability of dying of .0107, or 10.7 per thousand, again a figure close to the weighted mean death rate for all courts (11.55).

In logistic regression, when coefficients are exponentiated, they produce a relative risk. For example, the coefficient for average age in the mortality analysis, 0.056, is 1.058 when exponentiated. This implies that one additional year of age would increase the relative risk of death by 5.8 percent.

An ordinary least squares (OLS) version of the mortality regression produced results similar to those from the logistic analysis reported in table A6.3. The principal differences in the OLS version are that the proportion married and the ratio of people to houses acquire negative signs and are not significant.

28. This analysis can be understood as the preliminary step toward creating a parsi-

but not statistically significant effect. The density of people per statute acre, crowding within tenements, and some other variables do not emerge, in this analysis, as strong candidates for inclusion in a parsimonious model of determinants of sickness time. But these and other variables are worth further investigation in later analyses in order to see whether, in different circumstances, they might emerge as important factors. The same is true of some of the potential determinants of mortality.

Sickness Time

Limiting consideration only to the factors that exhibit both a large and a statistically significant effect, this analysis of the determinants of sickness time suggests that a few matter the most. Factors that tended, at higher levels, to promote greater sickness time were average age (AVERAGE), number of residents per house (PERHOUS and PERHOUS2), availability of health services and information (HEALTH), illiteracy (MARKS91), proportion of construction workers (CONSTRCT), dispersion of membership by age (SINCEDOF), and proportion of trade unionists (UNION). Factors that tended, at higher levels, to promote less sickness time were proportion of sanitation workers (SCAVN), size of town (TOWNPOP and TOWNPOP2), and the proportion of young members (INITRATE). In addition, a higher rate of population growth in a community, signaling infant births and an influx of young adult migrants, shows an association with lower sickness time, but at a low level of effect. Three regional variables, London, the southwest, and the South Midlands, suggest that unidentified factors associated with those areas played some role, albeit on a small scale.

Mortality

For mortality, too, a few factors matter the most. Those promoting greater mortality were average age (AVERAGE), dispersion of membership by age (SINCEDOF), wage level (WAGES92), proportion of workers in commerce and conveyance (COMCON), proportion of men married (MAR), number of residents per house (PERHOUS and PERHOUS2), proportion of construction workers (CONSTRCT), proportion of farmers (FARM), and proportion of trade unionists (UNION). Factors associated with lower rates of mortality were proportion of retailers (RETAIL).

In addition, several variables show relationships that are statistically significant at the 0.10 level but small in their implied effects. Four of these are occupational groups—workers in textiles, stone, glass, and lead—and a fifth is made up of railway workers, who may capture the added dangers associated with work in that trade or the more rapid communication of disease in areas with more extensive railway services. Two environmental variables also show up in this group, the ratio of people to land area and the size of the town in which AOF members lived. The mortality analysis shows further that three regions, the North Midlands, Monmouth and Wales, and the northern counties, have characteristics that remain to be identified. For these variables, the analysis suggests that any increase in their scale would lead to higher mortality. That is, for example, more stoneworkers, larger towns, and more people living in the North Midlands would likely produce higher death rates, on a small scale. And a higher initiation rate among AOF courts would reduce mortality, also on a small scale.

The meaning of these results depends on the direction of influence in both the sickness time and mortality analyses. Factors that promoted more sickness time should be viewed as favorable when they also promoted lower mortality, while factors that promoted less sickness time should be viewed as favorable only when they also promoted lower mortality.

These analyses suggest not only that different factors played the largest part in influencing sickness time and mortality but also that the differences are captured by types of variables. That is, the factors identified as influencing sickness time overlap only partially with factors influencing mortality. Socioeconomic factors such as the level of literacy, crowding in residential dwellings, and town size, in addition to the availability of health and public health services, play the largest role in the sickness time analysis, aside from the variables controlling for age. Yet the factors that play the largest role in the mortality analysis are occupations, the wage level, marital status, and membership in trade unions. Again leaving out the variables controlling for age, only four factors—the average number of residents per house, proportion of construction workers, town size, and membership in trade unions—emerge in both analyses as statistically significant. Only two of those—number of residents per house and share of construction workers—are statistically significant in both analyses and important in the scale of their effects. In sum, these separate analyses of determinants, which examine associations between the same group of determinants and the two separate outcome variables, sickness time and mortality, suggest that there is limited overlap. Most of the factors that are important in one analysis are not important in the other.

Sickness time was heightened—sicknesses were made more prolonged—especially as an effect of factors that can be interpreted in the following manner:

1. The proportion of people providing health services and information—doctors, nurses, chemists, and teachers—shows a strong positive association with sickness time and a negative association with mortality. Adding health workers to the community, these analyses suggests, would have reduced mortality (the negative sign suggests this effect, but the level of significance is not reassuring) while prolonging the average duration of sickness episodes. Members of the AOF survived their sicknesses for longer periods in communities of England and Wales where people providing health services and information were more numerous. This finding suggests that, while medical services and information may not have mattered a great deal for the course of mortality, in the circumstances of 1891, they did matter quite significantly for health. By implication, the people providing medical services and information in a community could do little to determine whether a sickness episode ended in death but a great deal to influence how long a sick person survived until death. Given that AOF members, as a rule, had access to doctors, this association suggests the added efficacy of easier access to medical services and information, as long as the purpose of those things is recognized as deferring the resolution of sickness in death.

2. Adding population to towns tended to increase mortality and reduce sickness time, the most unfavorable combination. Moreover, while the scale of the effect associated with mortality is small, that associated with sickness time is sizable. The addition of a hundred thousand inhabitants to a town's population, this analysis suggests, would cut average annual sickness time per capita by 0.347 days, while it would also increase mortality.

3. Crowding within residential dwellings (but not crowding in tenements as measured by census authorities) prolonged sickness, presumably capturing the effects of respiratory diseases with an elongated course, while adding to mortality risk. The contribution of crowding in housing is examined further in figure 9.4, which shows predicted sickness time and mortality in eight categories of crowding. More-crowded housing added in a substantial way to higher sickness time across most of the spectrum, up to 6–6.99 persons per house, before the relationship breaks down. For mortality, the association is sustained only to 5–5.49 persons per house.

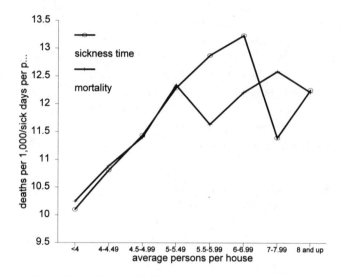

Fig. 9.4. Health and Crowding in Housing
Source: Data from AOF, *Directories*, 1872–1911; Great Britain, *Parliamentary Papers*, 1893–94, CIV, 31, 51–530; 1893–94, CV, v, xxxv–xxxvii, 3–1165; 1893–94, CVI, 9–545.

4. A higher proportion of public health workers, here represented by people employed as drainage workers and in collecting refuse and sweeping, paid generous health dividends. Areas with more public health workers enjoyed the most favorable outcome, lower mortality and less sickness time, although only the morbidity finding is statistically significant. The ratio of drainage workers and scavengers to all employed men was low in 1891, only 0.113 per thousand, and the effect of adding more workers large. This association implies further that filth diseases, which public health workers were meant to combat, played a significant role in the sickness profile of AOF members around 1891. Since such diseases do not loom large in the cause-of-sickness profiles reconstructed for 1902–19 in chapter 7, the implication is that they had declined sharply in importance during the 1890s.

5. Certain occupations played a strong role in health, so that the more, or the fewer, men who followed them in a community, the greater or the less the mortality or sickness risk.[29] Among these the most dramatic effects are associated with men working in the building trades. Additions to the number of men employed in construction in a community could be expected to produce

29. On specific risks associated with these and other jobs, see Hunter, *Diseases of Occupations;* for example, on the lead poisoning hazard of working in pottery, see 123 and 281; and Dupree, *Family Structure in the Staffordshire Potteries,* 84–86, 149. Dupree also points out that the North Staffordshire Potteries was a dangerous area because it combined coal mining and pottery work with dust and lead glazes. In these analyses pottery making is represented by the variable EARTH, for earthenware making.

unfavorable changes, increasing both mortality and sickness time. Similarly, communities where larger proportions of men mined and processed stone, worked in commerce and conveyance, worked with glass or lead or in the manufacture of textiles, or farmed all show statistically significant associations with higher mortality. To appearances, agricultural work itself bore greater risks that were compensated for by other features of rural life, which are controlled for here by such variables as population density (PERAREA). In contrast, areas with more retailers show an association with lower mortality.

These analyses indicate that the mixture of occupations in Britain mattered, but not in ways understood by friendly society actuaries. By indicating a coefficient for each factor, what these analyses do is to show the degree of association between that factor and the outcome, sickness time or mortality, net of all other factors. When coal mining and other mining trades do not show up as statistically significant, as they do not here, what is implied is that, in the actuary's analyses, mining coal and other minerals captured effects properly associated with other traits linked to mining rather than with mining itself. In the coalfields of northeast England, the Midlands, and south Wales, population and population density increased dramatically during the nineteenth century,[30] while the public health environment was degraded. Mining was a hazardous occupation, especially in the risks it posed of accidents and fatalities. But these socioeconomic factors played a larger role than the sickness hazards of mining in influencing the sickness outcome.[31]

6. These analyses indicate that, across England and Wales, higher wages were associated with more mortality and less sickness time, although the sickness association is not statistically significant.[32] Wages varied from job to job

---

30. Lawton, "Population," 10.

31. If this conclusion is accepted, an interesting puzzle is brought out. Does mining fail to stand out as a predictor of health outcomes because the sickness hazards of tuberculosis in the adult male population in general around 1891 equaled or outweighed the special hazards of mining associated with dust-related diseases, such as silicosis?

In an abridged form of the model, one specifying only the variables controlling for age, regional dummies, and occupations, adding these socioeconomic variables causes the variables for men working in mining to lose significance. However, it must be remembered that the conclusion that, in the sickness analysis, mining captures hazards more directly associated with socioeconomic characteristics of mining communities derives from analyses conducted at the aggregate level with ecological variables. Mining districts had unusually high concentrations of men in that occupation, which is reassuring about the integrity of these results. But it may be that individual-level data would show stronger associations between mining, on one hand, and morbidity and mortality risk, on the other. Furthermore, it is possible that mining fails to show strong health effects because those are captured by the greater discrimination associated with characteristics captured at the level of registration districts, whereas occupations, including mining, are represented only at the level of counties. That clearly does not impede other occupations in acquiring an association with mortality.

32. Friedlander et al., "Socio-economic Characteristics and Life Expectancies," argue that the relative importance of environmental variables in determining life expectancy diminished in England in the period 1851–1911 and the importance of factors of socioeconomic stratification, such as wages, increased. In the present analysis, environmental variables appear to have remained strong as late as 1891.

owing to market forces rather than to an overt appeal by working people to redress the ill effects of specific occupations, such as those shown by Ratcliffe's analyses.[33] To appearances, higher wages were meant to compensate the men who earned them for higher risks. But the added compensation was either insufficiently large or it was not spent in such a way as to counter the higher risks. In consequence, counties where wages were higher experienced more deaths among AOF members and possibly also sickness episodes curtailed early by death. County differences in wage levels are estimated here using A. L. Bowley's 1892 figures for agricultural laborers, which varied from county to county and are believed to reflect wage differentials in other trades.[34] Given the map of wage differences among agricultural laborers, where men in Lancashire, Northumberland, Cumberland, and probably also Durham earned the highest wages, it seems likely that the higher wages of agricultural workers in those counties reflect the high wages paid in mining and manufacturing. At the same time the combination of outcomes suggested by the analyses—higher mortality and less sickness time—suggests that accidents and injuries made up a large part of the added risk that these jobs posed.

7. Similarly, higher levels of membership in trade unions are associated with more sickness time and added mortality. Trade union members, by belonging, appear to have acquired less additional protection from health risks than the added hazards associated with the still narrow group of unionized jobs.

8. These analyses also suggest that areas where a higher proportion of men could not sign their names at marriage in 1891 experienced significantly higher sickness time and lower mortality, a favorable but unexpected outcome.[35] The sign on the coefficient for MARKS91 in the mortality analysis is negative and unstable, a characteristic that shows up when individual variables are dropped from the analysis. Hence it is difficult to interpret this finding, possibly because what is captured is the effect of illiteracy net of the proportion of teachers in a community, measured in the variable HEALTH.

9. Higher rates of population growth promoted less sickness time and perhaps also less mortality. Net of town size, crowding in housing, and population density, the effects of rapid growth were more beneficial than harmful. If anything is surprising about that result, it is only that the effect is small and unstable. Rapid growth meant that a locale was adding either infants or young adult migrants to its population and, except for infants, that meant more people with mortality and morbidity risks below those of the existing population.

33. See chapter 7.
34. Bowley, *Wages in the United Kingdom*, foldout after page 144. Bowley supplies data for most counties for 1892. For counties lacking data for that year, estimates have been supplied by using 1880 ratios with adjacent counties to estimate 1892 values. For London, Middlesex wages are used.
35. On the trend of literacy around 1891, see Mitch, *Rise of Popular Literacy in Victorian England*, 1 and passim.

IMPLICATIONS

Public health authorities in England and Wales, this analysis suggests, could have done much to reduce mortality and sickness time around 1891. Some of the policies available to them allowed actions in the same direction that promised beneficial effects for both sickness time and mortality. But the limited degree of overlap between factors that seem important in the two analyses suggests that for most possible actions the effects would have been advantageous for mortality or for sickness time but not for both. These possibilities stand out:

1. Crowded housing within communities, measured here by the average number of people per inhabited house, produced the most unfavorable outcome: higher mortality and higher sickness time.[36] Figure 9.4 shows that houses averaging more than five persons posed a high sickness risk (except in London, where the average number of inhabitants per dwelling is high and the association weaker).[37] Even a small reduction in the number of inhabitants per dwelling in the remainder of England and Wales, which averaged 5.32 people, would have promoted substantially better health and somewhat lower mortality. More-spacious housing would presumably have acted against the continuing importance of respiratory and other airborne diseases in the profile of causes of sickness, which persisted after respiratory diseases had begun to wane in importance in the profile of causes of death.[38] Late-nineteenth-century commentators who decried Britain's failure to build housing as rapidly as the population increased grasped a key problem in health policy.[39]

2. Cities the size of Liverpool and Manchester undermined the health of the nation. More-populous cities are associated in these analyses with higher mortality and sicknesses curtailed by death. Reducing the number or size of such cities promised to reverse these associations.

3. High wages and union membership are associated in both analyses with higher mortality. For public authorities the task was to identify the additional

36. Census authorities made no effort to estimate housing size, and the statistics used here combine spacious with small houses. Except for London, where spacious housing was more common, and perhaps for locales with crowded tenements, it is reasonable to suppose that differences in housing size balance out in the different categories. Census authorities did try for the first time in 1891 to measure overcrowding in tenements by counting tenements with an excessive number of people per room. That gauge fails to show an association with either outcome. It seems to be pushed aside both by its ineffectiveness as a measure, which census authorities acknowledged, and by the stronger force of crowding in space and in general housing.

37. London accounts for nearly all cases in the category of 7–7.99 persons per house.

38. See chapter 7.

39. E.g., Russell, *Public Health Administration,* 37.

risks faced by men who earned higher wages or belonged to trade unions, in order either to bring those risks under control or to shift men out of those jobs.

4. Communities with a large proportion of men engaged in construction show higher mortality and more sickness time. There, too, the task authorities faced was either to identify the added hazards associated with building or to forgo building. Ironically, these actions stand at odds with the first two policies that public authorities might have adopted to promote better health: building houses at a faster pace than the population grew and reducing the size of cities, which implies relocating people to towns and villages where accommodations for them would have to be built and where, therefore, the proportion of men employed in building trades would have to grow.

For the rest, however, these analyses suggest that public authorities needed to adopt parallel rather than coinciding policies. To reduce sickness time without undesirable mortality effects, it was most important to enlarge the supply of health and public health services. More doctors, nurses, chemists, and teachers, and more sanitation workers, promised the most generous payoffs. To reduce mortality, the most important additional action that public authorities might have taken was to review and reshape the mixture of occupations. Communities where too many men worked in dangerous trades—communications and conveyance, construction, farming, textiles, stone, glass, and lead—and too few in retailing showed the worse outcomes. To redress the effects associated with these occupations, public authorities needed to reflect on the human costs of an economic strategy that involved so many men practicing risky jobs.

In short, the actuaries failed to detect the at-times contradictory and at-times simply unrelated effects of forces affecting sickness time and mortality. Table 9.1 summarizes the results of these statistical analyses in a way that calls attention to this characteristic.[40] It includes all factors and calls attention to the sign associated with each in the two analyses. Read the mortality results down and the morbidity (sickness time) results across, looking at positive and negative associations. Table 9.1 shows the underlying antagonism in most of these relationships by distributing all explanatory factors among four possible cells. Two cells, the positive-positive cell in the upper left and the negative-negative cell in the lower right, represent agreement between outcomes: variables appearing in those cells act in the same direction in the sickness time and mortality analyses. Slightly more than half of the variables appear in these two cells, and slightly less than

40. The factors that appear with squared terms in the analysis of sickness time are considered here only for their net effect.

Table 9.1
DETERMINANTS OF SICKNESS TIME
AND MORTALITY

	Mortality	
	Positive	Negative
Sickness Time		
Positive	UNION	HEALTH
	PERHOUS	MARKS91
	PERAREA	CROWDED
	RRWKRS	RETAIL
	MONMWLS	OTHMNR
	TXTLES	LONDON
	COMCON	NW
	CNSTRCT	
	STONE	
	COALMNR	
	MACHINE	
	EARTH	
	FARM	
Negative	TOWNPOP	POPCHANG
	WAGES92	SCAVN
	MAR	PRTDISAB
	GLASS	SHIPS
	LEAD	FOOD
	ALCOHOL	EASTERN
	CHEMCLS	SMIDLAND
	FISH	YORK
	WMIDLAND	NMIDLAND
	SW	NORTHERN

half appear in the cells showing an inharmonious relationship.

The lower right cell represents the most desirable outcome, lower mortality and less sickness time. Its variables show the same sign in the two analyses, but none of them is statistically significant in both. The table suggests how comparatively easy it would have been for public authorities in England and Wales in 1891 to devise policies promoting higher morbidity and mortality. Indeed, they could merely have promoted many individual features of social and economic life that already existed. This figure also suggests the comparative ease of finding strategies to promote either better survival prospects or less sickness time. But its more important implication is about the difficulty that public authorities faced in devising a policy promoting both lower sickness time and lower mortality.

Friendly society actuaries seem to have jumped to conclusions. The factors they identified as the most hazardous—living in large towns and working as a miner—were risky. Yet each assumed the leading importance it took in actuarial studies not because it was a principal hazard by itself but because it captured the effects of other features of large cities and mining communities. In the analysis described here, where many additional factors have been studied, the result is inevitably to diminish the scale of effect associated with some variables, such as mining. The most important finding is not, however, that the actuaries were wrong in focusing on town size and hazardous trades. It is, instead, that those determinants stand as proxies for a wider array of forces that influenced sickness time and mortality. Town size stands as a representative of a group of socioeconomic and environmental factors, which, after age itself, exercised the chief influence on sickness time. And hazardous occupations stand for a larger group of occupations which, at the community level, played a leading role as determinants of mortality.

In recent times, according to the Black Report, both socioeconomic and occupational disparities still prevail in mortality and the incidence of sickness in Britain.[41] The growing access of workingmen to doctors in the nineteenth century did not equalize their experience with that of elites, nor has access to the National Health Service closed the divide.

IN THE EVENT

In fact, public authorities and private individuals alike pursued their own plans for reducing the risks of sickness time and death in England and Wales in the 1890s while they also pursued many other interests. Plans for better health were made explicit only in part, in the form especially of objectives set by public authorities. Another way to examine the health policies and plans that people actually executed, wittingly and unwittingly, is to look at how actual changes in the determinants of sickness time and mortality under study here influenced the course of health. The technique is a speculative simulation. This question is posed: how did the changes that actually occurred in all the variables considered in the regression analyses play out for England and Wales as a whole? Based on the estimates for coefficients derived for 1891, how do actual changes in these determinants between 1881 and 1901 appear to have driven sickness time

41. Great Britain, "Black Report," 1–2.

and mortality? The full results of this simulation appear in appendix 6, table A6.4.[42]

Results

In interpreting results, it is useful to think in terms of counterfactual trends. Every trend in a certain direction—for example, a decline in the proportion of men employed in one field or an increase in the degree of crowding in housing or spatial density—implies the possibility of a trend in the opposing direction, with opposing results. While this is a good heuristic device, it does not mean that just any alternative value can be plugged into the simulation model. In general, the regression results, upon which this simulation relies, should not be expected to hold up under sharply different values for any given variable.

Once again it is easiest to see how these things played out by making simple distinctions in four categories, two with positive effects and two with negative effects. On the positive side appear a reduction in sickness time and mortality and an increase in sickness time with a decrease in mortality (i.e., sicknesses ended later and less often in death). On the negative side appear a joint increase in sickness time with mortality and a reduction in sickness time associated with an increase in mortality (i.e., sicknesses ended earlier and more often in death). Cast in this way, some positive trends emerge along with a larger number of negative trends. The list below shows the changes in the variables that accompanied these four combinations of effects.

Sickness time and mortality declined
  proportion of sanitation, shipping, and food workers increased
  proportion of farmers and textile-manufacturing workers increased
  crowding in housing diminished
  proportion married diminished

42. George Alter suggested this approach. It has two steps. First, a predicted value for 1901 is estimated by multiplying the 1891 coefficients for each variable by the observed 1901 values of each variable, holding the age controls constant. Second, the effect associated with each variable is isolated by multiplying its 1891 coefficient by its 1881 value while holding all other variables to their 1901 values.

Values for one variable—average town size (using adjustment factors to derive estimates for 1881 and 1901 from the 1891 weighted average town size)—and values for three additional variables—literacy, unionization, and crowding in tenements—have been estimated by interpolation.

Unlike earlier estimates, the simulation will not accurately predict sickness time or mortality for a particular date, in this case 1901. Instead, it estimates the changes across the period 1881–1901 associated with each variable while predicting sickness time and mortality differences among AOF courts in 1891.

proportion living in North Midlands increased (slightly) and proportion living in Wales diminished

Sickness time increased and mortality declined
proportion of health workers increased
proportion of leadworkers and fishermen declined
proportion of Londoners increased

Sickness time and mortality increased
proportion of workers in several hazardous trades (commerce and conveyance, earthenware, stonework, machine and implement making, construction) increased
population grew and spatial density increased
proportion of the population with sensory handicaps and judged insane diminished
union membership rose
railway employment rose
proportion of people living in Yorkshire, the eastern counties, the South Midlands, and the northern counties diminished

Sickness time decreased and mortality increased
proportion of workers in several hazardous trades (glass, coal and other mining, chemicals) increased
proportion of retailers diminished
towns grew
crowding in tenements worsened
alcohol became more readily available
wages rose
illiteracy among young men declined
the northwest lost population while the southwest and the West Midlands gained

More often than not, the changes people made in these various ways threatened to cause health in England and Wales to deteriorate. Knowing that (holding age constant) sickness time increased among members of the AOF and that mortality declined among AOF members and the general population of England and Wales between 1881 and 1901—that is, knowing that the actual trends were positive—indicates the degree to which the relatively few positive trends outweighed negative shifts.

Good Effects

This simulation adds special, if possibly overstated,[43] force to the argument that investments in public health, here represented by the proportion

43. Close examination of how other variables change when this variable is dropped suggests that this variable may be capturing some of the effects associated with a bloc of large cities and densely settled areas in London and to a lesser degree in Lancashire and Yorkshire.

of men engaged as drainage workers and in refuse collection and sweeping, paid rich dividends in the period 1881–1901. Even though the 1891 differences in sickness time and mortality relate to the experience of adults rather than children and thus capture filth and water-borne diseases in only part of the population, and even though actual additions to the number of sanitation workers were small, this simulation suggests that the most efficacious action a community could take in the period around 1891 was to add sanitation workers. Such action reduced sickness time by the highest proportion of any factor under consideration while also lowering mortality by a small but significant proportion. Since many of the communities of England and Wales were in fact improving their facilities for supplying pure water and disposing safely of human waste and refuse in this period, this simulation suggests they had correctly identified and taken effective actions.

Between 1881 and 1901 the mean number of people per house in England and Wales dropped from 5.4 to 5.2 persons, a small but important decline after a long period in which little change had occurred. This simulation suggests that communities that added to the housing stock at a faster pace thereby reduced both sickness time and mortality. Less-crowded housing promoted better health, and the movement toward a higher ratio of dwellings to people represents one of the most substantial steps taken to improve health and the quality of life. Moreover, the shift to a higher ratio occurred within a part of the spectrum which, figure 9.4 indicates, made a substantial difference, because it fell at a point on the sickness time and mortality schedules where more crowding added unambiguously to poorer health quality. Scotland's failure to add to the stock of dwellings at a pace fast enough to diminish crowding provides one reason for its deterioration in sickness time and mortality, relative to England and Wales around 1900.[44]

However, communities with a higher proportion of construction workers added to sickness time and mortality. The parallel between the two variables is not, of course, exact. Communities could have a larger proportion of men engaged in constructing buildings other than houses. But these associations do suggest the need public authorities faced to balance the desirable effects of adding to the housing stock with the undesirable effects of adding to the ranks of construction workers.

The proportion of men working in two hazardous trades—textile manufacturing and farming—decreased sharply, while the share working in

44. See chapter 8.

the retail food trades increased. Further improvement would have oc-curred had the proportion of men working in other areas of retailing increased in the period 1881–1901. In sum, a shift toward retailing and away from mining, manufacturing, and farming promised to improve patterns of health, but that shift remained halting.

A rising proportion of people providing health services and informa-tion—doctors, nurses, chemists, and teachers—also shows strong effects in the simulation. These additions promoted longer sicknesses and lower mortality, signaling that sicknesses were ending later in their course and less often in death than in recovery.

London's gain in population, net of all other characteristics analyzed, emphasizes the city's status as a site of longer sicknesses and lower mortal-ity. Generally negative health effects are associated with living in large towns and cities, but London transcended some of these hazards.

Ill Effects

The statistical analyses discussed above suggest the usefulness, for pop-ulation health, of a reorientation of the economy, adding jobs in retailing while reducing the proportion of men engaged in a range of hazardous occupations including mining, commerce and conveyance, construction, farming, textile manufacturing, railway employment, and work with stone, glass, and lead. Although some positive trends in the occupational profile have been noted above, the negative signs are more numerous. Between 1881 and 1901 employment increased in a variety of hazardous trades. Against a small decline in the share of men occupied in lead making stands a larger increase in the proportion engaged in glass, stone, and earthenware work. Sharp growth in the share of men working in com-merce and conveyance and in making machines and implements also add-ed to health risks. Taking all changes in occupational distribution into account at once, this analysis suggests that England and Wales were mov-ing still toward poorer health. In their net effect, occupational shifts be-tween 1881 and 1901 added to sickness time by 5.17 percent and to mortality by 0.26 percent. Regional changes in population distribution were also negative in their net effects, but on a much smaller scale, adding 0.62 percent to sickness time and 0.05 percent to mortality.

Negative effects of industrial modernization were still being felt in En-gland and Wales at the end of the nineteenth century. Jobs associated with the modern industrial sector and employing large numbers of men still added sharply to health hazards around 1891. Although farming communities show up as having high health hazards, the risks associated with industrial work were often still larger. The long shift away from farming and into factory work and into jobs involving contact with hazardous materials aggravated health risks.

Within most of its spectrum, larger town size contributed to higher mortality risk and apparently to sicknesses ending earlier in death. Across the period 1881–1901, more of the population of England and Wales lived in urban than rural sanitary districts, the closest simple gauge provided by census authorities for deriving a trend of urbanization. That gauge shows a proportion rising from 67.9 percent in 1881 to 77.04 percent in 1901, and these proportions have been used to estimate how average town size for those dates varied from the 1891 figures for town size and proportion urban. Even controlling for spatial density and the ratio of people to houses, urban residence remained a strongly negative factor in 1891, to the point that continued urban growth, which rose sharply in the 1870s and thereafter, promoted poorer health.[45]

In 1898 Ebenezer Howard formulated a plan to export urban residents to constellations of new garden cities in the open countryside in hopes of helping people escape slums and air pollution.[46] Like other urban planners, Howard fretted especially about the poor, so that it is noteworthy that the association between cities and health shows up among members of the AOF, who included the working poor and many men who were not poor. Howard's specific plan was to create conurbations with individual towns of no more than thirty thousand people on a thousand acres of land surrounded by green belts. The analysis done here suggests that Howard's preferred density—thirty persons an acre—implied higher than average mortality. A smaller density would have worked better. But because Howard foresaw resettling people from the most unfavored neighborhoods of large cities, his plan would undoubtedly have reduced mortality, everything else being equal. In effect Howard wanted to resettle people from such cities as Liverpool and Manchester to new places resembling Nottingham.[47]

45. Harris, *Private Lives, Public Spirit,* 41–42, notes the sudden shift toward city living. Ward, *Birth Weight and Economic Growth,* 126, finds that, gauged by the birth weights of their infants, the health of poor mothers in several large western cities deteriorated.

46. Howard, *Garden Cities of To-morrow,* esp. 54–61; and Hall, *Cities of Tomorrow,* 8–19, 87–97.

47. Using regression to predict mortality while controlling for age and age dispersion, the death rate rises suddenly at densities greater than fifty per acre.

Changes damaging to health—higher mortality and sicknesses ending earlier in death—can also be attributed to crowding in tenements and a rising proportion of people selling alcoholic beverages, signaling presumably more alcohol consumption. Net of differing proportions of teachers in each county, the declining share of young men who could not sign their names at marriage also had unwanted health effects.

In the later nineteenth century, real wages and income rose and mortality declined. That coincidence has provided one of the strongest reasons to believe that improvements in the standard of living helped drive death rates downward. Here, in contrast, the simulation stresses regional differences in wages at a given moment and reveals a paradox. In counties where agricultural workers earned higher wages, sickness times tended to be lower and mortality higher. This suggests that sickness times were lower because episodes were more often curtailed by death in higher wage areas and that higher wages inadequately compensated men for higher risks, net of all other factors considered.

These findings imply the need to reinterpret the association between wages, on the one hand, and sickness time and mortality, on the other. Over time, rising real wages enabled workers to reduce mortality risks in their surroundings by buying more spacious housing, more nutritious and purer food, medical services, and other things, and paying taxes for public health improvements. Throughout, wages were distributed across regions in ways that compensated men to some degree for risks associated with work. Hence, miners earned more than farmworkers. Those differentials show up even when the comparison is made on agricultural wages, as it is here, since farmworkers in mining areas earned higher wages than farmworkers living elsewhere.[48]

As of 1891, the results reported in the statistical analyses suggest, compensation for risk still remained an important element in the association of wages with health, an element so strong that the secular trend of rising real wages was not yet powerful enough to overcome its effects. Between 1881 and 1901, amidst a trend toward wage equality across working-class trades, wages in agriculture and real wages in general rose sharply.[49] In the conventional interpretation, those rises are credited with helping reduce mortality. As Jeffrey Williamson argues, British workers were better off

48. Bowley, *Wages in the United Kingdom,* 29, shows the existence of two wage areas in Nottinghamshire, one near the county's mines and the other away from them, and finds the same effect in two other counties.
49. Mitchell, *British Historical Statistics,* 150–51, 158–59.

because of industrialization; it brought higher wages.[50] Given the trend toward lower mortality and higher sickness time, higher wages would be expected to have promoted longer sicknesses. But the cross-sectional analysis undertaken here shows opposite associations in the form of lower sickness time and higher mortality, which is evidence of deterioration in health. This association suggests that still, around 1891, the hazards that higher wages were meant to compensate still surpassed the beneficial, health-enhancing effects of greater pay, leaving better-paid workers with inadequate compensation for the risks they faced. The risk-premium wage associated with hazardous work was not yet as large as the risk itself.

Figure 9.1 shows that the relationship between cities and health was complex rather than simple and suggests the usefulness of further research on the distribution of growth among cities of different sizes. Certain patterns of urbanization—the growth of large cities, of 250 thousand to one million, with the characteristics of those cities in Britain in 1891—had greater negative effects on health than did the growth of cities of some other sizes. This analysis implies that air pollution, an important factor that cannot be quantified in the terms needed here, either did not dominate among city hazards or varied among cities on some other basis than population size and density. Spatial density also shows a close association with mortality. A sharply rising proportion of people to space in England and Wales between 1881 and 1901 tended to elevate death rates.

The rising rate of population growth in England and Wales promoted these undesirable effects. So, too, did a decline in the proportion of the population reported as impeded in sight, speech, hearing, or sanity. Communities with larger proportions of people disabled in these ways were not as prone to health problems as communities with other negative characteristics, such as crowded housing or hazardous occupations. But this group combines people born with sensory disabilities, who are unlikely to have joined friendly societies, with people who acquired such disabilities, who may have joined before they became disabled. More unionized workers added sickness time and mortality, suggesting the greater hazards linked to unionized, as opposed to non-unionized, jobs. Communities with larger proportions of people working for the railways also showed unfavorable health effects. Finally, and puzzlingly, a decline in the proportion of married men diminished sickness time and mortality. Modern theory leads to an expectation that communities with larger shares of married

50. Williamson, *Did British Capitalism Breed Inequality?* 30–31.

men would show longer survival in sickness, but this analysis produces the opposite finding.

If British authorities in 1891 could take advice from the analyses performed here, they would find that the same strategy could seldom be followed to reduce both sickness time and mortality. In one possible strategy, socioeconomic factors dominate, and in the other, occupational structure is most important. These results nevertheless suggest an optimal retrospective policy to improve health in England and Wales: realign large cities into small cities of one hundred thousand to two hundred fifty thousand; expand substantially each city's area, allowing for more space between residential housing units; and increase the pace of residential construction, lowering ratios of people per dwelling. At the level of smaller towns, an optimal policy would have promoted resettlement into villages with low rates of people per house, characteristics evidently strong enough to overcome the negative effect of farming itself on mortality. These policies would be costly in the necessary reallocation of workers toward the building trades, with their higher mortality and sickness time, and, consequently, with some deterioration in overall health owing to a more hazardous mixture of occupations. But the benefits to men in general would outweigh the costs to men added to the ranks of building craftsmen.

The quality of life in England and Wales, as measured by the patterns of health of AOF members, could best have been fostered, still at the century's end, by reversing the strongest features of nineteenth-century economic development. Deurbanization would have been more effective than urban sanitary reform in overcoming and correcting the noxious aspects of cities that were too numerous and were growing too rapidly. Deindustrialization, specifically in textiles, construction, and jobs in which people worked with hazardous materials, and a reorientation toward food preparation and retailing would have countered the tendency of the existing occupational structure to promote higher mortality.

These findings cast new light on the long-standing debate over the standard of living, which focuses on the period 1780–1850. In that debate a key argument has been about the timing of economic gains for working people as a class, specifically about when in the early decades of the nineteenth century workers gained enough more in real wages to improve their standard of living, rather than merely to maintain it or even to suffer deterioration.

The analyses discussed here suggest that, assessed in terms of vital statistics and the experience of AOF members in 1891, unfavorable effects of economic modernization continued to be felt at the end of the century, especially in large cities where people lived in crowded housing and worked in hazardous trades. In the cross-sectional analysis, higher wages seem to have carried mixed benefits, because they were tied to more hazardous occupations, and that association remained in place at the end of the nineteenth century. Thus, a male worker could gain quite substantially in real income without improving his quality of life, insofar as that is judged by the risks of sickness time and mortality. A time series analysis suggests that modern health circumstances—low death rates and protracted sicknesses—were gained through a long struggle in which the economic conditions of working people gradually improved. But this regional analysis suggests that structural changes were also important. What mattered was not merely the worker's individual capacity to buy a better standard of life but also the structural shift from an economy replete with hazardous occupations to one in which fewer people worked in life-threatening jobs and fewer people lived in health-threatening surroundings only partly alleviated by public health reforms.

Casting the issue more broadly, in terms of what this analysis suggests about time-worn determinants of sickness time and mortality, the most important conclusion is that different determinants, and different categories of determinants, influence the two outcomes. The most desired effect —lower mortality and less sickness time—is unlikely to be promoted by a single set of policies. Simultaneous programs may achieve each aim separately. But to some degree the two outcomes are inconsistent with one another, in that some policies which reduce one tend to increase the other. Furthermore, this analysis highlights the struggle over how to mitigate the health effects of economic modernization and industrialization. Public health reform emerges as an inadequate attempt to compensate for the economic changes that draw people to cities. It was the prime strategy of late-nineteenth-century health reformers, but not necessarily the best strategy.

In the end, Britain pressed mortality down, successfully lowering death rates among men and women, in the late nineteenth and early twentieth centuries. In that same period, sickness time increased, at least among men and women belonging to friendly societies. Recent sickness surveys show that sickness time in Britain increased also in the period 1971–87.[51] In

---

51. Riley, "Morbidity Trends in Four Countries."

retrospect it is apparent that British authorities promoted, and socio-economic changes accommodated, trends that favored lower mortality and longer sickness time, rather than the optimal mix of lower mortality and lower sickness time. To some degree the low mortality of the late twentieth century has been achieved at the expense of more protracted sickness.

Conclusion

How is the passage of health in the century and a quarter since 1870 to be interpreted in the light of findings presented in this book? None of the evidence or arguments given here challenges the central feature in the history of health in this period. Mortality declined. The average life lengthened from 41.4 years for an infant male in England and Wales in the 1870s to 73.2 years in 1989–91. In this era even many of the frailest among us—infants who previously had been unable to survive the earliest weeks of life—acquired the birthright of a long life. Health improved.

Beginning in the 1870s and lasting at least into the 1930s, however, the average amount of sickness time increased at each age. Although people fell sick less often, their sicknesses lasted longer. Those trends have been under way also in the era of the modern health survey, which in Britain started in the late 1960s. What began in the 1870s—a simultaneous lengthening of sickness time and curtailing of the number of sickness episodes in a life—seems to describe the modern form of morbidity trends. At once, then, health has evolved in three directions. Lives have been lengthened, the number of sickness episodes has been reduced, and the average duration of sickness episodes has increased. To live longer lives with fewer sickness episodes was a grand achievement, for it meant that workingmen survived longer when sick, rather than succumbing earlier, as they had done in the past. They were sick rather than dead. More often than in the past they also recovered from sicknesses and resumed work.

Sickness had been a grave personal and social problem in Britain in the mid-nineteenth century. People fell sick often and, compared to later experience, they died more often from their diseases and injuries. The mortality decline consisted of a trend not toward more wellness, however, but toward less lethal sickness. People traded short lives marked by frequent episodes of sickness for longer lives marked by:

fewer sickness episodes in the span that people had formerly lived,
more aggregate sickness episodes over the now longer life, and
more wellness time, but also
a proportionally greater increase in sickness time over wellness time.

What is the balance of these trends? It is, in the main, a triumph of good
health. People now live longer lives; they live through more wellness time;
and they experience fewer sicknesses at each age than did their counterparts in the past. But they also experience more sickness time than did their
counterparts in the past, at each age and altogether, too. In sum, this
analysis suggests why health has become a central preoccupation of modern life. It is not that people have discovered that they are sick when they
have what their forefathers used to take for trivial ailments. That is, it is
not that we fall sick more often because we define so many more things as
sickness. It is rather that we so much more rarely die from our sicknesses.
Our sicknesses last much longer than they did in the past. People legitimately need health care because of these prolonged maladies. The size of
the health establishment and the proportion of public and private resources allocated to it have grown under the impetus of lengthening sickness time.

The cost of health service has grown, too. In nineteenth-century Britain
workingmen negotiated cheap medical care for themselves and their families, using their superior organization in friendly societies and taking advantage of an oversupply of doctors. Working people dominated in setting
the terms under which they would first consult licensed practitioners about
their health problems, especially as regards cost. They spent more on tea
than they did for contract medical services. In a rhetorical battle over the
quality of care doctors would give friendly society members at cut-rate
prices, it was the workingmen who won. Doctors threatened to provide
less for contract than for private patients, but working people used their
apprehension of poorer care to negotiate the things they wanted: frequent
and convenient consultations and plentiful medications.

Toward the end of the nineteenth century, when the ratio of doctors to
patients shrank, the tide began to turn. The first sign of a new relationship,
in which doctors rather than working people held the upper hand, appears
in friendly society deliberations. Whereas formerly the members had often
challenged their doctors and other people occupying superior social or
professional positions, in the 1890s the men who belonged to sick clubs
became timid. They began to accept their doctors' excuses for care they

previously had rejected as inattentive or deficient. Later, in debates and discussions leading up to the National Insurance Act of 1911, the friendly societies failed to foresee that they could continue to pay so little for medical services only if they prevented the state from paying doctors more for treating beneficiaries newly enrolled under the act, as opposed to friendly society members already enrolled in sick clubs.

In the 1920s the terms of trade shifted decisively in favor of doctors. For nearly a century, workingmen, and increasingly their families, too, had treated doctors more as tradesmen to be bargained with than as learned social superiors and had hired doctors at fees adjusted to what working people could afford to pay, and sometimes for less than they could afford. Workingmen lost the upper hand in this relationship between the 1890s and the second decade of the twentieth century, first sacrificing the moral advantage and then losing the financial advantage. Since then the cost of care and the proportion of income devoted to it have increased even more than sickness time, making health services much costlier than they were.

In the nineteenth century workingmen took their sicknesses seriously enough to warrant saving in advance in order to compensate themselves for part of the wages they would lose when sick. They took the trouble, too, to organize schemes for doing this among themselves and to learn how to keep ledgers and do the other things needed to make a self-help system of insurance succeed. About the specific sicknesses they thought worthy of compensation, little information survives before the late nineteenth century, yet some scholars have come to strong conclusions about attitudes toward sickness in society in general.

In the past, Edward Shorter believes, people were made of sterner stuff; not until the 1960s did they take minor ailments seriously or share the modern anguish about health. Friendly society documents reporting causes of sickness and sources discussing attitudes toward sickness undermine Shorter's beliefs. In the late nineteenth and early twentieth centuries, the period best documented from sickness registers, men often took time off from work to recuperate from ailments which, by their diagnoses, seem to have been minor. What is more, they defined health broadly, in terms of the enjoyment of life, rather than narrowly, in terms of mere survival. They worried about discomfort as well as about pain. They acknowledged as sickness maladies that carried a significant chance of death and burden of pain and maladies that carried neither. Bronchitis counted as sickness for them, but so did minor colds and corns.

The epidemiologic transition describes a shift from infectious toward

degenerative diseases, which would show up in the kinds of records consulted here as an increase in the duration of sickness episodes. If the
findings of this study affirm the idea that such a transition took place, they
also qualify it. Among friendly society members the average duration of
sickness episodes began in the 1870s to increase, while the incidence of
sickness diminished. For those people, and perhaps also for all British
adults, the epidemiologic transition consisted not only of a shift toward
more prolonged organ and degenerative diseases but also of these important changes in sickness incidence and duration. Sickness registers suggest
a distinctive epidemiologic transition in sickness, one led by the earlier
retreat of fatalities from diseases and injuries than of the diseases and
injuries themselves. Men stopped dying as often as they had in the past
from respiratory diseases well before they stopped getting sick from those
same diseases.

Workingmen's sicknesses became more protracted at a time when they
were seeing doctors for more of their ailments. But the coincidence in time
is not marked. The workingmen who belonged to friendly societies began
to hire doctors under contract in the late eighteenth century and began to
do so in large numbers from the 1840s. The prolongation of their sicknesses did not emerge until the 1870s. Nevertheless, the eagerness of workingmen to hire doctors and, somewhat later, to enroll their family members
as contract patients suggests that they saw value in the medical care doctors gave. Their sense of the worth of doctors is borne out by statistical
analysis, which shows that sicknesses of AOF members lasted longer
around 1891 in locales of England and Wales where health providers were
more numerous. The point is not whether doctors cured them more quickly. They did not. The point is that doctors may have prevented them from
dying. This study implies that medical care can reclaim a position of
importance among factors responsible for mortality decline: health providers helped people manage their ailments and reduce the risk of dying
while sick. What seems to have mattered in the care that doctors provided
was not the twentieth-century-style intervention of antibiotics, vaccination, or reparative surgery but a traditional form of therapy, one that
diminished the lethality of sickness. Hence the crucial factor in the mortality decline was the expanding access of working people to licensed
practitioners.

A simultaneous decline in mortality and rise in sickness time is apparent
in the records of all the large friendly societies that compiled sickness
statistics, among the Oddfellows, who were not teetotalers, as well as the

Rechabites, who were. Only among the Foresters, however, can its course be plotted from year to year, and only among the Foresters is it possible also to discover regional differences in health experience. The maps of these differences show a Britain sharply divided. In mortality, favored and unfavored regions can be distinguished from one another along a north-south divide. But in sickness time the divide followed an east-west line. Scotland entered the 1870s at an advantage, and Wales at a disadvantage, compared to England. By the early twentieth century Wales's disadvantage had grown larger, and Scotland's advantage had been reversed. Whereas within England differences in patterns of health from county to county shrank between 1870 and 1910, between England and its adjacent lands the difference grew. Wales and Scotland fell behind. Within England the north was a region already unfavored.

Some manufacturing areas, notably Yorkshire and Lancashire, are conspicuous as areas of high mortality but low sickness time, a relation that reveals a central paradox of using time spent in sickness as a gauge of health patterns. There, men were sick less of the time because they died earlier in the course of their maladies rather than because they recovered earlier. On the gauge of sickness time alone, these regions would appear to have been healthy. When survival and health are considered jointly, however, they emerge as regions with a marked disadvantage, sharing the disadvantages of areas where men mined coal or, worse yet, where they made pottery.

Wales, Scotland, and the north of England fell behind, at least in part because they enjoyed smaller shares of factors that promoted better health and larger shares of factors that promoted poorer health than did England. In these regions housing was often more crowded, and workingmen were more likely to practice trades that carried substantial health risks and lower wages. In contrast, England's economy, especially in the south, was structured toward better health.

If the evidence extracted from friendly society records shows the existence, at least for the members of the societies themselves, of regional disparities in health, it shows also how complex was the problem of improving health. Changes in medicine, public health, the standard of living, and health habits were under way in Britain in the last part of the nineteenth century. But few of these changes promoted both lower mortality and less sickness time. A cross-sectional analysis linking AOF members to the characteristics of the locales in which they were situated suggests that mortality and sickness time responded to substantially different forces.

The strongest determinants of mortality—the occupations that men followed—contributed much less to sickness time than did socioeconomic conditions.

In the event, the British and their health authorities devised policies that promoted longer life rather than less sickness time. This analysis of determinants suggests that the authorities made an unwitting choice. They might instead have favored wellness. A hundred years later, sickness time looms larger as a public health concern than it did in the 1890s, and the long-run effects of trends toward lower mortality and more sickness time, which were under way in the 1870s, are evident. The decline of mortality was accompanied by an increase in the amount of time spent in sickness, an increase that has been traced here in Britain from the 1870s into the 1930s, and one in place in the 1970s and 1980s, too. The analyses done here suggest a leading reason why that should be so. Lower death rates have, over time, contributed to higher sickness time. One of the most important gains of the health transition has consisted of deferral of death for the sick. The unsolved task suggested by these analyses is to find policies that promote both lower mortality and less sickness time or that promote less sickness time without the cost of higher mortality. It is feasible to plan for the future a great morbidity decline, analogous to the great decline in mortality that has been under way since the late eighteenth century.

APPENDIX I

To Claim or
Not to Claim

M ANY ISSUES need to be considered in order to understand how the
friendly societies specified sickness and to see in what ways their
specifications led to more sickness or to less sickness, compared to what
would have obtained in the absence of such specifications. The overriding
difference can be explained as one between patterns of sickness and patterns of sickness claims: the friendly societies recorded claims rather than
sicknesses. The aim in this appendix is to explore limits to using the record
of claims, which can be observed, to reconstruct patterns of sickness,
which cannot be observed.

THE INTRODUCTION EFFECT

When compensation is introduced for wages forgone during sickness, even
though its level is low, some people who previously have not missed work
when sick will begin to miss work. Formerly, financial pressure prevented
them from taking time off for sicknesses that did not force them to bed or
during convalescence from such sicknesses, even when they displayed
symptoms that they and their workmates regarded as dangerous or un-
pleasant. With insurance, financial pressure is relieved, and more time is
missed from work because of sickness. The shift cannot be illustrated in
nineteenth-century experience, because no data are available comparing
insured to uninsured populations. But it can be illustrated by comparing
work absence before and after the introduction of the National Health
Service in 1948. Absence attributed to sickness increased sharply after that
date, due to the removal of financial pressures from previously uninsured

people, among other changes.[1] This "introduction effect" explains why absenteeism due to sickness rises when insurance is initiated or changed in a substantial way. But it provides little reason to expect absenteeism to continue to rise. Work absence jumped sharply when the National Health Service was introduced, but it did not continue to rise sharply.

Absence from work presumably increased when a club was formed or when new people joined. Because they belonged to sick clubs, workers could "afford" to miss work. But all the records available about sickness claims in the nineteenth century speak to circumstances in which compensation was already in place. Its continuing effect was limited to new members. In short, belonging to a friendly society allowed a person to take time off from work when sick at a certain level of inducement, that associated with the benefits offered. At a lower level of benefits, the average member would have taken less time off, and at a higher level, more.

COMPENSATION LEVELS AND THE THRESHOLD OF SICKNESS

The introduction of insurance increases the likelihood that a person will miss work because of sickness, and higher compensation augments that likelihood.[2] Friendly societies reacted to this inducement by offering to compensate members for part rather than all of the wages they lost. In the early years of the Hearts of Oak Friendly Society, applicants had to earn at least twenty-four shillings a week; claimants were paid eighteen shillings a week during the early part of any sickness episode and less later. There, the benefit ratio could be as high as 75 percent, although most members probably earned more than twenty-four shillings a week. In the less elitist societies, such as the Foresters, which set no wage minima, benefits totaled 40 percent or less of what workingmen earned. When a member's sickness lasted beyond six months, the club lowered benefits, first to half the standard level and then, for still more protracted sicknesses, to one-quarter. Full benefits usually amounted to eight shillings a week in the 1860s and 1870s, when unskilled workers earned fifteen to twenty shillings a week. Benefits were small enough to make it costly to miss work. When sick, a worker lost the difference between wages and benefits. This disincentive

1. Jones, *Absenteeism*, 37.
2. For an example, see Prins, *Sickness Absence*, 37–40.

increased as wages increased. For skilled workers earning twenty-five to thirty shillings or more a week, friendly society benefits ordinarily provided a smaller proportion of wages than they did for less skilled workers. Hence, more highly paid workers were somewhat less likely to enter or continue a claim than their lower-paid counterparts, since they got from it a smaller share of the wages lost. That disincentive remained in place over time, except for the rather small proportion of friendly society members who bought benefits in proportion to their wages rather than buying only the minimum. In sum, the introduction of friendly societies probably lowered the threshold of symptoms that people regarded as serious enough to force work absence, but it did not lower that threshold as far as would have occurred had daily benefits equaled daily wages.

Many modern commentators, observing that work absences increase when compensation is introduced or that absences rise further when benefit ratios are increased, create the impression that the sickness absences of the previous regime were real and those of the new regime are in some measure false. By implication, they would prefer the more rigorous sickness threshold that leads to less absenteeism, regardless of what independent sources of information, such as medical examinations, reveal about the health status of insured people. Where the threshold should be set is not an issue that can be resolved here, although it is one that troubles any comparison of the patterns of sickness suggested by friendly society records in the nineteenth and early twentieth centuries with more recent experience. As Ernest Ambrose remarked, recalling his village youth as a member of a friendly society: "There was precious little absenteeism in the early days—men couldn't afford to be off work, in fact they went on working many a time when they should not have done so."[3] Not every sickness became a claim, and it would be unrealistic to suggest that, over time, working people maintained exactly the same threshold for distinguishing illnesses worth making into claims from those not. Nevertheless, that threshold does not appear to have changed in major ways during 1872–1910, because leading features of the scheme of inducements remained the same. The Foresters and other friendly societies gradually increased benefits as wages rose, maintaining the ratio of benefits to wages. And they kept in place a system in which less well paid workers received a larger fraction of their wages in benefits than did better-paid workers.

3. Ambrose, *Melford Memories*, 114.

FORMS OF INSURANCE

Modern studies suggest further that the propensity to make a claim depends to some degree on the nature of insurance coverage. Workers are more likely to claim benefits when coverage is provided by private insurers, so that the relationship between the worker's financial interests and the cost of insurance is indirect, than when coverage is provided by the firm and the financial relationship is more direct.[4] Friendly societies, especially those, such as the Foresters, in which members insured themselves for sickness in village or neighborhood clubs, established a strong direct relationship, one made all the more apparent to members by their ongoing scrutiny of the club's assets and liabilities. The temptation that their insurance offered friendly society members to enter additional sickness claims was countered to a substantial degree by their financial stake in supplying the coverage.

CLAIMS AWARENESS

Once a system of insurance compensation is in place, there is also, for newly insured people, a period of learning, which insurance theorists discuss as a matter of "claims awareness." New friendly society members may not immediately have understood all the rules and practices that surrounded compensation. In particular, they may not immediately have understood how the availability of compensation invited them to behave differently. In the AOF each court funded its own sickness benefits. Since the members of a court monitored its financial position, they knew when the court could more readily afford to pay benefits and when it could not. Knowing that may have tempted them to enter more claims when the court was rich and fewer when it was poor. AOF directories report the size of each court's assets each year, and these data can be used to look for a statistical relation between the scale of court funds per member and sickness claims.

Four sample years, 1872, 1879, 1889, and 1899, have been analyzed. Considering only the relation between sickness and court reserves, statistical analysis shows that members were somewhat likelier to enter a sickness claim as reserves increased. But in this simple model the variable for reserves captures both their current size and some other effects, too. Reserves usually grew as a court aged. Hence, the size of a court's reserves

4. See Krueger, "Workers' Compensation Insurance," 21.

was simply a function of its history of sickness and burial claims and of the length of time that had passed since its formation. Consequently, a more complex model is needed, one that will take these several influences into account. In the more complex model,[5] the sign of the relation between sickness rates and the amount of reserves for each member changes. Members tended to enter not more but slightly fewer sickness and burial claims as reserves accumulated.[6] In 1899, for example, a one pound increase in assets per member was associated with a decrease in sickness time of 0.055 days and a decrease in the death rate of 0.076 deaths per thousand.

Since an increase in assets of one pound per member amounted to a very substantial gain that took years to achieve, the important point is not the minuscule scale of the change but the consistency of its sign in all the analyses with a complex model. Two explanations suggest themselves. First, the propensity to make a claim may have diminished slightly as a court aged and as it secured its financial position. If that is true, then what members learned in the friendly societies, in terms of claims awareness, was not more about how to make a sickness claim but more about how group esprit militated against making claims. Second, and more likely, the analysis shows that courts in which sickness and death claims were fewer in number tended to accumulate funds at a slightly higher rate than did courts where claims were more numerous. In either case, the scale of the effect was so small that it exerted little influence over sickness rates. AOF members did not to any significant degree base their decision to make a claim on the court's financial standing.

NINETEENTH-CENTURY WORRIES

Insurance logic dominated the views of those friendly society observers who believed that members were prone to overstate their sicknesses. These

5. For each sample year, sickness time and mortality appear separately as the dependent variable:
$$\text{ST (or DR)} = f(\text{AGE} + \text{INITRATE} + \text{SINCEDOF} + \text{FUNDSPER}),$$
where:
ST = the sickness time
DR = the death rate
AGE = the average age of court members
INITRATE = the rate at which new members joined
SINCEDOF = the court's age
FUNDSPER = the ratio of reserves to members
6. The signs for funds per member are negative in all eight estimates, and all are significant at the .01 level except for the 1872 estimate for sickness.

observers usually cited the incentive of benefits without noticing the disincentive of forgone wages. Or, if they noted the difference between wages and benefits, they suggested that workingmen might belong to more than one friendly society, a sly trick that would enable them to collect enough in benefits to make it worth their while to miss work. If benefits paid 40 percent of wages at their lower end among unskilled workers, then the wages could be matched by benefits if a man belonged to 2.5 societies at the same time. For skilled workers with higher wages, it would be necessary to join three or four societies.

No national register of membership was ever compiled, so it is not possible to determine whether a significant number of men ever did this. Some individual cases of dual membership are known. Timothy Mountjoy, a Gloucestershire miner, union organizer, and local political figure, belonged to two societies at the same time.[7] But for most people the higher premiums of multiple membership must be counted as a strong disincentive. True, they allowed a man to claim multiple benefits when sick. But they also required multiple premium payments when sick and well. Only men who were often sick and whose sicknesses were timed in a certain way could break even. For everyone else, and especially for men whose wages were low enough to make it necessary to pinch pennies, multiple memberships in ordinary friendly societies, such as the Foresters, made no sense.

In the long run and in a way especially noticeable in the 1920s and thereafter, the benefits paid by the AOF courts and other friendly societies lagged behind wages and prices. At the middle of the nineteenth century most clubs paid 8s. a week in benefits. In the 1870s many clubs hiked benefits to 10s. a week. Many of them kept benefits at that level well into the twentieth century; others raised them to 12s. or 15s., and by 1900 the most typical benefit was probably 12s. a week.[8] The proportion of wages that each benefit level comprised can be followed by interpreting these figures in the light of A. L. Bowley's estimates of adult male wages per

7. [Mountjoy], *Life, Labours, and Deliverances of a Forest of Dean Collier,* 38–40 and 52–53. In addition, the Ancient Order of Shepherds Friendly Society accepted as members only men who already belonged to another society. Men joined it to obtain higher benefits than those available from their initial club, and data on sickness histories were reported both to the initial club and the Shepherds. Information supplied by the AOF historian, Walter G. Cooper.

8. Data about benefit levels have been collected from these sources: AOF, Court Loyal Bodelwyddan papers, D/DM/510; AOF, Court Cock Royal papers, D1125/6/1–5; AOF, Court of Three Mary's papers, TU:10/7–8 and 13, and TU:97/1; AOF, Court Flower of the Forest papers, DFR 9(c); AOF, Abthorpe Court papers, rules, ZA1606 and ZA1692; High Pavement Chapel Provident Friendly Society papers, minutes, Oct. 9, 1876, HiF2.

Table A1.1
FRIENDLY SOCIETY BENEFITS AS A PERCENT OF WAGES

	Median wages	Friendly society benefits	Percent of wages
1860	18s.	8s.	44.4
1880	24s. 3d.	10s.	41.2
1914	31s. 6d.	12s.	38.1
1924	60s. 0.5d.[a]	12s.	20.0
1950	99s. 4d.[a]	12s.	12.1

Source: Data from Bowley, *Wages and Income in the United Kingdom,* 17 and 46; AOF, Court Loyal Bodelwyddan papers, D/DM/510; AOF, Court Cock Royal papers, D1125/6/1–5; AOF, Court of Three Mary's papers, TU:10/7–8 and 13 and TU:97/1; AOF, Court Flower of the Forest papers, DFR 9(c); AOF, Abthorpe Court papers, rules, ZA1606 and ZA1692; High Pavement Chapel Provident Society papers, minutes, Oct. 9, 1876, HiF2.
[a] Minimum rather than median wage.

week, in table A1.1, keeping in mind that poorly paid workers received somewhat larger proportions than did those earning high wages.[9] By 1950, when many clubs were still paying 10s. or 12s. a week and only a few as much as 15s., full benefits amounted to between 12.1 and 15.1 per cent of the average minimum wage of 99s. 4d.[10]

Protracted sicknesses earned reduced benefits. Thus, a man experiencing a prolonged sickness that kept him out of work for more than a year could by the 1950s earn as little as 2.5 per cent of the minimum wage from friendly society benefits. For some men such sums were not worth collecting. Benefits could most easily have been increased by augmenting the premiums that men paid for sickness insurance. Although there was often enthusiasm for raising benefits, there was seldom any for raising premiums.[11]

Working people invested a substantial part of their resources in the nineteenth century in a stream of future benefits that steadily lost value. They bought benefits of a certain value by paying premiums of a certain value. For example, in 1888 the AOF offered its members the chance of buying an annuity payable from age sixty-five at any of three levels, 2s. 6d., 7s. 6d., or 10s. a week. In 1888 those were marginally attractive potential retirement incomes for men who, in their active working life, earned 15s.

9. Bowley, *Wages and Income in the United Kingdom,* 17 and 46. Bowley supplies direct estimates of median wage levels for 1860, 1880, and 1914; the estimate for 1924 has been derived from his average figure for the increase in weekly earnings from 1914 to 1924.
10. Mitchell, *British Historical Statistics,* 163.
11. E.g., Kempston Friendly Society, DDX157/1, minutes, May 28, 1855.

to 20s. a week. But by the time a man aged thirty in 1888 reached age sixty-five, in 1923, not even the highest annuity was still attractive.

Beginning in 1781, men in the parish of Melchbourne, Bedfordshire, paid premiums for sickness and burial insurance. Their successors elected in 1913 to dissolve the club, dividing its assets of £72 4s. 6d., which had accumulated during 132 years, among about forty members. What would have been a substantial sum by the standards of the late eighteenth century—£72—was, by 1913, little more than beer money for the men who divided it.[12] The same story could be retold many times among clubs that dissolved in 1912 or 1913, when national insurance was introduced, and more forcefully still for those that broke up after the extension of national insurance in 1948. At the end of 1948 the AOF reported a net surplus of £3.2 million on assets of £20.4 million for 449,073 members.[13] Assets, which were still meant to pay all sickness relief and burial costs, totaled only £45.47 per member. Price changes had eroded the value of what working people held in the form of friendly society savings to the point where no one could count on those savings to pay a significant part of the costs of daily life. Like so many educational and charity endowments, the sick and burial endowments the friendly societies had accumulated no longer counted for much. It made more sense to break up a club and distribute its assets than to take the trouble to manage such piddling sums.

For the longer run, friendly society officials and members failed to anticipate price change and therefore failed to provide any easy means to adjust revenues and benefits if wages or prices did increase. Benefits were stipulated in each club's rules, and the rules were difficult to change even after wage and price increases had deprived eight or ten shillings a week of its appeal. But it is also true that the need to rely on friendly societies for sickness benefits waned as the benefits themselves lost value. Beginning with the Workmen's Compensation Act of 1906, the state assumed some of the friendly societies' liabilities. In the case of the 1906 act, such an effect was apparent by 1910 in a survey carried out by the National Conference of Friendly Societies.[14] More important effects followed from the Old Age Pensions Act of 1908, which provided weekly pensions of five shillings for workers over seventy with an income of less than £31 10s. a

12. Melchbourne Club, receipts and roster, P73/28/1.
13. AOF, *Report upon the Valuation of Assets and Liabilities* (London, 1951),4–5.
14. AOF, *Report of Delegates to the National Conference*, 6–7. The Oddfellows deducted benefits paid under this act, and the Employers' Liability Act of 1880, from what they paid. Independent Order of Odd Fellows Manchester Unity, *Rules of the Independent Order of Oddfellows* (Manchester, 1912), 124.

year, and the National Insurance Act of 1911. As friendly society benefits lost value, the state began to make transfer payments.

In the long run, the change in inducements was negative in its effect on sickness claims. It discouraged men from entering claims because the amount they received was, in real terms, progressively smaller. This disincentive to make a claim may have been present before the years of World War 1, but it does not show up in club ledgers. After the war, however, it is apparent in the form of unmade claims: men did not always take the trouble to claim benefits for every week of a sickness episode.

Up to the 1920s the principal change in inducements, what was still only a slight drift toward lower real benefits, tended to diminish the scale of sickness claims rather than to increase it. For the rest, what is most worthy of note from this review of inducements is the degree to which friendly societies in general, and the AOF in particular, adhered over time to the same construction of sickness and therefore sought, even if unwittingly, to keep the inducement to be sick at the same level. They maintained a benefit ratio close to 40 percent of the median wage, and thus they kept in place across the period 1872–1910 a scheme of stable inducements. If sickness rates within the AOF changed in that period, the changes cannot be explained as an effect of inducements.

THE WAITING PERIOD

Most friendly societies declined to pay claims for periods shorter than three days and sometimes for periods shorter than six days. When a member was sick for three days or longer, he could claim compensation for days one and two, but if he was sick only for a day or two, he could not make any claim. The members were sick, but no record of their sickness appears in friendly society accounts unless they also died. The AOF did not require its courts to apply any waiting period, but in practice the courts did apply one, usually a three-day period. The practical effect of the waiting period was to diminish or eliminate the incentive to use sickness as an excuse for taking a day off from work. Men still missed work for single days or short periods, Mondays especially, but those absences were rarely counted as sickness in the friendly society records.

How much sickness goes unobserved because of the waiting period? In the antibiotic era of the second half of the twentieth century, some medicines abbreviate the course of some diseases. Yet sickness is the most widely used excuse for work absences lasting only one or two days and is widely seen to be a false excuse.[15] In the nineteenth century, diseases and injuries took a "natural" course, which means not that they were unaffected by medical therapy but merely that they do not appear to have been shortened by it. Few of the drugs or other treatments doctors used then seem to have abbreviated sickness episodes, and some may, in fact, have prolonged them. This difference in the efficacy of therapeutic regimes implies that very short sickness episodes were less common in the nineteenth century than they would be later on.

Many individual sick club records survive to show the duration of claims lasting at least three days. From among those the records of an AOF court in the Northamptonshire village of Abthorpe have been selected, both because they are typical and because they extend over an unusually long period, from 1863 to 1922. For comparison, however, only one record set is available, the sickness register of the Great North of Scotland Railway for the years 1902–13.[16] The railroad's register shows both the date away from work and the date of return for most men who lost work time because of disease or injury. Some employees probably belonged to friendly societies, which means that their behavior was influenced by their club's rules. But the distinguishing feature of this sickness register is that it includes very short sickness episodes that did not qualify for compensation under friendly society rules as well as longer sicknesses that did qualify. However, it appears also to exclude long episodes; many employees sick for extended periods, longer than a half year, were apparently discharged. Therefore, the comparison is most useful for sicknesses of short and intermediate duration.

Figure A1.1 shows the distribution of sicknesses in the two groups, comparing the number of episodes lasting under one week with the number that lasted a full (six-day) workweek.[17] That is, the number of episodes

15. In a study of sickness and work absence among employees at the Bedford Hospital in 1968–74, J. D. Harte concluded both that episodes lasting three days or less were the most common and that their attribution to sickness often was suspect. Bedford Hospital Sickness Survey, Z625/19/8.
16. Only the ages of Abthorpe Foresters are known, and that distribution resembles the national average. It is reasonable to assume that the age distribution of the railroad employees, who included clerks as well as drivers and tenders, also resembled the national average for adult males.
17. It tends to understate slightly the number of friendly society episodes lasting for six days or less because the Abthorpe Foresters, like most friendly societies, kept records in working weeks of six days rather than in the calendar weeks in which the railroad kept its register. The effect is to disregard intervening Sundays. For the railroad workers, sicknesses lasting six and seven days are combined, which duplicates what the AOF did by disregarding Sundays.

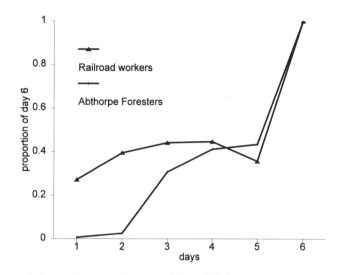

Fig. A1.1. Sickness Duration Compared, First Week
Source: Data from AOF, Abthorpe Court papers, ZA1600, benefits, 1896–
1910; Great North of Scotland Railway Passenger Department papers, registers
of staff off duty, vol. 2.

lasting one or two days was significantly lower than the number lasting a
week, but the number of episodes lasting three or four days approached
the number lasting six days. Very short episodes, lasting one or two days,
rarely received benefits in the Abthorpe court and therefore were rarely
counted. From the third day, however, and especially from the fourth, the
proportions are quite similar between the two groups. That is true also for
the distribution of episodes of two to thirteen weeks' duration, shown in
figure A1.2. As would be expected, the railroad workers' sicknesses were
on average somewhat shorter than those of the Abthorpe men; rail workers experienced more on-the-job injuries than did agricultural workers and
shoemakers, the occupations most common in Abthorpe, and the injuries
they suffered were resolved more quickly than the most commonplace
diseases of Abthorpe Foresters, which were respiratory ailments.[18]

Among railroad workers the modal length of a sickness episode was
three or four days, whereas among Abthorpe Foresters it was between one
and two weeks. In both groups men tended to return to work after full

18. Diagnoses of sicknesses among Abthorpe Court members are available only for the
period 1906–12.

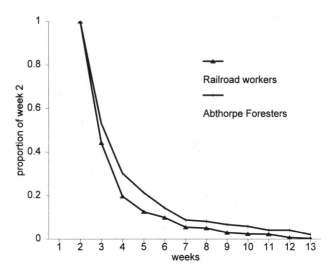

Fig. A1.2. Sickness Duration Compared, Weeks 1–13
Source: Data from AOF, Abthorpe Court papers, ZA1600, benefits, 1896–
1910; Great North of Scotland Railway Passenger Department papers, registers
of staff off duty, vol. 2.

weeks of sickness rather than after fractional weeks.[19] Among railroad
workers, 237 sicknesses lasted seven days, compared to only 150 that
lasted six days, and 102 lasted fourteen days, compared to 58 that lasted
thirteen days. A similar pattern obtains in the Abthorpe ledgers. Even
though the AOF, like other friendly societies, paid benefits on a daily basis,
for most of the period at 1s. 8d. a day, men tended to either extend or
curtail their convàlescence to full weeks. In the friendly societies a doctor's
certification of sickness, usually required each week for short sicknesses,
amounted to an authorization to miss work for a full week, despite the
financial disincentive. Benefits received from a friendly society fell far short
of the wages available from work, and each day a worker missed meant
that he had to absorb more of that benefit-wage gap. What is interesting is
that the railway workers, only some of whom belonged to friendly societies where they received any compensation for lost work time, show the
same tendency to miss full weeks as do the Abthorpe Foresters. If financial
considerations mattered more than health, the railway workers would be
expected to have timed their recoveries so that they returned to work

19. That proved to be true also of men insured under the National Insurance Act. Bradford
Hill, "Investigation of Sickness in Various Industrial Occupations," 220.

before a full week had passed rather than at the end of a full week. Workingmen convalesced with some deliberation.

That deliberation, plus the heavy burden of sicknesses lasting two weeks or more, means that, in terms of sickness time, the friendly society ledgers are dominated not by sickness episodes but by sickness time. Even though brief sicknesses were commonplace, at least in the experience of Scottish railway workers, they were not both frequent enough and long enough to exert a strong effect on the amount of sickness time. Using friendly society records to reconstruct the number of sickness episodes will undercount the actual number by leaving out sicknesses of only one or two days. But the undercounting occurs in a consistent way. Rules about the waiting period remained in place over time, and there is no reason to suppose that, during the period 1872–1910, the risk of sicknesses lasting only one or two days changed in a substantial way.[20] By applying a waiting period the friendly societies removed much of the contentiousness that would otherwise have surrounded the problem of distinguishing sickness from wellness, and they made some small savings on benefits.

CLAIMS FORGONE

In eighteenth-century Scotland, members of friendly societies did not always make claims when they were eligible to do so, because they considered the benefits more as charity than as insurance. In time, however, their attitude changed to the point where they made claims as a matter of course.[21] In nineteenth-century Britain, friendly society members made claims as a matter of course, but they did not claim for every sickness day. Some members neglected to enter claims. In the 1920s, when prices and wages rose sharply, some friendly society members no longer took the trouble to make claims because the amounts involved were too small. By the 1950s such negligence was commonplace, and a large and increasing differential between the level of benefits and that of wages made friendly societies unattractive to young adults. Such behavior was rare before the 1920s, although not unknown. Lord Snell, born the child of agricultural laborers and himself a member first of the AOF and later of the Hearts of Oak Friendly Society, claimed that he had never drawn on the funds,

20. Few therapies that might have sharply curtailed sickness were introduced in that period. Moreover, the consideration of causes of sickness, in chapter 8, suggests that there were no shifts in the disease profile capable of suggesting such a change.
21. Committee of the Highland Society of Scotland, *Report*, 42.

though he did not also claim that he had never been sick.[22] Men like Snell who became rich but remembered their working-class origins often did not make claims.[23] But they were so few in number, compared to the entire membership of a friendly society, that their indifference has a negligible effect. The overwhelming proportion of members paid friendly society premiums because they needed friendly society benefits, and they consistently collected their benefits in times of sickness. That can be seen in ledgers, which show payments to individuals.

MALINGERING

Friendly society members sometimes worried whether their peers would cheat by claiming to be sick when they were well. In the late-twentieth-century mind this hazard may appear at first glance to consist chiefly of short-term absenteeism attributed inaccurately to sickness. But because they required a waiting period, the friendly societies were little troubled by this form of malingering. They did, however, fret about other forms.

Benjamin Langton, a court secretary and thus someone well acquainted with the intricacies of court business, doubted that men who had been sick for many months could recover. He worried that members were declaring off extended part benefits not because they had recovered but because, after a year's hiatus and with a different diagnosis, they could become eligible again for full benefits. Some members, he feared, were "cute," meaning that they were willing to go without half or quarter benefits for a year in order to regain full benefits. And for doctors' diagnoses he felt scorn: "It is seldom the medical profession give the same diagnosis even of the same complaint after any lapse of time."[24] His fears were exaggerated. The benefits lost during the year required to regain eligibility for full benefits would have outweighed the potential gain.[25] And comparisons of doctors' certificates over time, such as can be done in the records of Court Equity in Cambridge, show that diagnoses were usually consistent.[26]

Friendly society members and officials were unable to identify specific forms of malingering that had a substantial impact on the number or

22. Snell, *Men, Movements, and Myself,* 19. Also Johnson, *Saving and Spending,* 74.

23. Snow, "Some Statistical Problems," 464.

24. *Foresters' Miscellany,* Apr. 1888, 191–92.

25. Furthermore, Langton's fears are contradicted by Wilkinson, *Friendly Society Movement,* 193.

26. AOF, Court Equity papers, R78/70. For further discussion of this court, see chapter 4.

duration of claims. Undoubtedly, some members claimed to be sick when they could have worked and fooled their doctors into giving them certificates, thereby adding artificially to the sickness rate. But friendly society observers also worried that members would return to work too soon, thereby endangering their ultimate recovery or adding to the chance of relapse. Judging from both the low volume of complaints and the difficulty of giving persuasive examples of it, malingering seems to have been a small rather than a large problem.

SELECTION

Insurance appeals especially to people who expect to need the coverage they buy, and insurers attempt to select the people they insure in order to protect themselves from this effect. The friendly societies operated on the premise that they needed to protect themselves from risk-prone individuals. Most societies tried to exclude candidates in bad health. By the 1870s they relied chiefly on medical examinations to distinguish those fit to join from those unfit.

In a comparatively elaborate statement about selection principles, the Abthorpe court of the AOF declared itself open only to candidates in sound health, of good character, and neither idle nor dissolute.[27] Such provisions might have prompted a refusal to admit many candidates. But the doctors' examination certificates suggest that the court was not selective in practice. In 1859 George Reeve joined; his medical certificate states: "He had several epileptic [sic] fits about 14 months ago, but has been in good health since. Possibly he may not have a recurrence of them." John Stokes was admitted even though he had had a disease of the elbow joint that disabled him for heavy labor.[28] A club in Wales held a special vote to judge a candidate who was in satisfactory health but deaf and dumb and decided to admit him.[29] The Shropshire Provident Society attempted from the moment of its foundation, in the 1850s, to exclude young men with tuberculosis and candidates who had medical complaints likely to be fatal to middle-aged men, providing an elaborate

---

27. AOF, Abthorpe Court papers, 1884 rules, ZA1692, 10.
28. Ibid., doctor's certificates, ZA1759–1810.
29. St. David's Unity of Ivorites, Bond of Hope Lodge papers, minutes, Aug. 24, 1889. See, to the same effect, Leicester Bond Street Friendly Society papers, DE1884/2, minutes, June 11, 1896.

list of conditions that should be asked about at the medical exam.[30] But their practice was inconsistent. For example, in 1871 they enrolled William Beamand even though he admitted in his application that his mother and sister had both died of consumption. Some applicants were refused, among them one of Elizabeth Roberts's respondents from Barrow, who remembered of his youth: "I was the only one who never passed for the Oddfellows. My sister took me by the hand to the doctor" who said: "You can take him back and tell your mother she should have drowned him when he was young and I'm not going to [pass him]."[31]

Minutes and medical certificates indicate that the friendly societies claimed the right to reject applicants in poor health but did little to apply that right. That interpretation is confirmed by quantitative evidence about the proportion of applicants who were rejected. In the Leicester Bond Street Friendly Society in the period 1829–59, 89.5 percent of applicants were accepted. Some of the remainder applied but did not follow up their applications to the point of actually being considered for membership. Of 561 applicants, only 30—5.3 percent—were refused admission.[32] Since reasons for the rejections are not given, those refusals may include both medical and social factors.

Military examiners applied far stricter standards than did the friendly societies. In the Boer War rejections ran as high as 60 percent. When a Scottish group looked into the issue, in the 1820s, it reported a military rejection rate of 17.5 percent and a friendly societies rate of 4.8 percent.[33] Other samples show similar or lower rates of rejection of friendly society applicants and often higher rates for the military, even in war time. Friendly societies often admitted people with hearing and speech defects, characteristics that did not disable them from work.[34] They did not reject applicants with bad teeth or flat feet, two of the principal grounds for rejection for military service,[35] or those with many other disabilities.

Furthermore, the degree to which friendly societies selected their members appears to have had little effect on their patterns of sickness. Most of the sicknesses that members suffered in the early years after admission

30. Shropshire Provident Society papers, minutes, 436/6727–6728, passim, and 436/1–960, the initial 960 proposals for insurance.
31. Roberts, *Woman's Place*, 164.
32. Leicester Bond Street Friendly Society papers, DE1884/1.
33. Committee of the Highland Society of Scotland, *Report*, 24–25.
34. Neison, *Observations*, 107.
35. Maurice, "National Health: A Soldier's Story," 41–56.

were not foreshadowed by their medical condition at admission.[36] Even a careful medical examination—and the Foresters required the medical examination of new members beginning in 1865—would not anticipate infectious maladies a man might contract in the future, organ damage, or a potential for muscular and skin diseases. In the first years after admission, Francis G. P. Neison, Jr., found that members newly admitted to the Foresters accumulated somewhat less sickness time than did established members of the same age. But the difference soon disappeared.[37] Medical selection had a short-lived effect. Club doctors could not predict the long-run health of candidates for friendly society membership, any more than their medical counterparts in the mid-twentieth century could predict the future health of job applicants.[38]

Actuarial investigations also showed that, to a disproportionate degree, the members who eventually withdrew had entered fewer claims than members who stayed in, and the Foresters had higher rates of secession than the Oddfellows.[39] That characteristic saved the societies some money, in that members who seceded had seldom made claims equal to their contributions. But the same investigations also showed that this disproportion mattered little, in terms of selection, because of the difficulty of anticipating future patterns of sickness.

Judging from the way they operated, friendly societies did not expect to be able to distinguish good risks from bad risks with much accuracy. It was possible, many observers noticed, to make distinctions that had some force for a few months. But, as time passed, the distinctions made had less and less merit. Although the societies continued to require the medical examination of new members, they avoided most of the problems associated with selection effects by requiring an initiation period. New members could not claim for benefits for six months or a year after joining, a rule that eliminated most of the problem of selection and most of the force of the selection effect, as Neison showed from AOF data.[40] The initiation period also guarded against insurance consciousness: people who buy

36. Geddes and Holbrook, *Friendly Societies*, 66–67.

37. Neison, *Rates of Mortality and Sickness, 1871–75*, 28.

38. E.g., Hinkle, Plummer, and Whitney, "Continuity of Patterns of Illness," 417–23; and Taylor, "Personal Factors Associated with Sickness Absence," 106–18. On the same point see also Alter and Riley, "Frailty, Sickness, and Death," 27–28.

39. Neison, *Rates of Mortality and Sickness, 1871–1875*, 81 and 86.

40. Ibid., 10–25. See also Hardy, "Friendly Societies," 291–92, who concluded that a selection effect existed but was small.

insurance are somewhat likelier to enter claims soon after their purchase than later.

Because the friendly societies did not force out members who fell sick, even if they remained sick for lengthy periods, the health pattern of their membership does not suffer from the "healthy worker effect,"[41] in which the workforce is healthier than the entire cohort because people with disabilities leave work. Friendly societies were made up of people who entered adulthood in good enough health to allow them to work. Their health remains under observation from that time forward.

In sum, the friendly societies applied a waiting period that reduced the number of sickness episodes that would be admitted as claims to those lasting three days or more, and in some societies to those lasting a week or more. The waiting period curtailed the number of claims and lowered what the societies had to pay in benefits. Waiting period rules were applied in the same form over time, so that the omission of short sicknesses occurs in a consistent way. It produces consistently lower rates of sickness incidence, compared to what would be found if all work absences due to sickness had been benefited. The attempt to select members also reduced friendly society liabilities and made claims lower than sicknesses. But the friendly societies rejected few applicants. They defined sickness in a specific way and sought to limit claims by using standard insurance devices. Their statistics tend to understate sicknesses and sickness time, compared to a regime in which benefits were offered without such limiting devices. But these effects applied in a consistent way across the period 1872–1910.

41. Fox and Collier, "Low Mortality Rates in Industrial Cohort Studies," 225–30.

Average Age and Age

AOF DIRECTORIES REPORT the average age of all members of a court rather than the exact ages of individual members. My aim is to compare sickness time between locales and across the years independently of age. In order to use the available information about average age to control for age, it is necessary to consider how courts differ in their age structures. This appendix explores these differences, showing why the regression model used in this analysis controls for age by including not only average age but also the number of years since the court was formed and the rate at which new members joined.

A COURT'S LIFE CYCLE AND AGE DISPERSION

The average is a measure of central tendency. Given that AOF members extended in age across the spectrum of adulthood, from eighteen up,[1] different courts usually had members within different ranges of age. Thus, as a measurement of central tendency, average age may mean different things for different courts. But the range of age structures that could occur is limited by AOF rules and practices. In the ordinary course of events, AOF courts were formed among youths and young adults (entrants were required to be between the ages of eighteen and forty) who lived in the same community.[2] Over time in the typical court's life cycle, the original members aged, some left the court or died, and new members joined. Each year existing members aged by one year, pushing the court's average age up. But the average age of all members did not advance by a year, because

1. The AOF also sponsored juvenile courts, which enrolled younger members, but their experience is not considered here.
2. Some courts were formed when independent friendly societies affiliated with the AOF, such as the Stonesfield Friendly Society did in 1912. That society, located in Oxfordshire, was organized in the eighteenth century.

new members were added at ages usually lower than the average age of existing members, and older members died. Sometimes the new members were young enough and numerous enough to pull the court's average age down. Over time, most courts added new members. In the five years from 1873 to 1877, for example, only twelve courts out of more than three thousand failed to initiate a single new member. Because courts ordinarily paid sickness benefits out of their own assets, there was a strong inducement for new courts to add members in order to fund benefits at the full allowance.[3] In the average year during 1873–77, courts with a mean of 124 members gained 12 initiates, adding nearly 10 percent to their membership each year.

In typical circumstances men joined and left AOF courts in patterns that produced a gradual rise in the average age. For example, the average age in 1871 of the 501 members in Court Sherwood Forest, formed in 1860 in Reading, was thirty-one. Thereafter, it rose gradually and stood at forty-seven years in 1922. The charter members aged, and some died or left the court, but much of the effect of their aging was counterbalanced by the addition of young recruits. By 1910, 1,213 men belonged to this court. The gains and losses were not smooth from year to year, but they were smooth over groups of years, so that the average age of the court evolved gradually. All courts did not evolve in this way. Court The Bough, formed in 1883 in Catterick, Yorkshire, managed to recruit only five new members in the period 1891–98, during which time seventeen men left the court and another died. An already small court shrank. If it had suddenly revived itself, by recruiting a large number of members around 1913, then its members would have been clustered around two quite different ages. The charter members from 1883, then about twenty-two, would have aged thirty years, making their average age in 1913 about fifty-two, but the 1913 recruits would have been young adults. In fact, however, this court ceased to report to the AOF and was either dissolved or consolidated. Its evolution was not smooth because the court failed to attract new members.

The typical pattern of recruitment is illustrated in figure A2.1, which shows the average ratio of recruits to existing members according to how many years had passed since a court's formation. In a court's first year, all members can be counted as recruits. Thus, courts paid sickness and death

---

3. Courts in distress could be assisted from funds accumulated by the district. Appeals and decisions about them were reported in the published minutes of district meetings, and those minutes show that such assistance was rarely given.

benefits in the first year of their existence only to a few members who had belonged long enough to become eligible and had experienced a claim. In the second year, courts typically added a high proportion of new members, totaling 46 percent of the number of their existing members. As time passed, the pace at which they added new members tapered off.[4] Whenever courts recruited new members in this pattern and lost only a small proportion of members through withdrawal and death, their average age rose gradually. Figure A2.2 shows the average ages reported in 1874 for all active courts in Britain. Throughout the period under study here, courts gained one-third of a year in average age for each year that passed.

In time, a typical court's membership would come to be stretched out across the spectrum of possible ages, so that a mature court might have some members aged eighteen and nineteen and some older than seventy. But in a younger court, one whose charter members had not yet reached old age and thus not yet begun to die out, and one also that had evolved in a smooth pattern of entrances and exits, the members would be concentrated in a single modal age group between the extremes. That mode would be comprised of the ages attained by the charter cohort: the men who joined in the earliest years after a court's formation, who constituted the largest bloc of members. Over time, average age would measure the central tendency of all ages across an expanding range, but under the strong influence of the tightly grouped ages of the charter cohort. The implications of this can be made clearer by reviewing average age and actual age in circumstances in which both are known. Neison, engaged by the AOF to study the order's sickness and mortality patterns during 1871–75, published his principal findings in the form of tables that related sickness and death rates at each age. Not all courts furnished information in the detail that Neison required, so his tables do not encompass the entire AOF membership. Nevertheless, Neison's findings about the distribution by age of AOF members as of January 1, 1871, can be compared with what the 1872 directory reports about membership at the end of 1871. Figure A2.3 shows two curves. One depicts the number of members as of January 1 at each age from 18 to 102. The other shows the number of members in courts with an average age ranging from nineteen, the lowest, to sixty-five, the highest. Even though the two curves do not deal with identical

---

4. The estimates shown here are based on the experience of courts formed in the period 1858–85 and under observation from 1873 through 1885. These recruitment patterns held up until 1912, when the National Insurance Act of 1911 went into effect.

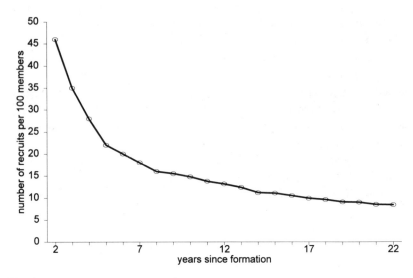

Fig. A2.1. Recruitment Rates in the AOF, 1873–1875
Source: Data from AOF, *Directories,* 1873–1876.

populations,[5] they show the leading difference in the way age is represented between individuals grouped by their ages and individuals formed
into subgroups and distributed by the average age of members in each
subgroup.

Figure A2.3 underscores what it means to say that the average is a
measure of central tendency. Average age is a summary statistic that com-
presses information. In any year, few courts had an average age as low as
21; those had been formed recently and as yet had few members. And few
courts had an average age over 55. Since Neison reported ages as high as
102, most of the compression occurred on the right side of figure A2.3.
Older members were rarely numerous enough in a court to dominate its
average age.

What is true of the order is true also of individual courts, albeit with
more variation. Consider the case of Court Princess of Hesse, located in
Newbury, Berkshire, for which the exact ages of entrances and exits can be
reconstructed beginning in 1892 from a roster the court secretary made

5. Court secretaries presumably had some difficulty in mastering the reporting require-
ments introduced for the 1872 directory, and thereafter new secretaries may also have had
some trouble understanding their responsibilities. But most secretaries served for extended
periods, partly because their service was paid, and seem to have learned their responsibilities
well.

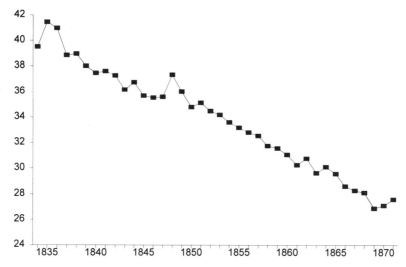

Fig. A2.2. Average Age of Court Members and Date of Court Formation, 1834–1871
Source: Data from AOF, *Directory,* 1874.

up.[6] Figure A2.4 shows this court's age structure in 1892 and periodically thereafter. In 1892 the members were clustered at ages 30–39, with only a few in their fifties or above. The modal age rose over time, reaching 45–49 by 1906, and the average age also increased, from 33.6 years in 1892 to 39.8 years in 1906.[7] Over time, the age structure of the AOF as a whole and of typical courts in it spread out, and the average age, in the early history of each court a value tightly surrounded by members, came to stand at the mean of an increasingly dispersed membership.

Because the average duration of sickness episodes rises with age at a slightly increasing rate—for any individual age rises in an arithmetic scheme but sickness risk in this form rises in a geometric scheme—

6. AOF, Court Princess of Hesse papers. The roster records date of initiation, age at entry, and the date at which membership ended, by death or withdrawal for members belonging in 1892 and those added in later years. These data have been used to distribute members by age group for each year from 1893 to 1906, a period in which data about the date of withdrawal or death is wanting for only thirteen members, who have been left out. This roster was kept into the 1970s, which means that information about the date of withdrawal is lacking for an increasing number of members, some of whom were still alive when this roster was taken out of service.

7. That is, the average age increased at a slightly faster pace, 0.44 years per year, than it did in the AOF as a whole. The pace was slower in the AOF as a whole than in existing courts because the data for the entire AOF include newly formed courts with the highest rates of recruitment.

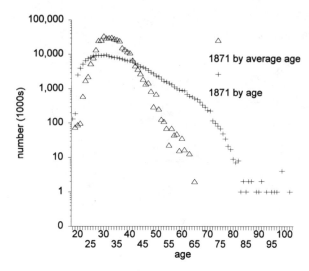

Fig. A2.3. Age Structures Compared, 1871
Sources: Data from Neison, *Rates of Mortality and Sickness, 1871–1875,* 35–36; AOF, *Directory,* 1872.

dispersal affects the sickness rate. A broader spectrum of ages produces higher sickness time even when the average age of court members remains the same. This is because the survival of a court for two or three decades means that it began to include some members who were old and particularly susceptible to prolonged sickness episodes. Even though their ages might be counterbalanced by the initiation of young adults, their sickness risk would not be counterbalanced. This can be called a dispersion effect. It shows up in frequency distributions of sickness rates among courts at each average age, and thus in the variance of sickness rates among courts. The problem posed by this feature of the available data is to find a satisfactory way to take dispersion into account, so that differences in the dispersion of members across the age spectrum do not produce their own illusion about the meaning of sickness rates.

In typical circumstances the average age of a court advanced as its charter cohort aged, and the average age sickness rate increased at a faster pace. Dispersion of members across the age spectrum is one of three stages in court evolution. Initially the court's membership was compressed within the ages eighteen to forty. In the second stage, the membership spread slowly across the age spectrum as charter members aged and the court added new members. Finally, the court achieved a mature age structure, with members ranging in age from eighteen to advanced old age. In the

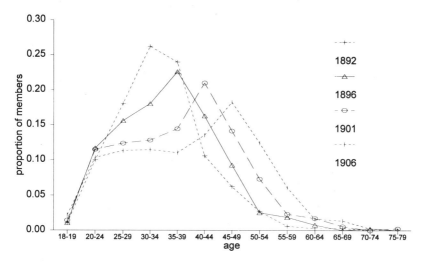

Fig. A2.4. Evolution of Court Princess of Hesse, by Average Age of Members, 1892–1906
Source: Data from AOF, *Directories,* 1873–1922.

typical circumstances of a smoothly evolving number of entrances and exits, a mature court no longer showed a strong modal age in its members because the charter cohort, which formed its mode in stages one and two, had died out. Thus the dispersion effect was felt in the years when a typical court was maturing, a period lasting about forty-five years, the time needed for its oldest charter members, aged thirty-five to thirty-nine, to reach eighty to eighty-four. At that age, so few charter members survived that their higher sickness risk ceased to have any effect except in very small courts. AOF courts formed in 1834 began to complete this maturation process around 1880, but, because new courts were formed every year, there were always many courts in the maturing stage. The AOF directories report the year in which each court was founded, and the court's age is used in the regression analysis to control for differences among courts in the dispersion of members by age.

BIMODAL AGE STRUCTURES

Not all courts evolved in a way similar to the AOF as a whole, regularly adding members, and adding more members than they lost. In some courts, atypical age structures emerged. For present purposes, where the point is to qualify average age as a measure of central tendency, the most important case occurred when courts recruited new members in such an irregular way that they developed bimodal age structures. A long period when few men joined followed by a period of heavy recruitment would produce an age structure with two modes, one made up of early members and the other of recent recruits. Yet the court's average age would fall somewhere between the two modes.

For example, hypothesizing two extreme cases, one court might have all its members evenly distributed between two age groups, some in their twenties and the others in their seventies. Another might have all its members evenly distributed between their forties and fifties. The two courts could have the same average age, but their sickness rates would probably be quite different. Using Neison's 1871–75 schedule of age-specific sickness rates and assuming that each hypothetical court has the same number of members, the bimodal court would have a sickness rate 3.7 times higher than the court with all of its members in their forties and fifties. Although the average age would be an accurate measure of central tendency, it would be a misleading indication of sickness risk. Depending on the proportions of new and old members, the recruits and their youthfulness might make a court appear to have an unusually low or high sickness rate for its average age. Thus, courts with bimodal age distributions might seem to have lower or higher sickness rates in comparison to the AOF as a whole while actually having sickness patterns that closely fit AOF experience at each age.

The 1873 directory adds information that had not appeared earlier in the form of the number of members initiated by each court in the previous year. Hence from that year the directories provide the information necessary to create a matrix of recruitment patterns consisting of the annual proportion of initiates to existing members. This matrix, too vast to show here, makes it possible to observe each court's recruitment pattern to see whether it was sufficiently irregular to produce a bimodal age structure. To raise the threat of bimodalism, a court had to have both an irregular recruitment pattern and three other characteristics: it had to have been in existence long enough for a sudden period of heavy recruitment to succeed a lengthy period of comparative inactivity; it had to have an average age high enough for the addition of a large number of youthful members to distort its age structure; and it had to recruit many new members within a short period.

Some courts meet these qualifications. For example, Court Father and Sons, formed in Whiston, Lancashire, in 1840, suddenly revived itself in

1878 and 1879, recruiting nine new members to add to its seventeen existing members. Before 1878 and after 1879, this court recruited few men. Its average age changed by three years, shifting down from forty-seven to forty-four. No conclusions should be drawn about whether this court's sickness rate was especially high or low without mentioning the likelihood that its age structure was bimodal.

The same steps that identify Court Father and Sons as probably having acquired a bimodal age structure also show how few courts each year meet the initial qualifications for being at risk to developing a bimodal structure. Across the period 1875–81, an average of only two courts a year meet these qualifications. Of those, fewer than half meet those qualifications and also show the requisite pattern of recruitment inactivity in previous years.

In sum, only a few courts developed bimodal age structures. Comparisons of the patterns of sickness of single courts with larger groups or the AOF as a whole should not be made without determining whether those courts may have had bimodal age structures. But bimodalism was so rare that it does not trouble comparisons made between groups of courts, which are the most common form of the comparison made in this study. Nevertheless, the information available about each court's annual ratio of initiates to existing members provides a further characteristic that can be used to qualify the court's experience relative to other courts.

Determinants of Sickness Time and Mortality

Table A3.1
DETERMINANTS OF SICKNESS TIME

Determinant	Constant					
	1.52*	−2.04	−1.85	−3.27	−5.36	−5.15
Lag1	.54***	.59***	.58***	.50***	.50***	.49***
Lag2	.34*	.43***	.41*	.32	.33	.32
AOF mortality		.17	.15	.20	.24	.24
Unemployment			.002*	.003*	.003*	.003*
Unemployment, lag1			−.002	−.002	−.002	−.002
Unemployment, lag2			.001	.002	.002	.002
Real wages				.03	.03	.03
Plaints					.01	.01
Prices 35 years earliers						−.003
Adjusted R-square	.87	.87	.88	.89	.89	.88

Sources: Data from Feinstein, *Statistical Tables,* T18–19, 42–43, 125–26, and 140; Feinstein, "New Look at the Cost of Living," 170–71; Johnson, "Small Debts and Economic Distress in England and Wales," 65–87 (with the series of plaints supplied by Johnson's collaborator, Humphrey Southall); Mitchell, *British Historical Statistics,* 12–13, 722–23; and AOF, *Directories,* 1872–1911.
*p < .05.
**p < .01.
***p < .001.

Table A3.2
DETERMINANTS OF AOF MORTALITY

Determinant	Constant					
	1.36	3.85	−.44	3.69	10.15	8.08
Lag1	.56***	.51**	.52*	.44*	.38*	.38*
Lag2	.32	.27	.46*	.36	.38*	.36*
Sickness time		−.11	.11	.41	.41	.47
Unemployment			−.001	−.002	−.002	−.002
Unemployment, lag1			−.002	−.002	−.001	−.001
Unemployment, lag2			−.001	−.002	−.003	−.003
Real wages				−.05	−.07**	−.08***
Plaints					−.04*	−.05**
Prices 35 years earlier						.03
Adjusted *R*-square	.67	.67	.69	.74	.78	.79

Sources: Data from Feinstein, *Statistical Tables,* T18–19, 42–43, 125–26, and 140; Feinstein, "New Look at the Cost of Living," 170–71; Johnson, "Small Debts and Economic Distress in England and Wales," 65–87 (with the series of plaints supplied by Johnson's collaborator, Humphrey Southall); Mitchell, *British Historical Statistics,* 12–13, 722–23; and AOF, *Directories,* 1872–1911.
*$p < .05$.
**$p < .01$.
***$p < .001$.

Table A3.3
DETERMINANTS OF MORTALITY AMONG ADULT MALES IN ENGLAND AND WALES

Determinant	Constant					
	1.94	5.48	2.93	3.71	18.60*	16.01
Lag1	.66***	.61**	.61**	.57**	.41*	.42*
Lag2	.23	.19	.26	.30	.30	.31
Sickness time		−.15	−.02	.51	.41	.48
Unemployment			.001	−.001	−.001	−.001
Unemployment, lag1			−.005	−.005	−.003	−.003
Unemployment, lag2			.002	−.0003	−.002	−.002
Real wages				−.07	−.09**	−.10**
Plaints					−.08*	−.09*
Prices 35 years earlier						.02
Adjusted *R*-square	.66	.66	.67	.70	.75	.74

Sources: Data from Feinstein, *Statistical Tables,* T18–19, 42–43, 125–26, and 140; Feinstein, "New Look at the Cost of Living," 170–71; Johnson, "Small Debts and Economic Distress in England and Wales," 65–87 (with the series of plaints supplied by Johnson's collaborator, Humphrey Southall); Mitchell, *British Historical Statistics,* 12–13, 722–23; and AOF, *Directories,* 1872–1911.
*$p < .05$.
**$p < .01$.
***$p < .001$.

APPENDIX 4

Boundary Problems
and Choices

IN THE PERIOD 1872–1910, Britain operated with multiple administrative systems, each with special responsibilities. That structure included at least three schemes of counties: the ancient (or civil) counties, the boundaries of which had been fixed since 1844 or, in many cases, much earlier, but in which some minor alterations were made during the period under study; the administrative counties, created by the Local Government Act of 1888; and the registration counties, formed in England and Wales in 1837 and in Scotland in 1855 as amalgamations of the registration districts in which births, marriages, and deaths were tallied. These three schemes (and a fourth, the parliamentary counties) used mostly the same names for counties, even though they did not always occupy the same geographic area.[1] While boundaries for the administrative and ancient counties were coextensive in most cases, registration counties were in several cases significantly different from either of the others. Since the nineteenth century, further changes have been made in county boundaries. Both the multiple systems of 1872–1910 and the changes in county boundaries threaten to confuse the issue of deciding which boundaries should be employed.

The AOF located courts within the ancient counties, which constitutes a powerful but in the end still ineffectual argument in favor of adopting the ancient counties as units of observation. For some of the data important to this study, census authorities amalgamated returns concerning civil parishes into the different county systems, in some census returns reporting totals of population, area, and houses for each. But they did not sustain that multiple system of reporting either across the entire period 1872–1910 or

1. Great Britain, Interdepartmental Committee on Social and Economic Research, *Census Reports*, 95–104, provides some information about the characteristics of each structure.

across all the questions on which census enumerators collected information. For a key part of the data they accumulated, information about occupations, the census authorities reported only by registration counties. Hence, there is no simple way to restructure Britain's administrative geography to overcome the problem of multiple administrative systems.

Other scholars who have faced this problem have recognized that, although the counties in each of these several systems were not coextensive, their boundaries were similar enough to maintain essential characteristics, especially in the categories in which the characteristics of counties can be specified from census information.[2] While that seems to be true of the administrative and ancient counties, it may not be true of the registration counties, for which boundaries were sometimes quite different, meaning that AOF courts situated in an administrative county of one name were sometimes located in a registration county of another name. In addition, a richer body of information is available from British censuses about the registration counties, and some of those data are broken down for smaller units, the registration districts. Overall, census information is reported about more characteristics for the registration than for the administrative counties.[3]

On one hand, therefore, analysis of the data may proceed on at least one and sometimes more than one of five levels:

1. Britain
2. England, Scotland, and Wales
3. administrative counties
4. registration counties
5. registration districts

On the other hand, it is useful to portray regional differences in maps, which give a visual impression and which also show in an economical way when pairs or groups of counties shared similar traits. But all five levels of analysis cannot be duplicated in maps, in part because of the unavailability of maps with the requisite characteristics to serve as a basis for drawing the maps shown in chapter 8.[4]

2. However, Baines, "Use of Published Census Data," 312–15, reallocated population to the system of ancient counties and added the administrative unit of London to his scheme. That adjustment was made necessary by his use of annual reports of vital events for the registration districts.
3. Census procedures and changes in them are discussed in Lawton, *Census and Social Structure.*
4. A detailed map of administrative counties against a background of longitude and lati-

The maps show patterns that differentiate among administrative counties. Map 8.1 shows the distribution of locales with at least one AOF court against a background of county boundaries comprised of the system of administrative counties created in 1888.[5] There is one major difference in court locations between the ancient county addresses given by the AOF and the counties to which courts are assigned in this map. In the ancient county system, London sprawled across Middlesex, Surrey, and Kent, whereas in the administrative system it was assigned its own territory, which was taken out of those three counties. In the other maps, court locations have been altered to the boundaries of the administrative counties. Most of the analysis in chapter 9 is based on registration counties and districts.

tude has been used to draw the national and county maps shown here. Similarly detailed maps for registration county and registration district boundaries as they existed in the period 1870–1920 would be needed to produce such maps.

5. Since each AOF court's location was given only for the system of ancient counties, that location had to be checked for each of the three other county systems.

APPENDIX 5

Factors Included in the Statistical Analysis

AGE AND ITS DISTRIBUTION

AVERAGE   the average age of court members

SINCEDOF   years since a court was formed, which is a proxy for the dispersion of membership by age

INITRATE   rate at which new members were added to each court

SOCIOECONOMIC FACTORS

POPCHANG   the rate of population growth per 1,000 in the registration district from 1881 to 1891, a proxy for health risks associated with large inflows of people

MAR and MAR2   the proportion per 1,000 of adult males in each registration district married at the 1891 census, included because modern analyses suggest that married people have lower death rates. A squared term (MAR2) appears also in the least squares equation to test for a nonlinear form

PERHOUS and PERHOUS2   the number of people per inhabited house in the 3,151 courts that could be assigned to municipal boroughs or civil parishes. This variable assesses the influence of crowding in general housing. A squared term (PERHOUS2) appears also in the least squares equation to test for a nonlinear form.

MARKS91   the proportion per 1,000 of men in each county marrying in 1891 and unable to sign the marriage register, a proxy for the relationship between low educational attainment and poor health

WAGES92   the average wage of agricultural laborers in each county in 1892, a proxy for variations in income

307

UNION   trade unionists as a proportion per 1,000 of the population in each county, a proxy for the degree to which union membership protected men from health hazards

TOWNPOP and TOWNPOP2   the number of people living in villages, towns, and cities for 3,151 courts that could be assigned to municipal boroughs or civil parishes. Studies of mortality in the nineteenth century find that it increased with town size.

PERAREA   the number of persons per statute acre in each registration district, a measure of spatial density

CROWDED   the proportion per 1,000 of persons living more than two to a room in tenements in the counties, a potential measure of crowding in housing

PRTDISAB   the proportion per 1,000 of the noninstitutionalized population in each county reported as having physical disabilities, a measure of the background level of disability

HEALTH   the proportion per 1,000 of doctors (physicians, surgeons, and general practitioners) plus nurses (nurses, midwives and invalid attendants) plus chemists plus teachers to each county's 1891 population, a proxy for the availability of health services and information

RRWKRS   the proportion per 1,000 of railway employees to the 1891 population of each county, a proxy for the integration of local with national infrastructures and thus for the speed at which infectious diseases spread; this variable may also capture risk in this occupation

ALCOHOL   the proportion per 1,000 of people employed in the sale of alcoholic beverages to the 1891 population of each county, a proxy for differences in alcohol consumption levels

SCAVN   the proportion per 1,000 of drainage workers, scavengers, and sweepers to the 1891 population of each county, a proxy for differences in sanitation facilities

OCCUPATIONS (all at county level and all per 1,000, males in the particular occupation as a proportion of the sum of males employed in all occupations, specified and unspecified)

LEAD   manufacturing lead substances

GLASS   glassmaking

EARTH   earthenware

STONE   stone

COALMNR and COALMNR2   coal mining

OTHMNR and OTHMNR2   other types of mining

MACHINE   making machines and implements

FISH   fishing

COMCON   merchants, bankers, insurance agents, and men engaged in carrying people, goods, and messages, i.e., commerce and conveyance

RETAIL   retail dealers in animal and vegetable substances, including tobacco

CNSTRCT   building and remodeling

SHIPS   shipwrights and others engaged in building or outfitting ships and boats

CHEMCLS   chemical making

TXTLES   textile fabrics

FOOD   retail food trades

FARM   farming

REGIONS

LONDON   London

SE   Surrey, Kent, Sussex, Hampshire, and Berkshire

SMIDLAND   Middlesex, Hertfordshire, Buckinghamshire, Oxfordshire, Northamptonshire, Huntingdonshire, Bedfordshire, and Cambridgeshire

EASTERN   Essex, Suffolk, and Norfolk

SW   Wiltshire, Dorsetshire, Devonshire, Cornwall, and Somersetshire

WMIDLAND   Gloucestershire, Herefordshire, Shropshire, Staffordshire, Worcestershire, and Warwickshire

NMIDLAND   Leicestershire, Rutlandshire, Lincolnshire, Nottinghamshire, Derbyshire

NW   Cheshire and Lancashire

YORK   West Riding, East Riding, and North Riding

NORTHERN   Durham, Northumberland, Cumberland, and Westmorland

MONMWLS   all Welsh counties

Results of Statistical Analysis

Table A6.1
WEIGHTED MEAN VALUES OF VARIABLES

Variable	Meaning	Mean
SICKRATE	sickness time, per member year	11.67 days
DEADRATE	death rate per year	11.552 per 1,000
AVERAGE	average age of court members	35.415 years
SINCEDOF	years since court formation	33.97 years
INITRATE	rate at which new members entered	63.87 per 1,000
POPCHANG	rate of population change, per Registration District	10.453 per 1,000
MAR	porportion married	648.084 per 1,000
PERHOUS	persons per inhabited house	5.324
MARKS91	proportion marrying and unable to sign register	67.354 per 1,000
WAGES92	average weekly agricultural wages	0.698 of a pound
UNION	proportion belonging to trades unions	35.47 per 1,000
TOWNPOP	size of municipal borough	451184.163
PERAREA	persons per statute acre	14.44
CROWDED	proportion in tenements that were crowded	95.106 per 1,000
PRTDISAB	proportion with physical disabilities	19.352 per 1,000
HEALTH	health care/information providers	10.447 per 1,000
RRWKRS	railroad workers	1.773 per 1,000
ALCOHOL	alcohol consumption levels	5.642 per 1,000
SCAVN	refuse collection labor force	0.113 per 1,000
LEAD	workers in lead	0.205 per 1,000
GLASS	workers in glass	1.62 per 1,000
EARTH	workers in earthenware	5.823 per 1,000
STONE	workers in stone	3.072 per 1,000
COALMNR	coal miners	39.735 per 1,000
OTHMNR	other miners	3.478 per 1,000
MACHINE	machine and implement makers	25.386 per 1,000
FISH	fishing	3.189 per 1,000
COMCON	workers in commerce and conveyence	117.212 per 1,000

(*continued*)

Table A6.1   (*Continued*)

Variable	Meaning	Mean
RETAIL	workers in retail trades	19.132 per 1,000
CNSTRCT	construction workers	74.615 per 1,000
SHIPS	workers in ships and shipbuilding	6.279 per 1,000
CHEMCLS	workers making chemicals	3.954 per 1,000
TXTLES	textile workers	28.687 per 1,000
FOOD	retail food workers	58.629 per 1,000
FARM	farmers	160.805 per 1,000
LONDON	London	0.087
SE	Southeast	omitted
SMIDLAND	South Midlands	0.087
EASTERN	Eastern counties	0.113
SW	Southwest	0.089
WMIDLAND	West Midlands	0.139
NMIDLAND	North Midlands	0.070
NW	Northwest counties	0.077
YORK	Yorkshire	0.075
NORTHERN	Northern counties	0.059
MONMWLS	Wales	0.045

Table A6.2
DETERMINANTS OF SICKNESS TIME

Factor	Coefficient	Elasticity	Level of Significance
AVERAGE	0.571	1.732	.000
SINCEDOF	0.065	0.188	.000
INITRATE	−0.011	−0.058	.000
POPCHANG	−0.012	−0.011	.075
MAR	−0.0006	−0.035	.986
MAR2	4.9E-06	0.176	.868
PERHOUS	3.310	1.510	.000
PERHOUS2	−0.205	−0.499	.000
MARKS91	0.047	0.272	.009
WAGES92	−2.642	−0.158	.398
TOWNPOP	−3.47E-06	−0.134	.009
TOWNPOP2	6.84E-13	0.012	.027
PERAREA	0.003	0.004	.487
CROWDED	0.006	0.052	.325
PRTDISAB	−0.086	−0.143	.282
UNION	0.026	0.079	.036
HEALTH	0.427	0.382	.047
RRWKRS	0.100	0.015	.623
ALCOHOL	−0.087	−0.042	.601
SCAVN	−21.255	−0.206	.008

(*continued*)

Table A6.2 (*Continued*)

Factor	Coefficient	Elasticity	Level of Significance
LEAD	−0.103	−0.002	.878
COMCON	0.002	0.017	.884
OTHMNR	0.031	0.009	.535
OTHMNR2	−0.0004	−0.0004	.511
EARTH	0.008	0.004	.463
SHIPS	−0.024	−0.013	.503
GLASS	−0.093	−0.013	.189
STONE	0.050	0.013	.327
MACHINE	0.010	0.021	.583
FISH	−0.014	−0.004	.807
CNSTRCT	0.041	0.264	.004
COALMNR	0.001	0.005	.939
COALMNR2	−2.75E-05	−0.004	.609
RETAIL	0.022	0.037	.646
CHEMCLS	−0.0003	−0.00009	.998
TXTLES	0.0005	0.001	.952
FOOD	−0.063	−0.316	.137
FARM	0.0009	0.012	.850
LONDON	5.030	0.037	.041
YORK	−1.502	−0.010	.230
EASTERN	−0.102	−0.001	.937
NMIDLAND	−2.071	−0.012	.119
NW	0.252	0.002	.902
MONMWLS	0.265	0.001	.867
SW	−1.824	−0.014	.074
SMIDLAND	−1.745	−0.013	.034
WMIDLAND	−0.111	−0.001	.920
NORTHERN	−0.548	−0.003	.712
CONSTANT	−25.734		.028

Source: Data from AOF, *Directories,* 1872–1911; Great Britain, *Parliamentary Papers,* 1893–94, CIV, 31 and 51–530; 1893–94, CV,v, xxxv–xxxvii, and 3–1165; 1893–94, CVI, 9–545; Great Britain, Registrar General of Births, Deaths, and Marriages, *Fifty-Fourth Annual Report* (1892), 64–67; Bowley, *Wages and Income in the United Kingdom,* table following 144; and Hunt, *Regional Wage Variations in Britain,* 355.
N = 2,930.
Dependent variable = days sickness per member year.
F = 55.718.
Adj. *R*-square = .473.

Table A6.3
DETERMINANTS OF MORTALITY

Factors	Coefficient	Elasticity	Level of Significance
AVERAGE	0.057	0.174	.000
SINCEDOF	0.012	0.036	.000
INITRATE	−0.0006	−0.003	.003
POPCHANG	−0.0003	−0.0003	.575
MAR	0.0004	0.022	.057
PERHOUS	0.030	0.014	.000
MARKS91	−0.0009	−0.005	.454

(*continued*)

Table A6.3   (*Continued*)

Factors	Coefficient	Elasticity	Level of Significance
WAGES 92	0.492	0.030	.017
TOWNPOP	2.52E-08	0.001	.050
PERAREA	0.002	0.003	.000
CROWDED	−0.0005	−0.004	.239
PRTDISAB	−0.005	−0.008	.415
UNION	0.003	0.009	.003
HEALTH	−0.006	−0.006	.677
RRWKRS	0.023	0.004	.043
ALCOHOL	0.020	0.010	.121
SCAVN	−0.020	−0.0002	.974
LEAD	0.055	0.001	.069
COMCON	0.003	0.025	.001
OTHMNR	−0.001	−0.0004	.338
EARTH	0.001	0.0006	.156
SHIPS	−0.0005	−0.0003	.826
GLASS	0.008	0.001	.088
STONE	0.010	0.003	.009
MACHINE	0.0002	0.0004	.880
FISH	0.005	0.001	.144
CNSTRCT	0.002	0.013	.052
COALMNR	0.0001	0.0003	.768
RETAIL	−0.010	−0.017	.003
CHEMCLS	0.0005	0.0002	.938
TXTLES	0.002	0.004	.001
FOOD	−0.0008	−0.004	.782
FARM	0.0007	0.010	.042
LONDON	−0.156	−0.001	.357
YORK	−0.061	−0.0004	.355
EASTERN	−0.087	−0.0009	.224
NMIDLAND	−0.184	−0.001	.006
NW	−0.108	−0.0007	.379
MONMWLS	0.172	0.0007	.062
SW	0.034	0.0003	.576
SMIDLAND	−0.014	−0.0001	.820
WMIDLAND	0.054	0.0007	.379
NORTHERN	−0.178	−0.0009	.080
CONSTANT	−8.085		.000

Source: AOF, *Directories,* 1872–1911; Great Britain, *Parliamentary Papers,* 1893–94, CIV, 31 and 51–530; 1893–94, CV, v, xxxv–xxxvii, and 3–1165; 1893–94, CVI, 9–545; Great Britain, Registrar General of Births, Deaths, and Marriages, *Fifty-Fourth Annual Report* (1892), 64–67; Bowley, *Wages and Income in the United Kingdom,* table following 144; and Hunt, *Regional Wage Variations in Britain,* 355.
N = 5,718.
Dependent variable = mortality; each court appears twice in the analysis, once as a 1 value weighted for members who died during the reference period and once as a 0 value weighted for members who survived.

Table A6.4
A Simulation: Percent Change, 1881–1901,
Due to Each Independent Variable

	Quantity		Percent change	
	1881	1901	Sickness time	Mortality
AVERAGE	35.415 yrs.	35.415 yrs.	0.0	0.0
SINCEDOF	33.97 yrs.	33.97 yrs.	0.0	0.0
INITRATE	63.87 per 1,000	63.87 per 1,000	0.0	0.0
POPCHANG	14.365 per 1,000	12.16 per 1,000	0.49	0.07
MAR and MAR2	657.975 per 1,000	636.898 per 1,000	−2.17	−0.85
PERHOUS and PERHOUS2	5.376 persons	5.195 persons	−3.72	−0.54
MARKS91	81.991 per 1,000	52.717 per 1,000	−24.93	2.60
WAGES92	£0.691	£.7678	−3.66	3.71
TOWNPOP and TOWNPOP2	408608.2 persons	463591.8 persons	−2.85	1.39
PERAREA	.6959 persons	.8714 persons	0.01	0.04
CROWDED	113.42 per 1,000	82.007 per 1,000	−3.59	1.56
PRTDISAB	5.325 per 1,000	4.705 per 1,000	0.97	0.30
UNION	33.899 per 1,000	36.755 per 1,000	1.34	0.80
HEALTH	9.589 per 1,000	10.901 per 1,000	10.11	−0.82
RRWKRS	1.276 per 1,000	2.674 per 1,000	2.51	3.20
ALCOHOL	8.793 per 1,000	9.398 per 1,000	−0.95	1.18
SCAVN	.1562 per 1,000	.4816 per 1,000	−124.81	−0.64
LEAD	1.183 per 1,000	.361 per 1,000	1.52	−4.62
COMCON	117.097 per 1,000	146.578 per 1,000	0.92	7.11
OTHMNR and OTHMNR2	3.718 per 1,000	2.854 per 1,000	−0.45	0.10
EARTH	5.003 per 1,000	5.149 per 1,000	0.02	0.02
SHIPS	5.756 per 1,000	6.994 per 1,000	−0.53	−0.06
GLASS	2.036 per 1,000	2.284 per 1,000	−0.42	0.20
STONE	3.835 per 1,000	4.677 per 1,000	0.75	0.80
MACHINE	83.221 per 1,000	96.196 per 1,000	2.24	0.26
FISH	3.157 per 1,000	1.955 per 1,000	0.31	−0.65
CNSTRCT	81.925 per 1,000	92.811 per 1,000	8.10	2.15
COALMNR and COALMNR2	47.014 per 1,000	62.041 per 1,000	−0.45	0.15
RETAIL	8.296 per 1,000	8.059 per 1,000	−0.10	0.24
CHEMCLS	6.696 per 1,000	8.401 per 1,000	−0.00008	0.09
TXTLES	51.762 per 1,000	40.561 per 1,000	−0.09	−1.69
FOOD	40.393 per 1,000	45.645 per 1,000	−5.96	−0.42
FARM	138.327 per 1,000	95.510 per 1,000	−0.69	−3.04
LONDON	0.140	0.148	0.73	−0.13
YORK	0.114	0.111	0.06	0.01
EASTERN	0.056	0.052	0.00008	0.04

(continued)

Table A6.4   (*Continued*)

	Quantity		Percent change	
	1881	1901	Sickness time	Mortality
NMIDLAND	0.063	0.063	−0.01	−0.00006
NW	0.161	0.158	−0.01	0.03
MONMWLS	0.062	0.061	−0.0006	−0.02
SW	0.059	0.070	−0.37	0.04
SMIDLAND	0.067	0.061	0.20	0.00008
WMIDLAND	0.113	0.119	−0.01	0.03
NORTHERN	0.065	0.062	0.03	0.05

Source: Mitchell, *British Historical Statistics,* 150–51 and 158–59; and Great Britain, *Parliamentary Papers,* 1881, XCVI, vi; 1883, LXXX, v, and appendix A, 60–71 and 99; 1901, XC, 20; 1903, LXXXIV, 1–6, and passim; and 1904, CVIII, 256–81 and 290.

Bibliography

SELECTED ARCHIVAL SOURCES

Aberdeen Medical Club. Papers, 1868–75. 2630. Aberdeen University Library, Aberdeen.

Admission Registers, Jan. 1, 1770–July 17, 1774, and 1869–74. MR 2/1 and MR 16/24. St. Bartholomew's Hospital Archives, London.

Amalgamated Society of Woodworkers. Papers, 1891–1900. Acc. 4685/1 and 112. Scottish National Library, Edinburgh.

Ancient Noble Order of United Oddfellows. Bolton Unity. Papers, 1871–72. FO/2/45. Bolton Metropolitan Borough Central Library, Bolton.

AOF (Ancient Order of Foresters). Abthorpe Court Brave Old Oak. Papers, 1842–1950. ZA1581–ZA1859. Northamptonshire Record Office, Northampton.

———. Beaminster Branch. Papers, 1897–1911. PC/BE:5/3. Dorset Record Office, Dorchester.

———. Court Anchor of Hope. Papers, 1898–1913. Minutes. Cooper Collection, formerly in possession of Walter Cooper, AOF historian. Now in possession of Ancient Order of Foresters Friendly Society, Southampton.

———. Court Ancient City. Papers, 1879–92. 37202–4. University of St. Andrews Library, Manuscripts Department, St. Andrews.

———. Court Cock Royal. Papers, 1871–1921. D1125/6/1–5. Gloucestershire Record Office, Gloucester.

———. Court Conqueror. Papers, 1926. KC40 8/1/1. West Yorkshire Archive Service, Huddersfield.

———. Court Equity. Papers, 1865–1951. R78/70. Cambridgeshire Record Office, Cambridge.

———. Court Flower of Suffolk. Papers, 1855–1915. Minutes. Cooper Collection, formerly in possession of Walter Cooper, AOF historian. Now in possession of Ancient Order of Foresters Friendly Society, Southampton.

———. Court Flower of the Forest. Papers. DFR 9(c). Neave Collection, University of Hull Archives, Hull.

———. Court Friendship. Papers, 1872–1909. GF 5/1. Suffolk Record Office, Ipswich.

———. Court Leiston Abbey. Papers. Rules, 1905 and 1916. Cooper Collection, formerly in possession of Walter Cooper, AOF historian. Now in possession of Ancient Order of Foresters Friendly Society, Southampton.

———. Court Loggerheads. Papers, 1877–1940. D/DM/217/1–16. Clwyd Record Office, Hawarden.

———. Court Loyal Bodelwyddan. Papers, 1864–1955. D/DM/510. Clwyd Record Office, Hawarden.

———. Court of Three Mary's. Papers, 1833–1905. TU:10/2, 7–8, and 13, TU:97/1. Calderdale District Archives, Halifax.

———. Court Perseverance. Papers, 1876–84 and 1899–1903. R78/70. Cambridgeshire Record Office, Cambridge.

———. Court Powis. Papers, 1884–1900. Minutes. National Library of Wales, Aberystwyth.

———. Court Pride of Walton. Papers, 1855–92. Minutes. Cooper Collection, formerly in possession of Walter Cooper, AOF historian. Now in possession of Ancient Order of Foresters Friendly Society, Southampton.

———. Court Prince of Wales. Papers, 1906–12. Minutes. Cooper Collection, formerly in possession of Walter Cooper, AOF historian. Now in possession of Ancient Order of Foresters Friendly Society, Southampton.

———. Court Princess of Hesse. Papers. Roster, 1892. Cooper Collection, formerly in possession of Walter Cooper, AOF historian. Now in possession of Ancient Order of Foresters Friendly Society, Southampton.

———. Court Prosperity. Papers, 1900–1910. GF 504/1/3. Suffolk Record Office, Bury St. Edmunds.

———. Court St. Helen's Pride. Papers, 1880–1916. Minutes. Cooper Collection, formerly in possession of Walter Cooper, AOF historian. Now in possession of Ancient Order of Foresters Friendly Society, Southampton.

———. District Management Committee. Papers, 1860–81. 4727/1. Shropshire Record Office, Shrewsbury.

———. Huddersfield District. Papers, 1880–1969. KC40. Kirklees Metropolitan Council Libraries and Arts Division, Local Studies and Archives Department, Huddersfield.

Appleby Original Friendly Society. Papers, 1780–1925. DE1508/8–15 and 15D55/20–21 and 24. Leicestershire Record Office, Leicester.

Ashford Female Friendly Society. Papers, 1788–1875. D747A/PZ1/1. Derbyshire Record Office, Matlock.

Ashford Men's Friendly Society. Papers, 1939–74. D2861 Z/2/1 and Z/4/1. Derbyshire Record Office, Matlock.

Ashley Female Friendly Society. Papers, 1830–66. D44/A/PZ. Stafford County Record Office, Stafford.

Ashton District Infirmary. Papers. Patients' Comment Book, 1906–8. DDH/1/133. Tameside Local Studies Library, Ashton-under-Lyne.

Beddoe, John. Collection. 1840–1907. DM2. Special Collections, University Library, University of Bristol, Bristol.

Bedford Hospital Sickness Survey. 1965–74. Z625/19/1–8. Bedfordshire Record Office, Bedford.

Binns, David. Autobiography, 1799–1883. 1203/4. Tyne and Wear Archives, Newcastle upon Tyne.

Blewbury Club. Papers, 1756–1912. D/ETy/Q5/1–16. Berkshire Record Office, Reading.

Bristol City Sick Benefit and Dividing Friendly Society. Papers, 1910–19. 40126. Bristol Record Office, Bristol.

British Medical Association. Papers, 1907–35. MP337/C102, MP578/C216, MP807/C277, MP556/C211, MP421/C148. Contemporary Medical Archives Center, Wellcome Institute for the History of Medicine, London.

Buchan Medical Society. Papers, 1862–1935. 1163/1/1A and 1163/2/1–10. Aberdeen University Library, Aberdeen.

Cambridge Friendly Societies' Medical Association. Papers, 1888–97. R78/70. Cambridgeshire Record Office, Cambridge.

Carrington Guild of St. George Friendly Society. Papers, 1837–1948. DDX 186/1–8. Cheshire Record Office, Chester.

County of Rutland Friendly Society. Papers, 1874–1975. DE 2048/1–11. Leicestershire Record Office, Leicester.

Dentist's Ledger, 1873–84. Box 1102. Northamptonshire Record Office, Northampton.

Doctors' Accounts, 1846–51. D/X 872/2. Durham Record Office, Durham.

Doctors' Accounts, 1898–1900. D/X 207/5. Durham Record Office, Durham.

Doctor's Ledger, 1875–85. Misc. Don 477/1. Lincolnshire Archives, Lincoln.

Doctors' Ledgers, Daybooks, and Other Items, 1869–89. Misc. Sq. I/1, III/1, IV/1–2. Oxfordshire Archives, Oxford.

Doncaster Medical Society. Papers, 1911. DS 22/1. Doncaster Archives, Doncaster.

Eaton Socon Club. Papers, 1785–1856. AD/563. Bedfordshire Record Office, Bedford.

Edwards, Dr. Ledger, 1904–12. D/DM/63/33. Clwyd Record Office, Hawarden.

Eversholt Friendly Society. Papers, 1860–1938. P42/28/3 and 7–10, X783/1–6. Bedfordshire Record Office, Bedford.

Francis and Co. Prescription Books, Registers, and Accounts, 1889–91 and 1911–15. DD/DM/196/1–2. Clwyd Record Office, Ruthin.

Friendly Society Rules, 1855–76. DDH 54/6–10. Nottinghamshire Archives Office, Nottingham.

Garioch and Northern Medical Association. Papers, 1854–1912. 1161/1/1–2. Aberdeen University Library, Aberdeen.

German Street Sunday School Sick and Funeral Society. Papers, 1829–1946. M12/7/1–7. Manchester Central Library, Manchester.

Glanau Rhyddallt Friendly Society. Papers, 1887. 10739B. National Library of Wales, Aberystwyth.

Glenfield Female Friendly Society. Papers, 1839–1913. 6D57/1–8. Leicestershire Record Office, Leicester.

Gloucester County Hospital. In-patient Records, 1834–44. 17563. Gloucester Library, Gloucester.

Gloucester Dispensary. Papers, 1915–26. Minute Book, 2122. Gloucester Library, Gloucester.

Grand United Order of Oddfellows, Charity Lodge. Papers, 1898. S/CL/4. West Yorkshire Archive Service, Huddersfield.

Grand United Order of Oddfellows, Huddersfield District. Papers, 1853–1964. KC 86/33–35. Kirklees Metropolitan Council Libraries and Arts Division, Local Studies and Archives Department, Huddersfield.

Great North of Scotland Railway Passenger Department. Papers, 1897–1926. OD.fL2GNS. Aberdeen University Library, Aberdeen.

Great Northern Railway Locomotive Friendly Society. Papers, 1878–1909. DS9/1–3; DS9/10/1–3. Doncaster Division, 1867–1906. Doncaster Archives, Doncaster.

Halford, Sir Henry. Papers, 1802–43. D/2252. Royal College of Physicians, London.

Hawarden Union District Medical Officer's Relief Book, 1908–16. D/DM/400/8. Clwyd Record Office, Hawarden.

High Pavement Chapel Provident Friendly Society. Papers, 1868–81. HiF 2. University of Nottingham, Department of Manuscripts and Special Collections, Nottingham.

Horsley Woodhouse Male Friendly Society. Papers, 1834–1968. D556G/1–18. Derbyshire Record Office, Matlock.

Independent Order of Rechabites. Papers, 1888–1961. D/IOR/48 and 56–57. Durham Record Office, Durham.

IOOF (Independent Order of Odd Fellows). Bedfordshire District. Papers, 1842–1941. OF1/1, OF1/10, OF4/5 and 12, OF 6/5. Bedfordshire Record Office, Bedford.

———. Duchesse of Bedford Lodge. Papers, 1846–1941. OF34/1–2. Bedfordshire Record Office, Bedford.

———. Duke of York Lodge. Papers, 1816–c.1840. DDX433/1. Lancashire Record Office, Preston.

———. Farmers' Friend Lodge. Papers, 1916–49. DDX433/18. Lancashire Record Office, Preston.

———. Farmers Refuge Lodge, Long Riston. Papers, 1859–78. DFR12. Neave Collection, University of Hull Archives, Hull.

———. Good Samaritan Lodge. Papers, 1843–55. R78/70. Cambridgeshire Record Office, Cambridge.

———. Idris Lodge. Papers, 1879–89. 8476D. National Library of Wales, Aberystwyth.

———. Loyal King William IV Lodge. Papers, 1831–91. DDX69/1–2. Lancashire Record Office, Preston.

———. Loyal Merton Hall Lodge. Papers, 1884–88. R78/70. Cambridgeshire Record Office, Cambridge.

———. Loyal Queen Adelaide Lodge, Chipping. Papers, 1841–1936. DDX814/1/1 and DDX814/2/1–2. Lancashire Record Office, Preston.

———. Loyal Star of the North Lodge. Papers, 1867–1949. D/IOO/1–39. Durham Record Office, Durham.

———. Loyal Steam Plough Lodge, Kirton in Holland Parish Council. Papers, 1898–1908 and 1924–33. Lincolnshire Archives, Lincoln.

———. Loyal Travellers Home Lodge, Blisworth. Papers, 1841–1904. B1.O.1–57. Northamptonshire Record Office, Northampton.

———. Loyal Vale of Clun Lodge. Papers, 1908–18. 1927/1. Shropshire Record Office, Shrewsbury.

———. Maiden Queen Lodge. Papers, 1884–1932. OF8/1–3, OF10/1, OF11/1–5, OF17/1–2, OF19/1. Bedfordshire Record Office, Bedford.

———. Pleasant Retreat Lodge. Papers, 1856–76 and 1881–92. DDX433/2 and 4, and DDX1400. Lancashire Record Office, Preston.

———. Preston District. Papers, 1859–69. DDX857/1. Lancashire Record Office, Preston.

———. Sir Walter Scott Lodge. Papers, 1881–1900. 2483/10. Tyne and Wear Archives, Newcastle upon Tyne.

———. Sir William Harpur Lodge. Papers, 1853–1942. OF36/1, OF42/1–2, OF48/1–8. Bedfordshire Record Office, Bedford.

———. St. Peter's Lodge, Lund. Papers, 1879–89. DFR 13. Neave Collection, University of Hull Archives, Hull.

———. Temple of Love Lodge. Papers, 1887–95. 3547C. National Library of Wales, Aberystwyth.

———. Whitchurch Lodge. Papers, 1926. 2794/14. Shropshire Record Office, Shrewsbury.

Johnston Papers. 1887–1900. ZJO/1/1, ZJO/1/14, ZJO/3/3–4. Bolton Metropolitan Borough Central Library, Bolton.

Johnstone, William C., Surgeon. Ledgers, 1844. CS96/93. Scottish Record Office, Edinburgh.

Kempston Friendly Society. Papers, 1840–1947. DDX157/1–3, 7–12, 14–15, 18. Bedfordshire Record Office, Bedford.

Ladyshore Colliery Co., Little Lever. Papers, 1863–1919. ZLA/18/1–3. Bolton Metropolitan Borough Central Library, Bolton.

Ladyshore Colliery Sick Club. Papers, 1863–1926. ZLA/17/3–4. Bolton Metropolitan Borough Central Library, Bolton.

Lamplugh Friendly Society. Papers, 1788–1949. D/SO/2/1–29. Cumbria Record Office, Carlisle.

Leicester Bond Street Friendly Society. Papers, 1829–1951. DE1884/1–21. Leicestershire Record Office, Leicester.

Leicester Mercury Sick Society. Papers, 1883–1923. Leicestershire Local Studies Library, Leicester.

Lincoln Oddfellows Medical Committee. Papers, 1897–1913. Misc. Dep. 96/2. Lincolnshire Archives, Lincoln.
Lincolnshire Medical Benevolent Society. Papers, 1823–1933. LMBS 1 and 3/2–3/5. Lincolnshire Archives, Lincoln.
Littlemore Pauper Lunatic Asylum. Papers, 1846–50. Oxfordshire Health Authority Archives, Oxford.
Litton Cheney Friendly Society. Papers, 1844–84. D524. Dorset Record Office, Dorchester.
Longley, J. A. N. Papers, 1892–1924. Diary, 35694/1–8. Bristol Record Office, Bristol.
Loughborough Friendly Societies' Medical Aid Association. Papers, 1899. Annual Report, Misc. 1061/1. Leicestershire Record Office, Leicester.
Louth Friendly Society. Papers, 1814–33. 1Falk1. Lincolnshire Archives, Lincoln.
Loyal Fane Friendly Society. Papers, 1840–1954. Loyal Fane I–V. Lincolnshire Archives, Lincoln.
Loyal Order of Ancient Shepherds. Heatherbell Lodge. Papers, 1910–12. Dundee Archive and Record Centre, Dundee.
———. Lorne Lodge. Papers, 1889–95. Dundee Archive and Record Centre, Dundee.
———. Robbie Burns Lodge. Papers, 1893–96. Dundee Archive and Record Centre, Dundee.
———. Wisbech District. Papers, 1839–81. R78/70. Cambridgeshire Record Office, Cambridge.
Lytham Sick Club. Papers, 1876–1912. RCLy/2/1. Lancashire Record Office, Preston.
Medical Diary (surgeon's ledger), 1862–84. D830. Stafford County Record Office, Stafford.
Melchbourne Club. Papers, 1781–1913. P73/28/1–2. Bedfordshire Record Office, Bedford.
Miscellaneous Items on Friendly Societies. 2794/14. Shropshire Record Office, Shrewsbury.
Montacute, Stoke, and Odcombe Medical Club. Papers, 1878. DD/SAS 5/1042. Somerset Archive and Record Service, Taunton.
Morcott Friendly Society. Papers, 1773–1914. DE1702/4–11. Leicestershire Record Office, Leicester.
Neave Collection. Nineteenth and Early Twentieth Centuries. DFR/2–21. University of Hull Archives, Hull.
Noot, Dr. William, of Cardigan. Papers, 1876. 12540D. National Library of Wales, Aberystwyth.
Ogleface Friendly Society. Papers, 1815–37. Acc. 3826. Scottish National Library, Edinburgh.
Order of the Sons of Temperance. Papers, 1903–12. DX/1871/2. University of Hull Archives, Hull.

Pharmacists' Prescription Books, 1847–1948, and Accounts, 1862–89. D/DM/273/12–14. Clwyd Record Office, Hawarden.

Philanthropic Order of True Ivorites, St. David's Unity. Papers, 1876–1955. Acc 4545/1–4. Dyfed Archive Service, Carmarthen.

Phillipson, Dr. Casebook, 1868–69. 1212/4. Tyne and Wear Archives, Newcastle upon Tyne.

Probart, Frank George, M.D. Personal Papers, 1826–56. 2753/4/20–27. Suffolk Record Office, Bury St. Edmunds.

Ratcliffe Infirmary. Papers, 1838–1910. RI/1/21, 46, and 101. Oxfordshire Health Authority Archives, Oxford.

Rochdale Lower Place Sick and Burial Society. Papers, 1842–65. DDX/261. Lancashire Record Office, Preston.

Royal Berkshire Friendly Society. Papers, 1874–1926. D/EBy/Q34. Berkshire Record Office, Reading.

Royal Foresters, Court Stone of Ezel. Papers, 1832–50. Cooper Collection, formerly in possession of Walter Cooper, AOF historian. Now in possession of Ancient Order of Foresters Friendly Society, Southampton.

Royal Standard Benefit Society. Papers, 1828–1952. A/RSB/1–43. Greater London Record Office, London.

Ruabon Doctor's Ledger, 1855–60. D/DM/301/3. Clwyd Record Office, Hawarden.

Ruddington Provident Society. Papers. DD 511/1–7. Nottinghamshire Archives Office, Nottingham.

Scott, William. Daybooks, 1837–50. MSS 6312–14. Scottish National Library, Edinburgh.

Shropshire Provident Society. Papers, 1840–1923. 436/1–960, 6720–24, 6727–28, 6730, and 6847. Shropshire Record Office, Shrewsbury.

Smith, James. Memoirs. GD/Mus 29/1. Dundee Archive and Record Centre, Dundee.

Stand Unitarian Sunday School and Chapel Sick and Burial Society, Whitefield. Papers, 1861–1931. L 31. Manchester Central Library, Manchester.

St. David's Unity of Ivorites, Bond of Hope Lodge. Papers, 1882–92. G1. University College of Swansea Library, Swansea.

Stonesfield Friendly Society. Papers, 1766–1913. Ston. 1–v. Oxfordshire Archives, Oxford.

Stutter, William Gaskoin, Surgeon of Brook Cottage, Wichambrook. Papers, 1839–74. Prescription Books and Patients' Ledgers, HC 517. Suffolk Record Office, Bury St. Edmunds.

Sudbury Friendly Society. Papers, 1885–1931. GF 505. Suffolk Record Office, Bury St. Edmunds.

Suffolk County Medical Benefit Society. Papers, 1825 and 1863–66. GF 6/4 and GF 401. Suffolk Record Office, Ipswich.

Surgeon's Ledger, 1860–86. HC 424/1/1/1. Suffolk Record Office, Ipswich.

Swarm Friendly Society. Papers, 1815–92. DD 959/1–6. Nottinghamshire Archives Office, Nottingham.

Taylor, John Stephen. Collection, 1888–1926. D/582, 597–601, 603–5. Royal College of Physicians, London.

Taylor, Shephard Thomas. Medical Diary, 1882–88. D/2437. Royal College of Physicians, London.

Waltham Friendly Society. Papers, 1837–1900. DE1163/2. Leicestershire Record Office, Leicester.

Watson, Dr. William McCulloch, of Montrose. Papers, 1870–87. MS Deposit 37. University of St. Andrews Library, Manuscripts Department, St. Andrews.

West Charlton Friendly Society. Papers, 1856–1908. D/P cha. ma. 23/2. Somerset Archive and Record Service, Taunton.

Whitcombe, George. "Suggestions Founded on the Recent Enquiry," June 1892. 4930. Gloucester Library, Gloucester.

Wiltshire Friendly Society. Papers, 1855–1935. Acc 2087. Wiltshire County Record Office, Trowbridge.

INTERVIEW

Walter Cooper, AOF historian. Interview by author. Woodbridge, Suffolk, May 25, 1991.

PUBLISHED AND SCHOLARLY SOURCES

[Abbott, Thomas, George Abbott, and Oswald Abbott]. *Report . . . on the 5th Quinquennial Valuation as at December 31st, 1900, of branches of the Loyal Order of Ancient Shepherds. . . .* Middlesbrough-on-Tees, 1903.

Abel-Smith, Brian. "The Rise and Decline of Early Health Maintenance Organisations: Their International Experiences." *Social History of Medicine* 2 (1989): 239–46.

Almond, G. W. "Sutton-in-the-Isle, 1912–1932." Cambridgeshire Central Library, n.d.

Alter, George, and James C. Riley. "Frailty, Sickness, and Death: Models of Morbidity and Mortality in Historical Populations." *Population Studies* 43 (1989): 25–46.

Ambrose, Ernest. *Melford Memories: Recollection of 94 Years.* N.p., 1972.

AOF (Ancient Order of Foresters') Friendly Society. *Directory of the Ancient Order of Foresters' Friendly Society.* Various sites, 1872–1922.

———. *Foresters' Miscellany.* N.p., 1848–94.

———. Ipswich District. *Half-Yearly Balance Sheets.* Ipswich, 1901–4.

———. Manchester District, *Quarterly Report.* Manchester, 1877–89. Various dates of publication.

———. *Quarterly Reports of the Executive Council,* 1875–89 and 1903. Various dates of publication. Cooper Collection, formerly in possession of Walter

Cooper, AOF historian. Now in possession of Ancient Order of Foresters Friendly Society, Southampton.

―――. *Report of Delegates to the National Conference of Friendly Societies.* Birmingham, 1910.

―――. *Report upon the Valuation of the Assets and Liabilities of the Order.* . . . Various sites and dates of publication, 1925–51. Cooper Collection, formerly in possession of Walter Cooper, AOF historian. Now in possession of Ancient Order of Foresters Friendly Society, Southampton.

―――. *Statement of the Valuations of the Districts and Courts.* . . . London, 1890, Norwich, 1897, and Manchester, 1902.

Anderson, Michael. *Family Structure in Nineteenth-Century Lancashire.* Cambridge, 1971.

Ansell, Charles. *A Treatise on Friendly Societies.* . . . London, 1835.

Arlidge, J. T. *The Hygiene, Diseases, and Mortality of Occupations.* London, 1892.

Armstrong, Alan. *Farmworkers in England and Wales: A Social and Economic History, 1770–1980.* Ames, Iowa, 1988.

Baernreither, J. M. *English Associations of Working Men.* Translated by Alice Taylor. London, 1893.

Baines, D. E. "The Use of Published Census Data in Migration Studies." In *Nineteenth-Century Society: Essays in the Use of Quantitative Methods for the Study of Social Data,* edited by E. A. Wrigley, 311–35. Cambridge, 1972.

Ballard, Edward. "Report to the Local Government Board on the Causation of the Annual Mortality from Diarrhoea." Great Britain, *Parliamentary Papers,* 1889, xxxv.

Barker, Theo, and Michael Drake, eds. *Population and Society in Britain, 1850–1980.* New York, 1982.

Barsky, Arthur J. *Worried Sick: Our Troubled Quest for Wellness.* Boston, 1988.

Bartholomew, J. G. *Gazetteer of the British Isles.* 9th ed. Edinburgh, 1966.

Bebbington, A.C. "The Expectation of Life without Disability in England and Wales: 1976–88," *Population Trends* 66 (1991): 26–29.

Becher, John Thomas. *The Constitution of Friendly Societies, upon Legal and Scientific Principles, Exemplified by the Rules and Tables of . . . the Southwell Friendly Institution.* . . . 5th ed. London, 1829.

Benjamin, Benjamin. *Health and Vital Statistics.* London, 1968.

Benson, John. *British Coalminers in the Nineteenth Century: A Social History.* New York, 1980.

―――. *The Penny Capitalists: A Study of Nineteenth-Century Working-Class Entrepreneurs.* New Brunswick, N.J., 1983.

―――. *The Working Class in Britain, 1850–1939.* London, 1989.

―――, ed. *The Working Class in England, 1875–1914.* London, 1985.

Berridge, Virginia. "Health and Medicine." In *The Cambridge Social History of Britain, 1750–1950,* edited by F. M. L. Thompson, 3:171–242. Cambridge, 1990.

Bickmore, D. P., and M. A. Shaw. *The Atlas of Britain and Northern Ireland.* Oxford, 1963.

Blaxter, Mildred. "Fifty Years On—Inequalities in Health." In *Population Research in Britain*, edited by Michael Murphy and John Hobcraft, 59–64. London, 1991.

Booth, Charles, ed. *Life and Labour of the People in London.* 2 vols. London, 1892.

Bowley, A. L. *The Change in the Distribution of National Income, 1880–1913.* Oxford, 1913.

———. *Wages and Income in the United Kingdom since 1860* Cambridge, 1937.

———. *Wages in the United Kingdom in the Nineteenth Century* Cambridge, 1900.

Bowser, Wilfred A. *Friendly Societies' Valuation and other Tables. . . .* London, 1896.

———. *Royal Berkshire Friendly Society: Report on the Quinquennial Valuation of Liabilities & Assets . . . and on the Sickness and Mortality Experience . . . 1883–97.* Newbury, 1898.

Boyer, George R. *An Economic History of the English Poor Law, 1750–1850.* Cambridge, 1990.

———. "What Did Unions Do in Nineteenth-Century Britain." *Journal of Economic History* 48 (1988): 319–32.

Brabrook, E. W. "On the Progress of Friendly Societies and Other Institutions. . . ." *Journal of the Statistical Society* 68 (1905): 320–42.

Bradford Hill, A. "An Investigation of Sickness in Various Industrial Occupations." *Journal of the Royal Statistical Society* 92 (1929): pt. 2, 183–238.

Brand, Jeanne L. *Doctors and the State: The British Medical Profession and Government Action in Public Health, 1870–1912.* Baltimore, 1965.

[Brodie, Benjamin C.], *Autobiography of the Late Sir Benjamin C. Brodie, Bart.* 2d ed. London, 1865.

Brown, A. F. J. *Meagre Harvest: The Essex Farm Workers' Struggle against Poverty, 1750–1914.* Chelmsford, 1990.

Bryder, Linda. *Below the Magic Mountain: A Social History of Tuberculosis in Twentieth-Century Britain.* Oxford, 1988.

Buckley, Anthony D. "'On the Club': Friendly Societies in Ireland." *Irish Economic and Social History* 14 (1987): 39–58.

Burn, James Dawson. *The Autobiography of a Beggar Boy.* Edited by David Vincent. London, 1978.

Burnett, John. *Idle Hands: The Experience of Unemployment, 1790–1990.* London, 1994.

Burnett, John, David Vincent, and David Mayall, eds. *The Autobiography of the Working Class: An Annotated Critical Bibliography.* 3 vols. New York, 1984–89.

Burrows, Victor A. "On Friendly Societies since the Advent of National Health Insurance." *Journal of the Institute of Actuaries* 63 (1932): 307–82.

Bynum, W. F. *Science and the Practice of Medicine in the Nineteenth Century.* Cambridge, 1994.

Calnan, Michael. *Health and Illness: The Lay Perspective.* London, 1987.

Cambridge Friendly Societies' Medical Association. *Rules.* 4th ed. Cambridge, 1896.

The Cambridge Victoria Friendly Societies' Asylum, Its Formation, Rise, and Progress.. . . . Cambridge, 1851.

Carley, James. "Friendly Societies in Meopham." *Bygone Kent* 4, no. 7 (1983): 393–99.

Chalmers, A. K. *The Health of Glasgow, 1818–1925: An Outline.* Glasgow, 1930.

Chamberlain, Mary. *Old Wives' Tales: Their History, Remedies, and Spells.* London, 1981.

Chamberlain, Mary, and Ruth Richardson. "Life and Death." *Oral History Journal* 11 (1983): 31–43.

Chancellor, Valerie E., ed. *Master and Artisan in Victorian England: The Diary of William Andrews and the Autobiography of Joseph Gutteridge.* London, 1969.

Chinn, Carl. *They Worked All Their Lives: Women of the Urban Poor in England, 1880–1939.* Manchester, 1988.

"Circumstances and Self Not Synonomous." *Foresters' Miscellany* (Jan. 1877): 286.

Combe, Dr. "The Preservation of Health." *Foresters' Miscellany* (Jan. 1872): 18–19.

Committee of the Highland Society of Scotland. *Report on Friendly or Benefit Societies, Exhibiting the Law of Sickness. . . .* Edinburgh, 1824.

Cooper, Walter G. *The Ancient Order of Foresters Friendly Society: 150 Years, 1834–1984.* Edited by Ken Anthony. Southampton, 1984.

Corfield, Carruthers. *A Handbook of Medical Terms.* Manchester, 1914.

Cornwell, Jocelyn. *Hard-Earned Lives: Accounts of Health and Illness from East London.* London, 1984.

Cox, Alfred. *Among the Doctors.* London, 1950.

Crossick, Geoffrey. *An Artisan Elite in Victorian Society: Kentish London, 1840–1880.* London, 1978.

Davis, Paul. *The Old Friendly Societies of Hull.* Hull, 1926.

Dickson, Walter. *On the Numerical Ratio of Disease in the Adult Male Community, deduced from the Sanitary Statistics of Her Majesty's Customs, for the Years 1857–1874.* London, 1876.

Digby, Anne. *Making a Medical Market: Doctors and Their Patients in English Society, 1720–1911.* Cambridge, 1994.

———. *Pauper Palaces.* London, 1978.

Digby, Anne, and Nick Bosanquet. "Doctors and Patients in an Era of National Health Insurance and Private Practice, 1913–1938." *Economic History Review* 41 (1989): 74–94.

Dupree, Marguerite W. *Family Structure in the Staffordshire Potteries, 1840–1880.* London, 1995.

Dyer, Alfred J. "Inadequate Contributions." *Foresters' Miscellany* (Dec. 1888): 373–74.

Earwicker, Ray. "Miners' Medical Services before the First World War: The South Wales Coalfield." *Llafur* III (1981): 39–52.

Eden, Frederick Morton. *Observations on Friendly Societies.* . . . London, 1801.

Eder, Norman R. *National Health Insurance and the Medical Profession in Britain, 1913–1939.* New York, 1982.

Edmonds, T. R. *Life Tables, Founded upon the Discovery of a Numerical Law Regulating the Existence of Every Human Being.* . . . London, 1832.

———. "On the Laws of Sickness, According to Age, Exhibiting a Double Coincidence between the Laws of Sickness and the Laws of Mortality." *Lancet,* no. 1 (1835–36): 855–58.

Edwards, Elizabeth. "The Friendly Societies and the Ethic of Respectability in Nineteenth-Century Cambridge." Ph.D. diss., Cambridgeshire College of Arts and Technology, 1987.

Elderton, W. Palin, and Richard C. Fippard. *The Construction of Mortality and Sickness Tables.* London, 1914.

England and Wales. Office of Population Censuses and Surveys. *Census 1971: Index of Place Names.* 2 vols. London, 1977.

———. *English Life Tables No. 14.* London, 1987.

———. *Parliamentary Papers.* Irish University Press Series. *Population.* 5 vols. Shannon, 1970.

———. Registrar General. *Supplement to the Annual Report.* London, 1885–1908.

———. Registrar General of Births, Deaths, and Marriages. *Annual Report of the Register-General of Births, Deaths, and Marriages in England.* London, 1855, 1888–94, and 1904.

———. *Mortality of Men in Certain Occupations in the Three Years 1910, 1911, and 1912.* Supplement to the Seventy-Fifth Annual Report of the Registrar General for England and Wales, pt. 4. London, n.d.

The Family Physician: A Manual of Domestic Medicine, by Physicians and Surgeons of the Principal London Hospitals. New ed. London, 1892.

Farr, William. *English Life Table.* London, 1864.

———. "On a Method of Determining the Danger and the Duration of Diseases at Every Period of their Progress." *British Annals of Medicine* 1 (1837): 72–79.

Faulkner, Edwin J. *Health Insurance.* New York, 1960.

Feinstein, Charles. "New Estimates of Average Earnings in the United Kingdom, 1880–1913." *Economic History Review* 43 (1990): 595–632.

———. "A New Look at the Cost of Living, 1870–1914." In *New Perspectives on the Late Victorian Economy: Essays in Quantitative Economic History, 1860–1914,* edited by James Foreman-Peck, 151–79. Cambridge, 1991.

————. *Statistical Tables of National Income, Expenditure, and Output of the U.K., 1855–1965.* Cambridge, 1976.

Feldman, Jacob J. "Work Ability of the Aged under Conditions of Improving Mortality." *Milbank Memorial Fund Quarterly/Health and Society* 61 (1983): 430–44.

Ferguson, Thomas. *Scottish Social Welfare, 1864–1914.* Edinburgh, 1958.

Finlayson, Geoffrey. *Citizen, State, and Social Welfare in Britain, 1830–1990.* Oxford, 1994.

Fissell, Mary E. *Patients, Power, and the Poor in Eighteenth-Century Bristol.* Cambridge, 1991.

Flinn, M. W. Introduction to *Report on the Sanitary Condition of the Labouring Population of Gt. Britain,* by Edwin Chadwick. Edinburgh, 1965.

————. "Medical Services under the New Poor Law." In *The New Poor Law in the Nineteenth Century,* edited by Derek Fraser, 45–66. New York, 1976.

Floud, Roderick. "Medicine and the Decline of Mortality: Indicators of Nutritional Status." In *The Decline of Mortality in Europe,* edited by R. Schofield, D. Reher, and A. Bideau, 146–57. Oxford, 1991.

Floud, Roderick, Kenneth Wachter, and Annabel Gregory. *Height, Health, and History: Nutritional Status in the United Kingdom, 1750–1980.* Cambridge, 1990.

Fogel, Robert W. "The Conquest of High Mortality and Hunger in Europe and America: Timing and Mechanisms." In *Favorites of Fortune: Technology, Growth, and Economic Development since the Industrial Revolution,* edited by Patrice Higonnet, David Landes, and Henry Rosovsky, 33–71. Cambridge, Mass., 1991.

————. "Nutrition and the Decline of Mortality since 1700: Some Preliminary Findings." In *Long-term Factors in American Economic Growth,* edited by Stanley L. Engerman and Robert E. Gallman, 439–555. Chicago, 1986.

Foreman-Peck, James, ed. *New Perspectives on the Late Victorian Economy: Essays in Quantitative Economic History, 1860–1914.* Cambridge, 1991.

Foster, Andrew. "Are Cohort Mortality Rates Autocorrelated?" *Demography* 28 (1991): 619–37.

Foster, Janet, and Julia Sheppard. *British Archives: A Guide to Archive Resources in the United Kingdom.* Detroit, 1982.

Fox, A. J., and P. F. Collier. "Low Mortality Rates in Industrial Cohort Studies Due to Selection for Work and Survival in the Industry." *British Journal of Preventive and Social Medicine* 30 (1976): 225–30.

Fox, Daniel M. *Health Policies, Health Politics: The British and American Experience, 1911–1965.* Princeton, 1986.

Freeman-Grenville, G. S. P. *Atlas of British History.* London, 1979.

Friedlander, D., Jona Schellekens, E. Ben-Moshe, and Ariela Keysar. "Socio-economic Characteristics and Life Expectancies in Nineteenth-Century England: A District Analysis." *Population Studies* 39 (1985): 137–51.

Fry, John. *Profiles of Disease: A Study in the Natural History of Common Diseases.* Edinburgh, 1966.

Fuller, Margaret D. *West Country Friendly Societies*. Lingfield, 1964.

Gage, Timothy B. "The Decline of Mortality in England and Wales 1861 to 1964: Decomposition by Cause of Death and Component of Mortality." *Population Studies* 47 (1993): 47–66.

Garrett, Eilidh, and Alice Reed. "Satanic Mills, Pleasant Lands: Spatial Variation in Women's Work, Fertility, and Infant Mortality as Viewed from the 1911 Census." *Historical Research* 67 (1994): 156–77.

Geddes, Peter, and John P. Holbrook. *Friendly Societies: A Text-Book for Actuarial Students*. Cambridge, 1963.

Gilbert, Bentley B. *The Evolution of National Insurance in Great Britain: The Origins of the Welfare State*. London, 1966.

Goadby, Edwin. "Trade and Health." *Foresters' Miscellany* (July 1878): 158–63; (Oct. 1878): 200–204.

Gosden, P. H. J. H. *The Friendly Societies in England, 1815–1875*. Manchester, 1961.

———. *Self-Help: Voluntary Associations in Nineteenth-Century Britain*. New York, 1973.

Gray, Robert. *The Aristocracy of Labour in Nineteenth-Century Britain, c. 1850–1900*. London, 1981.

———. *The Labour Aristocracy in Victorian Edinburgh*. Oxford, 1976.

Great Britain. *Annual Abstract of Statistics: 1994*. London, 1995.

———. Interdepartmental Committee on Social and Economic Research. *Census Reports of Great Britain, 1801–1931*. London, 1951.

———. *Parliamentary Papers*. London, 1881, XCVI; 1883, LXXVIII–LXXX; 1890–91, XCIV; 1893–94, CIV–CVII; 1901, XC; 1903, LXXXIV.

———. Working Group on Inequalities in Health. "The Black Report," by Douglas Black, Peter Townsend, Nick Davidson, and Margaret Whitehead. In *Inequalities in Health*, edited by Peter Townsend and Nick Davidson, 29–213. London, 1988.

———. Working Group on Inequalities in Health. "The Health Divide," by Margaret Whitehead. In *Inequalities in Health,* edited by Peter Townsend and Nick Davidson, 215–400. London, 1988.

Green, David G. "Doctors versus Workers." *Economic Affairs: Supplement* 5(1984): i–xii.

———. *Working-Class Patients and the Medical Establishment: Self-Help in Britain from the Mid-Nineteenth Century to 1948*. Aldershot, 1985.

Greenbaum, Susan D. "Economic Cooperation among Urban Industrial Workers: Rationality and Community in an Afro-Cuban Mutual Aid Society, 1904–1927." *Social Science History* 17 (1993): 173–93.

Greenhow, E. H. *Papers Relating to the Sanitary State of the People of England*. London, 1858; n.p., 1973.

Greenwood, Arthur. *The Health and Physique of School Children*. London, 1913.

Greer, A. W. *Tubbs: A Nineteenth-Century G.P.* King's Lynn, 1988.

Grey, Edwin. *Cottage Life in a Hertfordshire Village: "How the Agricultural La-*

bourer Lived and Fared in the Late '60's and '70's". St. Albans, [1935].

Grimes, Sharon Schildein. *The British National Health Service: State Intervention in the Medical Marketplace, 1911–1948*. New York, 1991.

Gruenberg, Ernest M. "The Failures of Success." *Milbank Memorial Fund Quarterly/Health and Society* 55 (1977): 3–24.

Guha, Sumit. "The Importance of Social Intervention in England's Mortality Decline: The Evidence Reviewed." *Social History of Medicine* 7 (1994): 89–113.

Haines, Michael R. "Conditions of Work and the Decline of Mortality." In *The Decline of Mortality in Europe*, edited by R. Schofield, D. Reher, and A. Bideau, 177–95. Oxford, 1991.

Haley, Bruce. *The Healthy Body and Victorian Culture*. Cambridge, Mass., 1978.

Hall, Peter. *Cities of Tomorrow: An Intellectual History of Urban Planning and Design in the Twentieth Century*. Oxford, 1988.

Hamilton, David. *The Healers: A History of Medicine in Scotland*. Edinburgh, 1981.

Hannah, Leslie. *Inventing Retirement: The Development of Occupational Pensions in Britain*. Cambridge, 1986.

Hanson, C. G. "Welfare before the Welfare State." In *The Long Debate on Poverty: Eight Essays on Industrialisation and 'the Condition of England,'* 118–25. London, 1972.

"Happy and Healthy Old Men." *Foresters' Miscellany* (Oct. 1879): 458–60.

Hardwick, Charles. *The History, Present Position, and Social Importance of Friendly Societies. . . .* London, 1859.

Hardy, Anne. *The Epidemic Streets: Infectious Disease and the Rise of Preventive Medicine, 1856–1900*. Oxford, 1993.

Hardy, George F. "An Enquiry into the Methods of Representing and Giving Effect to the Experience of a Friendly Society." *Journal of the Institute of Actuaries* 31 (1894): 86–154.

———. "Friendly Societies." *Journal of the Institute of Actuaries* 27 (1888): 245–348.

Harris, Jose. *Private Lives, Public Spirit: A Social History of Britain, 1870–1914*. Oxford, 1993.

Hart, J. Y. "An Investigation of Sickness Data of Public Elementary School Teachers in London, 1904–1919." *Journal of the Royal Statistical Society* 85 (1922): 349–411.

Hatton, William. *A Treatise on Friendly Societies, with Tables*. London, 1874.

Hennock, E. P. *British Social Reform and German Precedents: The Case of Social Insurance, 1880–1914*. Oxford, 1987.

Henriques, Ursula R. Q. *Before the Welfare State: Social Administration in Early Industrial Britain*. London, 1979.

Higgs, Edward. "Disease, Febrile Poisons, and Statistics: The Census as a Medical Survey, 1841–1911." *Social History of Medicine* 4 (1991): 465–78.

Highet, Robert. *Rechabite History: A Record of the Origin, Rise, and Progress of the Independent Order of Rechabites (Salford Unity) Temperance Friendly Society . . . 1835 to . . . 1935.* Manchester, 1936.

Hinkle, Lawrence E., Norman Plummer, and L. Holland Whitney. "The Continuity of Patterns of Illness and the Prediction of Future Health." *Journal of Occupational Medicine* 3 (1961): 417–23.

Hobsbawm, E. J. "The Labour Aristocracy in Nineteenth-Century Britain." In *Labouring Men: Studies in the History of Labour,* 272–315. London, 1964.

———. *Workers: Worlds of Labor.* New York, 1984.

Hodgkinson, Ruth G. *The Origins of the National Health Service: The Medical Services of the New Poor Law.* Berkeley, 1967.

Hoffman, Frederick L. *National Health Insurance and the Friendly Societies.* Newark, N.J., 1921.

———. *Poor Law Aspects of National Health Insurance.* Newark, N.J., 1920.

Hollingsworth, J. Rogers, Jerald Hage, and Robert A. Hanneman. *State Intervention in Medical Care: Consequences for Britain, France, Sweden, and the United States, 1890–1920.* Ithaca, 1990.

Horn, Pamela. *Labouring Life in the Victorian Countryside.* Dublin, 1976.

Howard, Ebenezer. *Garden Cities of To-morrow.* London, 1960.

Howkins, Alun. *Reshaping Rural England: A Social History, 1850–1925.* London, 1991.

———. "The Taming of Whitsun: The Changing Face of a Nineteenth-Century Rural Holiday." In *Popular Culture and Class Conflict, 1590–1914: Explorations in the History of Labour and Leisure,* edited by Eileen Yeo and Stephen Yeo, 187–209. Brighton, 1981.

Hudson, Derek. *Munby, Man of Two Worlds: The Life and Diaries of Arthur J. Munby, 1828–1910.* N.p., 1972.

Hudson, Pat, and Lynette Hunter, eds. "The Autobiography of William Hart, Cooper, 1776–1857: A Respectable Artisan in the Industrial Revolution." *London Journal* 7 (1981): 144–60; 8 (1982): 63–75.

Hudson, Samuel. *Supplementary Tables of Annuities, Sickness, & Mortality Values.* Burton-on-Trent [1911].

Huggett, Frank. *A Day in the Life of a Victorian Farm Worker.* London, 1972.

Hunt, E. H. "Industrialization and Regional Inequality: Wages in Britain, 1760–1918." *Journal of Economic History* 46 (1986): 935–66.

———. *Regional Wage Variations in Britain, 1850–1914.* Oxford, 1973.

Hunter, Donald. *The Diseases of Occupations.* 5th ed. London, 1975.

Independent Order of Odd Fellows Manchester Unity. *Attack by Lord Albemarle on the Manchester Unity Friendly Society; with the Reply in Defense of the Order by Samuel Daynes. . . .* Norwich, 1857.

———. *Report of the Actuaries upon the Twentieth Valuation.* Heanor, n.d.

———. *Rules of the Independent Order of Oddfellows Manchester Unity Friendly Society.* Manchester, 1908, 1912.

Inkster, Ian. "Marginal Men: Aspects of the Social Role of the Medical Community in Sheffield, 1790–1850." In *Health Care and Popular Medicine in Nine-*

teenth Century England, edited by John Woodward and David Richards, 128–63. New York, 1977.

Instructions for the Establishment of Friendly Societies. London, 1837.

"In the Law Courts." *Foresters' Miscellany* (Dec. 1887): 402.

"An Investigation into the Economic Conditions of Contract Medical Practice in the United Kingdom." *British Medical Journal,* supplement 2 (1905).

"Is Insanity Sickness?" *Foresters' Miscellany* (Apr. 1870): 112–13.

Jackson, Brian. *Working-Class Community: Some General Notions Raised by a Series of Studies in Northern England.* London, 1968.

Jewson, N. D. "The Disappearance of the Sick Man from Medical Cosmology, 1770–1870." *Sociology* 10 (1976): 225–44.

Johansson, S. Ryan. "The Health Transition: The Cultural Inflation of Morbidity during the Decline of Mortality." *Health Transition Review* 1 (1991): 39–68.

———. "Measuring the Cultural Inflation of Morbidity during the Decline in Mortality." *Health Transition Review* 2 (1992): 78–89.

Johnson, Paul. "The Employment and Retirement of Older Men in England and Wales, 1881–1981." *Economic History Review* 47 (1994): 106–28.

———. *Saving and Spending: The Working-Class Economy in Britain, 1870–1939.* Oxford, 1985.

Jones, Dot. "Did Friendly Societies Matter? A Study of Friendly Societies in Glamorgan, 1794–1910." *Welsh Historical Review* 12 (1985): 324–49.

———. "Self-Help in Nineteenth-Century Wales: The Rise and Fall of the Female Friendly Society." *Llafur* 4 (1984): 14–26.

———. "Women and Computers: Llangeitho Female Benefit Society, 1842–1930." Paper prepared for History Research Seminar, University of Wales, Aberystwyth, 1993.

Jones, Richard. *Absenteeism.* London, 1971.

Jordan, Thomas E. *The Degeneracy Crisis and Victorian Youth.* Albany, N.Y., 1993.

Joseph, Keith. "Friendly Societies that Smile on Self-Help." The *Independent* (London), Feb. 2, 1994.

Kearns, Gerry. "Biology, Class, and the Urban Penalty." In *Urbanising Britain: Essays on Class and Community in the Nineteenth Century,* edited by Gerry Kearns and Charles W. J. Withers, 12–30. Cambridge, 1991.

———. "An Inductive Approach to Cause of Death Analysis." Paper prepared for Conference on the History of Registration of Causes of Death, Bloomington, Ind., 1993.

Kiesling, L. Lynne. "Duration of Downturns and Self-Insurance: Cumulative Distress and Income Assistance in Victorian Lancashire." Unpublished paper, Feb. 1994.

Kirk, Neville. *The Growth of Working-Class Reformism in Mid-Victorian England.* Chicago, 1985.

Klein, Rudolf. *Complaints against Doctors: A Study in Professional Accountability.* London, 1973.

Kmenta, Jan. *Elements of Econometrics*. New York, 1971.

Krueger, Alan B. "Workers' Compensation Insurance and the Duration of Workplace Injuries." National Bureau of Economic Research Working Paper 3,253. Cambridge, Mass., 1990.

Lane, Joan. "Eighteenth-Century Medical Practice: A Case Study of Bradford Wilmer, Surgeon of Coventry, 1737–1813." *Social History of Medicine* 3 (1990): 369–86.

———. "The Provincial Practitioner and His Services to the Poor, 1750–1800." *Society for the Social History of Medicine Bulletin* 28 (1981): 10–14.

Laqueur, Thomas Walter. *Religion and Respectability: Sunday Schools and Working-Class Culture, 1780–1850*. New Haven, Conn., 1976.

Lawton, Richard, ed. *The Census and Social Structure: An Interpretative Guide to Nineteenth-Century Censuses for England and Wales*. London, 1978.

———. "Population." In *Atlas of Industrializing Britain, 1780–1914*, edited by John Langton and R. J. Morris, 10–29. London, 1986.

Lee, C. H. *British Regional Employment Statistics, 1841–1971*. Cambridge, 1979.

———. "Regional Inequalities in Infant Mortality in Britain, 1861–1971: Patterns and Hypotheses." *Population Studies* 45(1991): 55–65.

Lee, Clive. "Regional Structure and Change." In *Atlas of Industrializing Britain, 1780–1914*, edited by John Langton and R. J. Morris, 30–33. London, 1986.

———. "Services." In *Atlas of Industrializing Britain, 1780–1914*, edited by John Langton and R. J. Morris, 140–43. London, 1986.

Leeds Amalgamated Friendly Society. *The Friendly Societies' Journal*. Edited by T. Ballan Stead. 1875–90.

Leneman, Leah. "Lives and Limbs: Company Records as a Source for the History of Industrial Injuries." *Social History of Medicine* 6 (1993): 405–28; 7 (1994): 175–76.

Levine, A. L. *Industrial Retardation in Britain, 1870–1914*. London, 1967.

Levitt, Ian, and Christopher Smout. *The State of the Scottish Working-Class in 1843: A Statistical and Spatial Enquiry Based on the Data from the Poor Law Commission Report of 1844*. Edinburgh, 1979.

Levy, Hermann. "The Economic History of Sickness and Medical Benefit before the Puritan Revolution." *Economic History Review* 13 (1943): 42–57; 14 (1944): 135–60.

Lewchuck, Wayne. "Industrialization and Occupational Mortality in France prior to 1914." *Explorations in Economic History* 28 (1991): 344–66.

Loudon, Irvine. *Medical Care and the General Practitioner, 1750–1850*. Oxford, 1986.

Mackenzie, F. M. "The Battle of the Clubs and How to Win It." *British Medical Journal* (July 4, 1896): 8–10.

MacKinnon, Mary. "English Poor Law Policy and the Crusade against Outrelief." *Journal of Economic History* 47 (1987): 603–25.

Manton, Kenneth G., and Eric Stallard. *Recent Trends in Mortality Analysis*. Orlando, Fla., 1984.

Marcroft, William. *The Marcroft Family and the Inner Circle of Human Life.* Rochdale, 1888.

Marland, Hilary. *Medicine and Society in Wakefield and Huddersfield, 1780–1870.* Cambridge, 1987.

Marr, Vyvyan. "Notes on an Investigation of the Sickness and Mortality Experience of a Friendly Society," *Transactions of the Faculty of Actuaries* 4 (1908): 153–71.

Marshall, Charles. "Charles Williams's Accident." *Foresters' Miscellany* (July 1893): 477–79.

———. "Do You Belong to a Benefit Society?" *Foresters' Miscellany* (July 1871): 389–95.

Matsumura, Takao. *The Labour Aristocracy Revisited: The Victorian Flint Glass Makers, 1850–80.* Manchester, 1983.

Maunsell, J. "The New Era of Medical Aid: A Rejoinder." *Foresters' Miscellany* (Oct. 1884): 205–10.

Maurice, Frederick. "National Health: A Soldier's Story." *Contemporary Review* 83 (1903): 41–56.

McKeown, Thomas. *The Modern Rise of Population.* London, 1976.

McKibbin, Ross. *The Ideologies of Class: Social Relations in Britain, 1880–1950.* Oxford, 1990.

Meacham, Standish. *A Life Apart: The English Working Class, 1890–1914.* London, 1977.

Mitch, David F. *The Rise of Popular Literacy in Victorian England: The Influence of Private Choice and Public Policy.* Philadelphia, 1992.

Mitchell, Allan. "The Function and Malfunction of Mutual Aid Societies in Nineteenth-Century France." In *Medicine and Charity before the Welfare State*, edited by Jonathan Barry and Colin Jones, 172–89. London, 1991.

Mitchell, B. R. *British Historical Statistics.* Cambridge, 1988.

Moffrey, R. W. *A Century of Oddfellowship.* Manchester, 1910.

Morris, R. J. "Clubs, Societies, and Associations." In *The Cambridge Social History of Britain, 1750–1950*, edited by F. M. L. Thompson, 3:395–443. Cambridge, 1990.

———. "Voluntary Societies and British Urban Elites, 1780–1850: An Analysis." *Historical Journal* 26 (1983): 95–118.

[Mountjoy, Timothy]. *The Life, Labours, and Deliverances of a Forest of Dean Collier. . . .* N.p., 1887.

Mulcaster, Samuel. *Tables for Friendly Societies Agreeable to Their Old Usage and Customs. . . .* London, 1833.

Mullin, James. *The Story of a Toiler's Life.* Dublin, 1921.

National United Order of Free Gardeners. *Directory and General Reference Book for 1916.* Hull, 1916.

Neave, David. *Mutual Aid in the Victorian Countryside: Friendly Societies in the Rural East Riding, 1830–1914.* Hull, 1991.

Neison, Francis G. P., Sr. *Contributions to Vital Statistics: being, a Development of the Rate of Mortality and the Laws of Sickness. . . .* 3d ed. London, 1857.

———. *Observations on Odd Fellow and Friendly Societies*. 14th ed. London, 1867.

Neison, Francis G. P., Jr. *The Rates of Mortality and Sickness According to the Experience for the Five Years, 1871–1875, of the Ancient Order of Foresters Friendly Society*. . . . London, 1882.

———. *The Rates of Mortality and Sickness According to the Experience for the Ten Years, 1878–1887, of the Independent Order of Rechabites*. . . . Manchester, 1889.

———. *Report upon the Additional Statistics Deduced from the Original Records of the Sickness Experience (1871–1875) of the Order*. . . . Leeds, 1886.

———. "Some Statistics of the Affiliated Orders of Friendly Societies (Odd Fellows and Foresters)." *Journal of the Statistical Society* 40 (1877): 42–89.

Newsholme, Arthur. *Fifty Years in Public Health*. New York, 1935.

Niven, James. "The Cost of Disease." *Transactions of the Manchester Statistical Society* (1910–11): 139–69.

North, Fiona. "Explaining Socioeconomic Differences in Sickness Absence: The Whitehall II Study." *British Medical Journal* 306 (1993): 361–66.

Northey, J. W. "Sane or Insane?" *Foresters' Miscellany* (Apr. 1873): 430–38.

Oddy, D. J. "The Health of the People." In *Population and Society in Britain, 1850–1980*, edited by Theo Barker and Michael Drake, 121–39. New York, 1982.

Oliver, Thomas, ed. *Dangerous Trades: The Historical, Social, and Legal Aspects of Industrial Occupations as Affecting Health*. . . . London, 1902.

Omran, Abdel R. "The Epidemiologic Transition: A Theory of the Epidemiology of Population Change." *Milbank Memorial Fund Quarterly* 49 (1971): 509–38.

An Open Letter to the Working Men of Birmingham on their Relations to the Medical Profession. . . . Birmingham, 1900.

Oppenheim, Janet. *Shattered Nerves: Doctors, Patients, and Depression in Victorian England*. New York, 1991.

The Ordnance Survey Gazetteer of Great Britain. London, 1987.

Orloff, Ann Shola. *The Politics of Pensions: A Comparative Analysis of Britain, Canada, and the United States, 1880–1940*. Madison, Wis., 1993.

Paget, James. "National Health and National Work." In *Selected Essays and Addresses*, edited by Stephen Paget, 381–97. London, 1902.

Parry, Noel, and Jose Parry. *The Rise of the Medical Profession: A Study of Collective Social Mobility*. London, 1976.

Parsons, Talcott. *The Social System*. N.p., 1951.

Pelling, Henry. "The Concept of the Labour Aristocracy." In *Popular Politics and Society in Late Victorian Britain*, 37–61. London, 1968.

Pennington, C. I. "Mortality, Public Health, and Medical Improvements in Glasgow, 1855–1911." Ph.D. diss., University of Stirling, 1977.

Peterson, M. Jeanne. *The Medical Profession in Mid-Victorian London*. Berkeley, Calif., 1978.

Phelps Brown, E. H. *The Growth of British Industrial Relations: A Study from the Standpoint of 1906–14.* London, 1959.

Phillips, Edward. "The Battle of the Clubs: The Coventry Public Medical Service." *British Medical Journal* (July 11, 1896): 96–97.

Pope, Rex, ed., *Atlas of British Social and Economic History since c. 1700.* New York, 1989.

Porter, Dorothy, and Roy Porter. *Patient's Progress: Doctors and Doctoring in Eighteenth-Century England.* Cambridge, 1989.

Porter, Roy, and Dorothy Porter. *In Sickness and in Health: The British Experience, 1650–1850.* New York, 1988.

Potter, Warren, and Robert Oliver. *Fraternally Yours: A History of the Independent Order of Foresters.* London, 1967.

Preston, Samuel H., and Michael R. Haines. *Fatal Years: Child Mortality in Late-Nineteenth-Century America.* Princeton, 1991.

Price, Richard. *Masters, Unions, and Men: Work Control in Building and the Rise of Labour, 1830–1914.* Cambridge, 1980.

Prins, Rienk. *Sickness Absence in Belgium, Germany (FR), and the Netherlands: A Comparative Study.* [Amsterdam], 1990.

Prinzing, Friedrich. *Handbuch der medizinischen Statistik.* 2d ed. Jena, Germany, 1931.

"The Proposed Advance of Twenty-five Per Cent." *Foresters' Miscellany* (Nov. 1888): 329–32; (Dec. 1888): 368–69.

Purvis, Martin. "Popular Institutions." In *Atlas of Industrializing Britain, 1780–1914,* edited by John Langton and R. J. Morris, 194–97. London, 1986.

Quadagno, Jill S. *Aging in Early Industrial Society: Work, Family, and Social Policy in Nineteenth-Century England.* New York, 1982.

Radley, C. J. "Superannuation." *Foresters' Miscellany* (July 1889): 196–200.

Ratcliffe, Henry. *Observations on the Rate of Mortality & Sickness Existing among Friendly Societies. . . .* Manchester, 1850.

———. *Observations on the Rate of Mortality and Sickness Existing amongst Friendly Societies. . . .* Colchester, 1862.

[Ratcliffe, Henry]. *Independent Order of Odd-Fellows, Manchester Unity Friendly Society: Supplementary Report, July 1st, 1872.* N.p., n.d.

Reeves, [Mrs.] Pember. *Family Life on a Pound a Week.* London, 1912.

Reid, Alastair. "Intelligent Artisans and Aristocrats of Labour: The Essays of Thomas Wright." In *The Working Class in Modern British History: Essays in Honour of Henry Pelling,* edited by Jay Winter, 171–86. Cambridge, 1983.

Reid, Douglas A. "The Decline of Saint Monday, 1766–1876." *Past & Present,* no. 71 (1976): 76–101.

Richardson, Ruth. *Death, Dissection, and the Destitute.* London, 1987.

Riley, James C. "From a High Mortality Regime to a High Morbidity Regime: Is Culture Everything in Sickness?" *Health Transition Review* 2 (1992): 71–78.

———. "Height, Nutrition, and Mortality Risk Reconsidered." *Journal of Interdisciplinary History* 24 (1994): 465–92.

———. "Ill Health during the English Mortality Decline: The Friendly Societies' Experience." *Bulletin of the History of Medicine* 61 (1987): 563–88.

———. "The Risk of Being Sick: Morbidity Trends in Four Countries." *Population and Development Review* 16 (1990): 403–32.

———. "The Risk of Being Sick at Higher Ages." Paper read at meeting of the Population Association of America, Washington, D.C., Mar. 22, 1991.

———. *Sickness, Recovery, and Death: A History and Forecast of Ill Health.* Iowa City, 1989.

———. "Working Health Time: A Comparison of Preindustrial, Industrial, and Postindustrial Experience in Life and Health." *Explorations in Economic History* 28 (1991): 169–91.

Riley, James C., and George Alter. "The Epidemiologic Transition and Morbidity." *Annales de démographie historique* (1989): 199–213.

Ritter, Gerhard A. *Social Welfare in Germany and Britain: Origins and Development.* Translated by Kim Traynor. Leamington Spa, 1986.

Roberts, Elizabeth. "Oral History Investigations of Disease and Its Management by the Lancashire Working Class, 1890–1939." In *Health, Disease, and Medicine in Lancashire, 1750–1950: Four Papers on Sources, Problems, and Methods,* edited by J. V. Pickstone, 33–51. Manchester, 1980.

———. *A Woman's Place: An Oral History of Working-Class Women, 1890–1940.* Oxford, 1984.

Roberts, Robert. *The Classic Slum: Salford Life in the First Quarter of the Century.* Manchester, 1971.

Rodger, Richard G. "The Invisible Hand: Market Forces, Housing, and the Urban Form in Victorian Cities." In *The Pursuit of Urban History,* edited by Derek Fraser and Anthony Sutcliffe, 190–211. London, 1980.

Rose, Sonya O. *Limited Livelihoods: Gender and Class in Nineteenth-Century England.* Berkeley, Calif., 1992.

Rowntree, B. Seebohm. *Poverty: A Study of Town Life.* New York, 1980.

Routh, Guy. *Occupation and Pay in Great Britain, 1906–60.* Cambridge, 1965.

Rule, John. *The Experience of Labor in Eighteenth-Century Industry.* New York, 1981.

Rumsey, Henry W. *Essays and Papers on Some Fallacies of Statistics concerning Life and Death. . . .* London, 1875.

———. *Essays on State Medicine.* New York, 1977.

Rusher, Edward A. "The Statistics of Industrial Morbidity in Great Britain." *Journal of the Statistical Society* 85 (1922): 27–86.

Russell, James Burn. *Life in One Room: or, Some Serious Considerations for the Citizens of Glasgow.* Glasgow, 1888.

———. *Public Health Administration in Glasgow.* Edited by A. K. Chalmers. Glasgow, 1905.

Schofield, Eunice M. *Medical Care of the Working Class about 1900.* [Lancaster], 1979.

Scott, Fred. *The Condition and Occupations of the People of Manchester and Salford.* London, 1889.

Scull, Andrew. *The Most Solitary of Afflictions: Madness and Society in Britain, 1700–1900.* New Haven, Conn., 1993.

Sendrail, Marcel, Georges Baudot, Guy Mazars, Pierre Huard, Joan Bossy, Pierre Hillemand, Emile Gilbrin, Emile Aron, and Paul Freour. *Histoire culturelle de la maladie.* Toulouse, 1980.

Shaw, Gareth. "Retail Patterns." In *Atlas of Industrializing Britain, 1780–1914,* edited by John Langton and R. J. Morris, 180–84. London, 1986.

Shorter, Edward. *Bedside Manners: The Troubled History of Doctors and Patients.* New York, 1985.

————. *From Paralysis to Fatigue: A History of Psychosomatic Illness in the Modern Era.* New York, 1992.

"Sick Clubs." *Foresters' Miscellany* (Apr. 1871): 354–55.

[Siddall, T. W.] *Manchester Unity Independent Order of Oddfellows: Story of a Century, 1824–1924 [Sheffield District].* N.p., n.d.

Smith, F. B. "Health." In *The Working Class in England, 1875–1914,* edited by John Benson, 36–62. London, 1985.

————. *The People's Health, 1830–1910.* New York, 1979.

Smout, T. C. *A Century of the Scottish People, 1830–1950.* London, 1986.

Snell, Henry. *Men, Movements, and Myself.* 2d ed. London, 1938.

Snow, E. C. "Some Statistical Problems Suggested by the Sickness and Mortality Data of Certain of the Large Friendly Societies." *Journal of the Statistical Society* 76 (1913): 464.

Sontag, Susan. *Illness as Metaphor.* New York, 1978.

Southall, Humphrey R. "Morbidity and Mortality among Early Nineteenth-Century Engineering Workers." *Social History of Medicine* 4 (1991): 231–52.

————. "Neither State nor Market: Mutual Societies and Welfare Provision in Pre-1914 Britain." Unpublished paper, 1993.

————. "The Origins of the Depressed Areas: Unemployment, Growth, and Regional Economic Structure in Britain before 1914." *Economic History Review* 41 (1988): 236–58.

————. "Poor Law Statistics and the Geography of Economic Distress." In *New Perspectives on the Late-Victorian Economy: Essays in Quantitative Economic History, 1860–1914,* edited by James Foreman-Peck, 180–217. Cambridge, 1991.

————. "The Tramping Artisan Revisits: Labour Mobility and Economic Distress in Early Victorian England." *Economic History Review* 44 (1991): 272–96.

————. "Unionization." In *Atlas of Industrializing Britain, 1780–1914,* edited by John Langton and R. J. Morris, 189–93. London, 1986.

Southall, Humphrey R., and D. M. Gilbert. "A Good Time to Wed: Marriage and Economic Distress in England and Wales, 1839–1914." *Economic History Review* 49 (1996): 35–57.

Spree, Reinhard. *Health and Social Class in Imperial Germany: A Social History of Mortality, Morbidity, and Inequality.* Translated by Stuart McKinnon-Evans and John Halliday. Oxford, 1988.

Stead, T. Ballan. "The New Era in Medical Aid." *The Foresters' Miscellany* (Apr. 1884): 83–91.

Stephens, W. B. *Education, Literacy, and Society, 1830–70: The Geography of Diversity in Provincial England.* Manchester, 1987.

Stern, J. "The Relationship between Unemployment, Morbidity, and Mortality in Britain." *Population Studies* 37 (1983): 61–74.

"Stimulants." *Foresters' Miscellany* (Oct. 1876): 199.

Stollberg, Gunnar. "Health and Illness in German Workers' Authobiographies from the Nineteenth and Early Twentieth Centuries." *Social History of Medicine* 6 (1993): 261–76.

"Superannuation." *Foresters' Miscellany* (Oct. 1882): 201–8; (Jan. 1883): 273–76.

Supple, Barry. "Legislation and Virtue: An Essay on Working-Class Self-Help and the State in the Early Nineteenth Century." In *Historical Perspectives: Studies in English Thought and Society,* edited by Neil McKendrick, 211–54. London, 1974.

Susser, Mervyn, William Watson, and Kim Hopper. *Sociology in Medicine.* 3d ed. New York, 1985.

Sutton, William. *Special Report on Sickness and Mortality Experienced in Registered Friendly Societies. . . .* Sessional Papers, 1896, LXXIX, 1–1181.

Swan, J. S. "Hints upon Some of the Advantages of Friendly Societies." *Foresters' Miscellany* (Jan. 1878): 18–21.

Szreter, Simon. "The Importance of Social Intervention in Britain's Mortality Decline c. 1850–1914: A Reinterpretation of the Role of Public Health." *Social History of Medicine* 1 (1988): 1–37.

Taylor, Harry Pearson. *A Shetland Parish Doctor: Some Recollections of a Shetland Parish Doctor during the Past Half Century.* Lerwick, 1948.

Taylor, P. J. "Personal Factors Associated with Sickness Absence." *British Journal of Industrial Medicine* 25 (1968): 106–18.

Thackrah, Charles Turner. *The Effects of Arts, Trades, and Professions on Health and Longevity.* London, 1832; Canton, Mass., 1985.

Tholfsen, Trygve R. *Working-Class Radicalism in Mid-Victorian England.* New York, 1977.

Thompson, E. P. *The Making of the English Working Class.* New York, 1963.

Thompson, F. M. L. *The Rise of Respectable Society: A Social History of Victorian Britain, 1830–1900.* Cambridge, Mass., 1988.

Thompson, Pishey. *The History and Antiquities of Boston. . . .* Boston, 1856.

Treble, James H. *Urban Poverty in Britain, 1830–1914.* New York, 1979.

Turner, Bryan S. *Medical Power and Social Knowledge.* London, 1987.

Twaddle, Andrew C. *Sickness Behavior and the Sick Role.* Boston, 1979.

Vincent, David. *Bread, Knowledge, and Freedom: A Study of Nineteenth-Century Working-Class Autobiography.* London, 1981.

Waddington, Ian. "General Practitioners and Consultants in Early-Nineteenth-Century England: The Sociology of an Intraprofessional Conflict." In *Health*

Care and Popular Medicine in Nineteenth Century England, edited by John Woodward and David Richards, 164–88. London, 1977.

———. *The Medical Profession in the Industrial Revolution.* Dublin, 1984.

Waitzkin, Howard. "A Critical Theory of Medical Discourse: Ideology, Social Control, and the Processing of Social Context in Medical Encounters." *Journal of Health and Social Behavior* 30 (1989): 220–39.

Wall, Richard, ed. *Mortality in Mid-Nineteenth-Century Britain.* N.p., 1974.

Wallis, Thomas Wilkinson. *Autobiography of Thomas Wilkinson Wallis, Sculptor in Wood. . . .* Louth, 1899.

Ward, Peter. *Birth Weight and Economic Growth: Women's Living Standards in the Industrializing West.* Chicago, 1993.

Watkins, William. *Statistical Notes on the Rate of Mortality and Sickness Existing among the Members of the Ancient Order of Foresters. . . .* Brighton, 1855.

Watson, Alfred W. *An Account of an Investigation of the Sickness and Mortality Experience of the I.O.O.F. Manchester Unity . . . 1893–1897.* Manchester, 1903.

———. "The Analysis of a Sickness Experience." *Journal of the Institute of Actuaries* 62 (1931): 12–61.

———. *Friendly Society Finance Considered in its Actuarial Aspect: A Course of Lectures.* London, 1912.

———. "National Health Insurance and Friendly Societies during the War." In *War and Insurance,* edited by James Shotwell, 171–225. London, 1927.

———. "National Health Insurance: A Statistical Review." *Journal of the Royal Statistical Society* 90 (1927): 449–50.

Watson, Reuben. *The Causes of Deficiencies in Friendly Societies, and Some Remarks on Hazardous Occupations.* Manchester, 1889.

———. *An Explanatory Treatise on the Valuation of Friendly Societies with a Full Description of the Method Employed in the Calculations. . . .* Brighton, 1878.

Watterson, Patricia A. "Infant Mortality by Father's Occupation from the 1911 Census of England and Wales." *Demography* 25 (1988): 289–306.

Webb, Katherine A. *'One of the Most Useful Charities in the City': York Dispensary, 1788–1988.* Borthwick Papers 74. [York], 1988.

Wells-Smith, Henry. *The Rate of Mortality and Sickness (. . . 1901–5 . . .) of the Independent Order of Rechabites. . . .* Manchester, 1918.

Weindling, Paul. *The Social History of Occupational Health.* London, 1985.

Whiteside, Noel. "Counting the Cost: Sickness and Disability among Working People in an Era of Industrial Recession, 1920–39." *Economic History Review* 40 (1987): 228–46.

———. "Private Agencies for Public Purposes: Some New Perspectives on Policy Making in Health Insurance between the Wars." *Journal of Social Policy* 12 (1983): 165–94.

WHO (World Health Organization). *The First Ten Years of the World Health Organization.* Geneva, 1958.

———. *International Statistical Classification of Diseases and Related Health Problems.* Tenth revision. 3 vols. Geneva, 1992.

Wiener, Martin J. *English Culture and the Decline of the Industrial Spirit, 1850–1980.* Cambridge, 1981.

Wilkinson, John Frome. *The Friendly Society Movement: Its Origin, Rise, and Growth.* . . . London, 1886.

Williamson, Jeffrey G. *Did British Capitalism Breed Inequality?* Boston, 1985.

Winslow, Forbes. "A Doctor's Opinion." *Foresters' Miscellany* (Oct. 1872): 172.

Winter, J. M. *The Great War and the British People.* Cambridge, 1986.

———. "Unemployment, Nutrition, and Infant Mortality in Britain, 1920–1950." In *Influence of Economic Instability on Health*, edited by J. John, D. Schwefel, and H. Zöllner, 169–99. Berlin, 1983.

Wohl, Anthony S. *Endangered Lives: Public Health in Victorian Britain.* London, 1983.

———. *The Eternal Slum: Housing and Social Policy in Victorian London.* London, 1977.

Wood, Peter. *Poverty and the Workhouse in Victorian Britain.* Wolfeboro Falls, N.H., 1991.

Woods, Robert. "The Effects of Population Redistribution on the Level of Mortality in Nineteenth-Century England and Wales." *Journal of Economic History* 45 (1985): 645–51.

Woods, Robert, and P. R. Andrew Hinde. "Mortality in Victorian England: Models and Patterns." *Journal of Interdisciplinary History* 18 (1987): 27–54.

Woods, R. I., P. A. Watterson, and J. H. Woodward. "The Causes of Rapid Infant Mortality Decline in England and Wales, 1861–1921." *Population Studies* 42 (1988): 343–66; 43 (1989): 113–32.

Woods, Robert, and John Woodward. "Mortality, Poverty, and the Environment." In *Urban Disease and Mortality in Nineteenth-Century England*, edited by Robert Woods and John Woodward, 19–36. London, 1984.

Wrigley, E. A., and R. S. Schofield. *The Population History of England, 1541–1871: A Reconstruction.* Cambridge, Mass., 1981.

Yeo, Stephen. "Working-Class Association, Private Capital, Welfare, and the State in the Late Nineteenth and Twentieth Centuries." In *Social Work, Welfare, and the State*, edited by Noel Parry, Michael Rustin, and Carole Satyamurti, 48–71. Beverly Hills, Calif., 1980.

Youngson, A. J. *The Scientific Revolution in Victorian Medicine.* Canberra, 1979.

Index

343

Chipping Oddfellows, 103
Chronic Bright's disease, 191
cities, health hazards of, 235–41, 249,
    255, 263, 265–66
claims, for sickness benefits: duration of,
    283–87; propensity to submit, 287–88;
    and sickness, 7–8, 23, 98–123, 275–92.
    See also sickness
claims awareness, 278–79
Clarke, Dr., 114
colds, 10, 193, 201–2, 210, 271
Combs, Oliver C., 56
contract practice, 49–56, and private prac-
    tice, 75, 83–86, 89–97
Corfield, Carruthers, 138, 192
Cornwell, Jocelyn, 135
Court Equity, 77–78, 282, 288
Court Father and Sons, 300–301
Court Loggerheads, 82
Court Loyal Bodelwyddan, 55, 82
Court Powis, 118–19
Court Princess of Hesse, 296
Court Sherwood Forest, 294
Court The Bough, 294
Cox, Alfred, 51
Crackwell, G. M., 114
Crook, P. S., 138
Crossick, Geoffrey, 30, 37, 121

death. See mortality
death, profile of causes, 188–97
Defoe, Daniel, 27
Derbyshire, 230
Dickson, Walter, 195n. 13
Digby, Ann, 3, 121
dispensaries, 49, 85
diseases, profile of causes, 23, 142, 186,
    188–89, 193–98, 201–2, 210, 252, 255.
    See also sickness; and names of specific
    diseases
dividing societies, 36n. 37. See also names
    of friendly societies
doctors, 48, 77, 98, 171–72; advice to
    sick, 50, 133–34; charges, 51, 59, 66–
    67, 75–97, 122–23; duties, 100–104;
    and elites, 62, 88, 96; and friendly soci-
    eties, records, 83–85, 200; numbers of,
    49; and restraint of trade, 72; type and
    quality of services, 48, 98–123; and
    workingmen, 46, 59, 67–73. See also

British Medical Association; contract
    practice; family clubs; surgeons; works
    clubs
Duke of York Lodge, IOOF, 138
Durham, 215–16, 229, 254
duration of sickness, 8–9, 11, 154–56,
    162, 170–74, 189, 193–95, 199, 238,
    272, 280–82, 290

Eden, Frederick Morton, 28
Edmonds, T. R., 171
Edwards, Elizabeth, 31, 40–41
elites, views of working people, 134–35
England: determinants of sickness time and
    mortality, 241–68; distribution of AOF
    courts, 214; health patterns, 23, 162–
    69, 179–85, 216–32, 273; mortality de-
    cline, 179–85. See also Britain
epidemiologic transition, 195–97, 271–72
Eversholt Friendly Society, 202

family clubs, 49n. 16, 57–58
Family Physician, The, 50–51, 192, 199,
    202
Farr, William, 171–72, 177, 235
Foresters. See AOF; and names of individu-
    al courts
Foresters' Miscellany, 37–38, 50, 57, 107,
    136, 140–41, 192, 199, 200
frailty, of population, 13, 153, 185–87
friendly societies, 4, 17, 121, 139; age lim-
    its, 159, 288–90, 295; assets and induce-
    ment to submit a claim, 10–11, 41,
    131n. 10, 147–50, 278–79, 282; bene-
    fits, 132; characteristics of members, 15–
    16, 30–36, 44; and churches, 16–17;
    and claims awareness, 278–79; and con-
    tract medical practice, 49–50, 75–83;
    and doctors, 19, 47–74, 104–5, 98–
    123; ethos, 37, 40–44; functionalism,
    129; group culture, 129–30; and hazard-
    ous occupations, 202–9; and health pat-
    terns, 167–69; history, 27–28; initiation
    and initiation period, 73, 122, 152, 161,
    215–16, 250, 284; and insanity, 138,
    140–42, 151; life cycle, 293–301; meth-
    ods of valuation, 147–50; and morals,
    135–40; and poor law, 86–89; and qual-
    ity of medical care, 62, 68–73; records
    of, 6–7, 14, 191; and retirement, 145–

LIBRARY OF CONGRESS CATALOGING-IN-PUBLICATION DATA

Riley, James C.
  Sick, not dead : the health of British workingmen during the mortality decline /
James C. Riley.
      p.   cm.
  Includes bibliographical references and index.
  ISBN 0-8018-5411-3 (alk. paper)
    1. Medicine, Industrial—Great Britain—History.   2. Blue collar workers—Health
and hygiene—Great Britain—History.   I. Title.
RC963.3.R55   1997
616.9'803'0941—dc20   96-26961
                                                                      CIP